Philosophical Perspectives on Technology and Psychiatry

International Perspectives in Philosophy and Psychiatry

Series editors: Bill (K.W.M.) Fulford, Katherine Morris, John Z Sadler, and Giovanni Stanghellini

Volumes in the series:

Mind, Meaning, and Mental Disorder
Bolton and Hill

What is Mental Disorder?
Bolton

Postpsychiatry
Bracken and Thomas

The Philosophical Understanding of Schizophrenia
Chung, Fulford, and Graham (ed.)

Nature and Narrative: An Introduction to the New Philosophy of Psychiatry
Fulford, Morris, Sadler, and Stanghellini

The Oxford Textbook of Philosophy and Psychiatry
Fulford, Thornton, and Graham

Dementia: Mind, Meaning, and the Person
Hughes, Louw, and Sabat

Body-Subjects and Disordered Minds
Matthews

Talking Cures and Placebo Effects
Jopling

Schizophrenia and the Fate of the Self
Lysaker and Lysaker

Rationality and Compulsion: Applying Action Theory to Psychiatry
Nordenfelt

The Metaphor of Mental Illness
Pickering

Trauma, Truth, and Reconciliation: Healing Damaged Relationships
Potter (ed)

The Philosophy of Psychiatry: A Companion
Radden

Feelings of Being
Ratcliffe

Values and Psychiatric Diagnosis
Sadler

Disembodied Spirits and Deanimated Bodies: The Psychopathology of Common Sense
Stanghellini

Essential Philosophy of Psychiatry
Thornton

Empirical Ethics in Psychiatry
Widdershoven, McMillan, Hope and Van der Scheer (eds)

Forthcoming volumes in the series:

Philosophy, Psychoanalysis, and the A-rational Mind
Brakel

Philosophical Perspectives on Technology and Psychiatry

Edited by

James Phillips

OXFORD
UNIVERSITY PRESS

OXFORD
UNIVERSITY PRESS

Great Clarendon Street, Oxford OX2 6DP

Oxford University Press is a department of the University of Oxford.
It furthers the University's objective of excellence in research, scholarship, and education by publishing worldwide in

Oxford New York

Auckland Cape Town Dar es Salaam Hong Kong Karachi
Kuala Lumpur Madrid Melbourne Mexico City Nairobi
New Delhi Shanghai Taipei Toronto

With offices in

Argentina Austria Brazil Chile Czech Republic France Greece
Guatemala Hungary Italy Japan Poland Portugal Singapore
South Korea Switzerland Thailand Turkey Ukraine Vietnam

Oxford is a registered trade mark of Oxford University Press
in the UK and in certain other countries

Published in the United States
by Oxford University Press Inc., New York

First published 2009

A catalogue record for this title is available from the British Library

Data available

Library of Congress Cataloging in Publication Data

Philosophical perspectives on technology and psychiatry / edited by James Phillips.
p. ; cm. — (International perspectives in philosophy and psychiatry)
Includes bibliographical references and index.
ISBN 978–0–19–920742–8 (alk. paper)
1. Psychiatry—Philosophy. 2. Psychiatry—Technological innovations.
I. Phillips, James, 1938- II. Series.
[DNLM: 1. Psychiatry. 2. Philosophy. 3. Technology. WM 100 P5678 2008]
RC437.5.P4356 2008
616.89001—dc22

2008025820

Typeset by Cepha Imaging Private Ltd., Bangalore, India
Printed and bound in the United Kingdom by
Biddles Ltd., King's Lynn, Norfolk.

ISBN 978–0–19–920742–8

10 9 8 7 6 5 4 3 2 1

Contents

Contributors *vii*

Introduction *1*

Part 1 **Technical reason in psychiatry**

1 The instrument metaphor, hyponarrativity, and the generic clinician *23*
John Z. Sadler

2 Technological rationality in psychiatry: immanent critique, critical theory, and a pragmatist alternative *35*
Peter Zachar and Scott Bartlett

3 Technological reason and the regulation of emotion *55*
Louis C. Charland

Part 2 **Critical approaches to technology in psychiatry**

4 Technology, aesthetic explanation, and psychoanalysis *73*
Miguel Uribe

5 Focusing the lenses of feminist theories to reflect on technology and psychiatry *87*
Sue V. Rosser

6 The critical theory of psychopharmacology: the work of David Healy and beyond *115*
Douglas Porter

7 Toward a post-technological information theory *135*
Donald Mender

Part 3 **Technology and psychiatric disorders**

8 Technology and mental disorders: a clinical probe into the differential impact on individuals *153*
Douglas W. Heinrichs

9 Frontal fatigue: how technology may contribute to mental illness *167*
Mark D. Rego

10 Bored to tears? Depression and Heidegger's concept of profound boredom: a postpsychiatry contribution *181*
Phillip Sinaikin

Part 4 **Technological instruments and psychiatry**

11 Psychiatric rehabilitation and the notion of technology in psychiatry *203*
Abraham Rudnick

12 Drugs, not hugs: antidepressant medication trials and suicidality in children—a case history in the philosophy of science as an argument for the need for improved technology in psychiatry *215*
Stuart L. Kaplan

13 Philosophical considerations of an internet-enabled telephone and computer psychiatric symptom monitoring system: maintaining the balance between subjectivity and objectivity in research *231*
Karen Iseminger and Dale Theobald

14 The assessment of emotional awareness: can technology make a contribution? *249*
Robert S. Kruger

Part 5 **Ethical issues in technology and psychiatry**

15 Thinking about the repair manual: technique and technology in psychiatry *263*
Jennifer Radden

16 Beyond repugnance: human enhancement and the President's Council on Bioethics *279*
Michael A. Cerullo

17 The reflectively anxious and depressed: psychotropics and lives worth living *293*
Mark P. Jenkins

Index *309*

Contributors

Scott Bartlett

Michael A. Cerullo

Louis C. Charland

Douglas W. Heinrichs

Karen Iseminger

Mark P. Jenkins

Stuart Kaplan

Robert Kruger

Donald Mender

Douglas Porter

Jennifer Radden

Mark D. Rego

Sue V. Rosser

Abraham Rudnick

John Sadler

Phillip Sinaikin

Dale Theobald

Miguel Uribe

Peter Zachar

Introduction

1. The faces of technology

As we move into the twenty-first century, our lives are dominated by technology. We live with and through its achievements. For immediate examples I need look no further than the computer on which I am writing this text, the Internet through which I will send it out, and (to revert to older technology) the worldwide postal system through which I will convey a hard copy. What is true of the rest of life is of course true of medicine. Beyond a certain age, most of us owe our existence and our continued vigor to some achievement of medical technology. And what is true in a major way of general medicine is to a significant degree true of psychiatry. Prozac has long since arrived, and in its wake an ever-growing armamentarium of new psychotropics; beyond that, neuroscience promises ever more technological advances for the field.

As will be reflected in the papers in this volume, the effect of technology on the field of psychiatry remains highly ambiguous. On the one hand there are the achievements, both in the science and practice of psychiatry; on the other hand technology's influence on the field threatens its identity as a humanistic practice. In this ambiguity psychiatry is not unique. As will be apparent in later sections of this Introduction, major thinkers have for a long time been highly ambivalent and concerned about the technological order that now defines modern society.

For a representative example of the role of technology in psychiatry—and of the upbeat attitude of official psychiatry—let me a cite a recent appearance on the 'Today' show of the then president of the American Psychiatric Association, Steven S. Sharfstein, defending the field of psychiatry against attacks by the Church of Scientology. Describing his appearance Sharfstein wrote in a column in *Psychiatric News*:

> What is the message for the audience of not only the 'Today' show but of all the spinoff media events that occur as a result of this opportunity?
>
> First and foremost, we can tell the world about psychiatry—that psychiatrists are physicians and that our field is backed by science like other branches of medicine. In recent years, thanks to advances in neuroscience, brain secrets at the molecular and genetic levels are being revealed, identifying the close links between nature and nurture.
>
> (Sharfstein 2005)

Sharfstein's message is reasonable, but it does remind us how tightly we have yoked the fate of our field to achievements in neuroscience, genetics, and other cutting-edge scientific areas made possible by newly acquired instruments in our technological tool box.

Science and technology as exemplified by Sharfstein's statement are topics that will occupy us at length in this volume, although technology in its capacity to further basic scientific research is not the only way we will approach our theme of technology and psychiatry. The relationship of technology and science is a reciprocal one that moves in both directions. Through technological instruments we are able to study the brain, but through science we discover technological treatments. Magnetic resonance imaging is an investigatory instrument; an antidepressant is a therapeutic technique.

Technology, in fact, has several sides or faces, of which I will emphasize three. On the one hand there are the achievements, as indicated above, the conquests of air, earth, and illness—all of which have a tendency to mutate into commodities (Borgmann 1984). Analysis of this side of technology moves in the direction of a description of our lives *as lived* by commodities, as dominated by an endless quest (indeed, greed) for ever more technological *things*. Such analysis leads to further description of how the commodities begin to redefine our sense of ourselves. Prozac in this sense is not just a technological advance; it becomes a commodity that we cannot do without.

A second face of technology, that emphasized by Sharfstein, has to do with reality as it is revealed by technological instruments. With this dimension of technology the real becomes that which is made visible through the lens of technology (Idhe 1991). The most dramatic examples are to be found in nuclear physics, where the ultimate building blocks of reality are completely the products of the most sophisticated reactors, etc. In psychiatry, with our advancing imaging technology we probe ever deeper into the structures of the brain. And at the level of more simple technology, the psychiatrically real becomes that which can be seen, the symptom, and especially that which can be measured. Disorders and treatments are reduced to what can be defined by diagnostic criteria and to what can be mapped out on a scale.

Finally, there is a third face of technology, not the technology of things and commodities and not the technology of instruments, but rather the way of thinking that is inherent in the technological approach to life. Many philosophers have attempted to analyze the technological attitude, the most well-known certainly being Martin Heidegger (1976), who reversed the customary interpretation of technology as applied science and determined pure science to be the handmaiden of technology.

2. Historical background

Major historians and philosophers of technology agree that what we think of as the technological revolution began in the seventeenth century, although in fact major technological accomplishments did not take off until the latter part of the eighteenth century. What came first was the new style of thinking in the seventeenth century that we denominate the 'scientific revolution'. Hans Jonas has described this change well:

> The scientific revolution changed man's ways of thinking, *by* thinking, before it materially changed, even affected, his ways of living. It was a change in theory, in world-view, in metaphysical outlook, in conception and method of knowledge. It did not at first—and for a long time—concern itself with the realm of practice, even though some of its most eloquent philosophical prophets assigned to it this role early enough: that assignment itself was in the realm of thought... Technology, historically speaking, is the delayed effect of the scientific and metaphysical revolution with which the modern age begins.
>
> (Jonas 1974: 47)

Jonas is quick to add, however, that technology is not an afterthought or later application of the scientific revolution, but rather embedded as possibility in the new scientific metaphysics. Thus the scientific and technological revolutions were intimately intertwined, although historically the latter followed the former.

The new thinking was embodied in figures like Bacon, Descartes, and Galileo; and, consistent with the point just made, what we see in these individuals is not a series of technological discoveries but rather a change in attitude toward investigation of the external world. Although he did not define the methodology, Francis Bacon articulated the program of the new approach, overturning the Aristotelian goal of knowledge as contemplation of the truth and redefining it as mastery of nature for human ends.

> I would address one general admonition to all: that they consider what are the true ends of knowledge, and that they seek it not either for pleasure of mind, or for contention, or for superiority to others...but for the benefit and use of life, and that they perfect and govern it in charity... [From the marriage of the Mind and the Universe] there may spring helps to man, and a line and race of inventions that may in some degree subdue and overcome the necessities and miseries of humanity...or the matter in hand is no mere felicity of speculation, but the real business and fortunes of the human race, and all power of operation...And so those twin objects, human knowledge and human power, do really meet in one.
>
> (From the Preface to The Great Instauration, cited by Jonas 1966: 189)

It is implicit in Bacon's program that if knowledge is to become practical and turn nature to human ends, it will have to begin with an understanding of how nature works. Only in that way will it be possible to exercise power over nature and redirect its' workings toward human utility. Descartes and Galileo were the pivotal figures in outlining the methodology that would make Bacon's program possible. Heirs to Copernicus' first step in the scientific revolution a half century earlier, his overthrow of the Aristotelian, geocentric cosmos, they formulated the principles that would allow an understanding of Copernicus' discoveries. What were required were laws of mechanics that would apply anywhere in the cosmos, both on the earth and with heavenly bodies. Galileo transformed the understanding of motion and subjected it to mathematical analysis. Both Galileo and Descartes articulated a geometrizing of nature and a mathematization of physics. Descartes provided a dramatic philosophic articulation of this new view with his notion of the entire physical world as *res extensa*, nature as extended substance subject to analysis through geometry and mathematics. He invented analytical geometry as a tool for analysis of the new view of motion. With this vision he reduced the difference between man-made and natural mechanics. He wrote, for instance, '*…the example of certain bodies made by art was of service to me, for I can see no difference between these and natural bodies…And it is certain that there are no rules in mechanics which do not hold good in physics, of which mechanics forms a part or species (so that all that is artificial is also natural…)*' (Descartes 1955 [1644] IV, art. 203, 299).

Although technology as instrument of scientific inquiry was present from the beginning of the scientific revolution (e.g. Galileo's telescopes), major technological breakthroughs did not occur until the late eighteenth and nineteenth centuries. Beginning with relatively simple inventions like James Watt's steam engine, the technological revolution was fully launched with applications of the new sciences of chemistry and electromagnetics. We continue to live in the era inaugurated by the technological advances stemming from those sciences. In the past one and half centuries the rate of technological advance has only continued to accelerate, resulting in what Ellul has famously termed the 'technological society'.

In concluding this section let me add one relevant footnote to this brief historical review of the technological revolution: namely that the field of medicine represents something of an exception to the theme that technological innovations have lagged behind their scientific precursors. To quote Jonas once more:

> Medicine alone, and naturally, was always an intimate fusion of theory and practice, and the increasingly scientific inquiries into the human body were never undertaken without regard to their use in the art of healing (and indeed never by other than medical men). To the extent, then, that medicine can be called a 'technology' (a moot point), evolving modern medicine would be the first case of a scientific technology.
>
> (Jonas 1974: 73)

3. Philosophic analysis

In this introductory sketch it is only possible to touch on some of the major figures who have attempted an analysis of technology, the technology revolution, and the impact of technology on contemporary life. I need also add that in the effort to analyze the meaning of technology, it is not possible to draw fine distinctions between philosophical, historical, sociological, and other analyses. Because I cannot in a few pages cover all the individual figures who have played a role in the philosophical evaluation of technology, for more comprehensive accounts I must refer the reader to some of the surveys of this field (Achterhuis 1999; Bunge 1972; Dusek 2005; Feibleman 1972; Jarvie 1972; Kaplan 2004; Mitcham and Mackey 1972; Olsen and Selinger 2007; Scharff and Dusek 2003; and Skoliminoski 1972).

3.1 First-generation analyses

As a first participant in this discussion of the philosophical foundations of modern technology, I will invoke Lewis Mumford (1963, 1972, 1973), whose analysis is historical and sociological as well as philosophic, and who, unlike most of the analysts of technology, pushes the origins of technology to well before the modern era. In his analysis of technology, Mumford locates the critical turning point not in the seventeenth century but at the dawn of history when humans first turned to the development of '*monotechnics, devoted to the increase of power and wealth by the systematic organization of workaday activities in a rigidly mechanical pattern*' (1972: 81), and in that way developed the first embodiments of the '*Megamachine*,' Mumford's metaphor for a technologically dominated society. For Mumford the ensuing centuries witnessed the ever-expanding dominion of the *Megamachine*. Monotechnics has from the beginning alienated man for his more organic, biologically based existence, and this has reached an extreme point in the modern era, when '*the whole process of technical development has become increasingly coercive, totalitarian, and—in its direct human expression—compulsive and grimly irrational, indeed downright hostile to more spontaneous manifestations of life that cannot be fed into the machine*' (ibid.: 83).

To bring us back to the modern era, we do well to begin with our main analyst of the previous section, Hans Jonas, whose investigation is even more philosophical than historical. As indicated above, Jonas argues that although technological achievement followed scientific advance historically, technological possibility was present in the new science from the beginning: both in the literal sense that the new science required technological instruments, and in the 'metaphysical' sense that the treatment of nature as a mathematically analyzable mechanical system has built into it the possibility of manipulating nature in manifold ways. '*Practice in the service of theory, which is what experiments are, is readily converted into theory, in the service of practice, which by now most of 'science' almost automatically becomes*' (Jonas 1974: 71).

Discussion of Jonas' analysis leads us readily to Martin Heidegger, the philosopher who has provided the most penetrating analysis of technology, and who was also the teacher of Jonas and undoubtedly an influence on the latter's thought. If Jonas, with his insistence on the unity of science and technology, rejects the notion of technology as simply applied science, Heidegger (temporally, of course, prior to Jonas), takes this train of thought much further in claiming an ontological priority of technology over modern science. In his justly acclaimed study, 'The Question Concerning Technology (1976),' Heidegger rejects the customary interpretations of technology as means to end (instrumental interpretation) and as human activity (anthropological interpretation) and argues that technology is an original form of the revealing of Being that characterizes the modern era. Technology reveals or uncovers Being as 'standing-reserve' (*Bestand*): '*Modern technology, as a revealing which orders, is thus no mere human doing. Therefore we must take that challenging, which sets upon man to order the real as standing-reserve, in accordance with the way it shows itself. That challenging gathers man into ordering. This gathering concentrates man upon ordering the real as standing-reserve*' (1976: 300). What this means is that technology involves a basic vision of the world as a reserve of material to be manipulated and forced to convert itself into whatever potential lies hidden in it. Heidegger is quick to point out that man, in this supposed position of power over material nature, is himself vulnerable to being interpreted as so much more standing-reserve. '*As soon as what is unconcealed no longer concerns man even as object, but exclusively as standing-reserve, and man in the midst of objectlessness is nothing but the orderer of the standing-reserve, then he comes to the very brink of a precipitous fall, that is, he comes to the point where he himself will have to be taken as standing-reserve*' (ibid.: 308).

In his renowned work, *The Technological Society* (Ellul 1964), Jacques Ellul performed a sociological analysis of modern technology that is consistent with Heidegger's philosophical analysis. In tracing the development of technology into the twentieth century, Ellul describes a totalizing effect of technology that comes to dominate our culture. In describing his work, Mitcham and Mackey write: '*The technological society is created when technique becomes its central component; technique defines our epoch the way Catholicism defined the Middle Ages or Buddhism the Age of Asoka*' (Mitcham and Mackey 1972: 5). As with

Heidegger, Ellul sees the technological order as a historical phenomenon that defines the individual and over which he has limited control.

> It [technique] is not the result of a plot or plan by any one man or any group of men who direct it or apply it or shunt it in new directions. The technical phenomenon is impersonal, and in following its course we have found that it is directed toward man. In investigating its preferred loci, we find man himself. This man is not the man in the mirror. Nor is he the man next door or the man in the street. Proceeding at its own tempo, technique analyzes its objects so that it can reconstitute them; in the case of man, it has analyzed him and synthesized a hitherto unknown being...Until recently, we were obliged to think of man as divided in his relation to the technical world. One part of him was given over completely to the monster and subjected to the interior and exterior rules; but the other part he could keep for himself: his inner life, his family life, his psychic life. He suffered from this division, but nonetheless he retained a very considerable measure of freedom...Many more aspects of the human personality have been exposed to the technical society, and today very nearly the entire human race is experiencing this progressive cleavage of personality.
>
> (Ellul 1964: 387–410)

3.2 **Contemporary analyses**

The above analyses have, each in its own way, been critical of the dominance of technology in modern life. Each of the thinkers, all members of an older generation, has also suggested mediating responses to the technological threat, albeit in the context of a primarily skeptical attitude toward technology. I have emphasized these individuals because of their prominence in the philosophical discussion of technology. There is, however, a younger generation of philosophers who have expanded the discussion of technology, at times in a more balanced and less critical manner than their forbears.

More than any living philosopher, Albert Borgmann has provided a nuanced analysis of the role of technology in contemporary life. For that reason I will highlight his foundational work. As in the case of the philosophers discussed above, Borgmann assumes a critical posture toward the effects of technology, but he is quite concrete in his suggestions for dealing with the technological threat.

Borgmann describes the technology order in which we live as one dominated by the *device paradigm*, his term for the technological objects that populate our daily lives. The device is the hidden machinery that makes products or commodities readily available. A watch provides time, an automobile transportation, the heating/cooling system heat or air conditioning. In each case the mechanism (or means) making the product (or end) available is out of sight, and for most of us incomprehensible. All we need know is how to press the relevant buttons or levers to make the apparatus work. Borgmann distinguishes such devices from primitive technologies such as heating by means of a hearth in which the mechanism is both visible and directly connected to the human beings who are using it. Discussing the device paradigm Borgmann writes:

> ...these features become visible when we learn to see how the presence of things is replaced with the availability of commodities and how availability is procured through devices. Devices...dissolve the coherent and engaging character of the pretechnological world of things. In a device, the concealed, and the commodities, which are made available by a device, are enjoyed without the encumbrance of or the engagement with a context.
>
> (Borgmann 1984: 47)

In his effort to find a way back to a world less dominated by devices and more connected to pretechnological things, Borgmann points us to what he describes as focal things and practices. His immediate examples are basic activities such as running, cooking, and family meals. In all such activities the individual's involvement in the natural human world is direct and not mediated through technological objects and devices.

In psychiatry the most obvious examples of technological things or commodities are psychopharmacological agents. They are treatment means that produce a product, namely symptom reduction in the patient. Analyzed from Borgmann's perspective, what is interesting about pharmaceuticals is that we know *that* they work but in fact do not know exactly *how* they work. Unlike the watch or the heating system, even expert pharmacologists do not know the precise device mechanisms of the common psychotropic medications.

Following Borgmann's analysis, psychotropics raise many of the broader questions of the device paradigm beyond the basic issue of our ignorance of their exact mechanism. On the one hand they are extremely useful and represent a major accomplishment of psychiatric science. On the other hand they readily transmute into commodities that at their worst can distort patients' self-perceptions. Contemporary society often descries the doctor or psychiatrist as pill-pusher, but it is now a common experience for the patient to present herself as a biological thing to be fixed with the right pill. In this self-perception the patient is viewing herself as one more system or commodity, not that different from the heating system or the plumbing system: push the right button, pull the right lever, take the right pill, and the machine works.

Other contemporary thinkers have pursued the analysis of technology in other directions, and space does not allow an analysis of all of them. In a series of books (1981, 1991, 1995, 1999), Andrew Feenberg engages the dystopian views of earlier-generation analyses and actively dialogues with figures from the Frankfurt school. In his work (1977, 1986) Langdon Winner analyzes technology in the context of its socio-political context. Hubert Dreyfus, drawing on Heidegger's analysis of the human individual's embeddedness in the world, contrasts this Being-in-the-world with the artificial rationality of artificial intelligence (1972, 1992). Don Ihde emphasizes the way in which technological devices have altered our perception of reality (1991). As mentioned above, further information on these and other figures can be found in review articles and surveys of the field (Achterhuis 1999; Bunge 1972; Dusek 2005; Feibleman 1972; Jarvie 1972; Kaplan 2004; Mitcham and Mackey 1972; Olsen and Selinger 2007; Scharff and Dusek 2003; Skoliminoski 1972).

3.3 Technical reason

Finally, a dimension of the philosophical analysis of technology that warrants separate, explicit treatment—albeit implicit in much of the above discussion—and that is quite applicable to the philosophical discussion of technology and psychiatry, is what I will call technical reason—a way of thinking also referred to as instrumental reasoning or technological reasoning. With the use of technical reason knowledge is structured in an instrumental, means/ends manner. For any problem there is a stock of knowledge that can be ordered in formulaic fashion so that once the problem is presented, the correct solution (the means) can be applied to fix (the end) the problem. A particular problem is always an instance of a general type, and for the type there is a typical solution. The formula in medicine goes: if patient has condition A, apply treatment B. The currently popular evidence-based medicine and treatment algorithms, as well as manualized treatment primers, are examples of this kind of technical thinking.

It hardly needs stating that treatment algorithms, the evidence-based approach, and treatment manuals are useful tools in psychiatric practice. What issue is then being addressed in referring to them as examples of technical reason? The issue is that they, and other examples of the technical approach, can at their worst turn psychiatric treatment (or medical treatment, for that matter) into a mechanical procedure. The patient becomes an instance of a diagnostic category, and the treater becomes a generic treater. Follow the technicized approach too literally and one schizophrenic becomes interchangeable with the next, and one psychiatrist with another. In this situation of the fungible patient and the fungible treater, the individuality of both is lost, and the need for individual judgment on the part of the psychiatrist is rendered obsolete. The competent, generic psychiatrist need only recognize that the patient is an example of the general disease category and be capable applying the generic treatment for that category. As I wrote on another occasion: '*This technical approach to diagnosis and treatment is not that different from the technical attitude in other problem domains, where the image of broken object and repair manual prevails. With the technicist strategy in psychiatry we are close to seeing the patient as something broken that can be fixed with a correct use of the psychiatric repair manual*' (Phillips 2002*a*: 77).

What is of course missing in the technical model is the practical experience of the seasoned practitioner. To use another language, the *science* of psychiatry has replaced the *art* or *craft* of psychiatry. The technical model implies that the former will supersede the latter. In the scientific, technical future, the wise, seasoned practitioner will be a superannuated remnant of the past.

The origins of technical reason have been traced by, among others (an analysis of technical reason is strongly implied in Jonas' treatment of technology, as described above), Stephen Toulmin. In *Cosmopolis* (1990) and especially *Return to Reason* (2001) Toulmin describes the early decades of the seventeenth century as a pivotal period in which, for a variety of historical and social reasons (the Thirty Years War being prominent among them), the thinking public reacted strongly against the broad humanism and skepticism of the sixteenth century and longed for a kind of knowledge that would be certain and reliable. As I indicated above, Galileo supplied a method and Descartes gave it a full philosophical articulation. Through the use of geometric and mathematical analysis, nature could be understood with the rigor of mathematical certainty.

As Toulmin traces this intellectual history, seventeenth-century rationalism abrogated the distinction between 'rationality' and 'reasonableness,' two forms of thinking or argumentation, indeed two forms of science, with which thinking people were comfortable in previous times.

From the mid-seventeenth century on an imbalance began to develop. Certain methods of inquiry and subjects were seen as philosophically serious or 'rational' in a way that others were not. As a result, authority came to attach particularly to scientific and technical inquiries that put those methods to use. Instead of a free-for-all of ideas and speculations—a competition for attention across all realms of inquiry—there was a hierarchy of prestige, so that investigations and activities were ordered with an eye to certain intellectual demands. Beside the *rationality* of astronomy and geometry, the *reasonableness* of narratives came to seem a soft-centered notion, lacking a solid basis in philosophical theory, let alone substantive scientific support. Issues of formal consistency and deductive proof thus came to have a special prestige, and achieved a kind of *certainty* that other kinds of opinions could never share. As time went on, academic philosophers came to see literary authors like Michel de Montaigne—an essayist who had little use for 'disciplines' and put equally little reliance on formal logic—as not being philosophers at all, let alone scientists (Toulmin 2001: 15).

As Toulmin describes it, modern rationalism, with its insistence on abstract, formal language and argumentation, readily developed into what I am describing as technical reason or instrumental thinking. '*Theory acquired the dominant role, and Practice came to be spoken of as merely a way of applying Theory. Even in clinical medicine, where a fresh concern with practical, concrete, and particular issues has arisen beginning in the 1960s, prestige still tends to attach to academic studies that focus on abstract, universal theories*' (ibid.: 23).

Toulmin is on target in tracing this discussion back to Aristotle and to the subsequent fate of his ideas. On the one hand the development of modern science required a rejection of Aristotelian science (Copernicus' revolution in astronomy and Galileo's analysis of motion are the two immediate examples). On the other hand, seventeenth-century rationalism also, and without warrant, dismissed Aristotle's distinction between theoretical and practical knowledge, his forerunners of Toulmin's rationality and reasonableness. For Aristotle different subject matters require different styles of thinking. While mathematics allows for universal, context-free principles, questions about how to live require practical knowledge (*phronesis*). Practical knowledge involves generalities or 'universals', but these are always context-dependent and subject to reformulation to fit the particular occasion. In dealing with human behavior we use generalities of the sort: 'in this kind of situation, people will usually act in such-and-such a manner'. As Toulmin reminds us, '*...in real-life situations, many universals hold generally rather than invariably. So, in medicine and other human disciplines, we must remember the difference between the general factual assumptions that support 'reasonable' arguments in the practical arts, and the 'rational' deductions that are the stock-in-trade of mathematically formulated theories*' (ibid.: 111).

The legacy of seventeenth-century rationalism is thus a general disparagement of Aristotelian practical knowledge. '*The idea that all the practical arts owe a debt to the skills Aristotle calls phronesis was not especially welcome to rational-minded thinkers in the modern period*' (ibid.: 114). Although practical knowledge might seem a natural approach to psychiatric practice, it tends to be pushed aside as insufficiently scientific and not up to the standards of scientific, technical thinking. The treatment algorithms and manuals that should be useful *aids* in practice are inflated into the *science* of practice, and the consequence is a dumbed-down psychiatry with a patina of science.[1]

4. Dimensions of philosophy and technology in psychiatry

The chapters of this volume will be organized around five different themes. There is clearly some overlapping among the sections, as many of the chapters touch on more than one of the organizing themes. The first section will focus on the theme just discussed, technical reason. Other sections will be devoted to critical approaches to technology and psychiatry, technology and psychiatric disorders, technological instruments in psychiatry, and ethical issues in technology and psychiatry. A central question running through all of these sections and chapters is that of final judgment about the impact on technology and psychiatry: technology as blessing, technology as curse. Obviously technology is both, and the various chapters deal with this question each in its own way.

4.1 Technical reason in psychiatry

The three chapters in the first section of this volume address technical reason in psychiatry from different perspectives. All express concern that along with the achievements of technology there has been too great an emphasis on technical reason and that that has led to an imbalance in the field. In 'The Instrument Metaphor, Hyponarrativity, and the Generic Clinician,' John Sadler argues that instrumentalist thinking has thoroughly invaded psychiatric practice and thereby transformed the field. He describes several 'cultural artifacts' such as diagnostic and treatment manuals to exemplify the 'instrument metaphor' that now defines psychiatric practice. The consequence of this trend in psychiatric practice is the 'generic clinician' who applies the same techniques as any other clinician and is readily interchangeable with other generic clinicians.

Peter Zachar and Scott Bartlett offer a different slant on this theme in 'Technological rationality in psychiatry: immanent critique, critical theory, and a pragmatist alternative.' They emphasizes the difference between specific techniques and what they term technological rationality. Techniques are specific procedures and instruments that are useful in resolving concrete problems. The success of such techniques, however, leads to unrealistic expectations about what technology can accomplish. These expectations are embodied in technological rationality which, in the extreme, argues that technology is the solution for everything. The authors argue for a dialectical relationship between productive, problem-based techniques and global, unrealistic technological rationality—a relationship in which the benefits of technology are preserved without leading to unrealistic expectations. In their analysis they invoke the 'immanent critique' of the Frankfurt school as well as John Dewey's version of pragmatism as dynamic instrumentalism.

Finally Louis Charland's 'Technological reason and the regulation of emotion' focuses on a specific area, that of the emotions, in which he sees a problematic dominance of the technical attitude. He argues that our technologically oriented psychiatry has taken an instrumentalist approach to regulation of emotion that severely limits and distorts the role of emotion in psychiatric practice. A prominent example is the exclusion of moral judgments and values, emotion-laden aspects of experience, from psychotherapy because they do not fit the technical model. To illustrate his point, Charland both contrasts the modern notion of emotion with the traditional notion of passion, and our contemporary practice of technically regulated emotion with the 'moral treatment' of the nineteenth century.

4.2 Critical approaches to technology in psychiatry

The chapters in this section of the volume overlap somewhat with those of the first section in that some of them touch again on the problems engendered by technical rationality. They are, however, a more diverse group, each offering a critical analysis of some aspect of technology in psychiatry. As with the chapters of the first section, the authors do not engage in a whole scale condemnation of technology ('critical' should not be taken as equivalent to 'criticism') but rather, in the context of recognizing the real accomplishments of technology in psychiatry, focus on particular issues in psychiatry's relationship to technology.

In 'Technology, aesthetic explanation, and psychoanalysis,' Miguel Uribe contrasts technical, mechanistic explanations of clinical phenomena with the very different kind of 'explanation' provided by the interpretations used in psychoanalysis and psychoanalytic psychotherapy. In developing this contrast he invokes Wittgenstein's views on aesthetic explanation to suggest that psychoanalysis, while failing to meet the standards of instrumentalist thinking, is better understood (and defended) in the context of aesthetic explanation. He argues that there is a proper place for both kinds of explanation in clinical practice.

A very different discussion comes into play in Sue Rosser's 'Focusing the lenses of feminist theories to reflect on technology and psychiatry.' She reviews a comprehensive number of feminist theories to demonstrate how the various feminist perspectives reveal aspects of the relationship between science and society in the areas of biology and technology. To make the discussion more immediately relevant to the area of psychiatry, she focuses, in each feminist perspective, on the examples of serotonin reuptake inhibitors (SSRIs) and functional magnetic resonance imaging (fMRI) to demonstrate what the particular perspective might reveal about those technological modalities in psychiatry.

Shifting focus to another area of the field, in 'The critical theory of psychopharmacology: the work of David Healy and beyond,' Douglas Porter invokes the work of David Healy to address the cultural and sociological dimensions of a particular psychiatric technology, namely psychopharmacology.

He argues that the evolution of this technology has not followed an inevitable, progressive course but rather has been determined by several contingent, cultural factors. A focus on the cultural context in which pharmacological research and practice have developed allows for a critical approach to this technology, one more nuanced than either a blanket embrace or rejection.

Finally, addressing still another technological dimension of contemporary psychiatry, its increasing effort to translate clinical phenomena into informational data that can be processed by computer software, Donald Mender questions this effort in 'Toward a post-technological information theory.' He argues that information theory is unsuited to deal with phenomena like meaning and subjectivity that are at the heart of human psychology and psychiatric practice. Any reduction of the mind to a 'data-processing instrument equated with a computer-like brain' will inevitably leave out much that is important in understanding psychopathology and clinical work. In a technically difficult discussion Mender argues that with the aid of post-Newtonian concepts classical information theory can be revised in a way that escapes the reductionism of standard computer models.

4.3 Technology and psychiatric disorders

A third section of the volume deals with the impact of technology on psychiatric disorders. This if of course a broad area, and the number of chapters could be great. There are very many aspects of modern technology that arguably could have an impact on psychopathology and clinical practice. The three chapters in this section provide a fair representation of ways in which technology influences psychiatric phenomena: the first, in the case of specific technologies on psychiatric conditions, in some instances positive, in some instances negative; the second, in the broader effect of a technological culture on human stress; and the third, in another speculation on the broader consequences of a technological age on how we view one common disorder, depression. (The use of particular technologies to assist in psychiatric treatment will be covered in the next section.)

In 'Technology and mental disorders: a clinical probe into the differential impact on individuals', Douglas Heinrichs details the impact of technology on three psychiatric disorders. In the first situation he describes the interactions of an individual suffering from attention deficit disorder with a complex phone menu. In a second situation he points to the benefits of communication through e-mail for patients with Asperger syndrome who have limited tolerance for direct human contact. In a final example Heinrichs describes the complex impact of technologically driven expectations of efficient, machine-like performance on patients with volatile mood disorders.

Mark Rego undertakes a large question in 'Frontal fatigue: how modernization and technology may produce mental illness.' Starting from the documented increase in mental disorders in recent decades and its putative relation to the increase of stress in modern life, he argues that these phenomena can best be understood as the effect of modern technology's excessive demands on the prefrontal cortex.

Finally, in another effort to understand the global effect of technology on the mental health of modern society, Phillip Sinaikin invokes Heidegger in 'Bored to tears? Depression and Heidegger's concept of profound boredom: a postpsychiatry contribution.' Citing Heidegger's work on technology as well as his notion of fundamental mood as disclosive of human existence, he argues that depression and profound boredom are the characteristic mood of our technological epoch. In his analysis he offers of critique of recent investigations of the efficacy of antidepressants that could have easily been included in the second section of the volume.

4.4 Technological instruments in psychiatry

A fourth section of the volume covers the dimension of technology as therapeutic instrument. The four chapters offer examples of ways in which specific technologies can aid in psychiatric practice. These four chapters dialogue and often contrast with chapters from earlier sections as we continue to hover around the central dilemma: technology as problem, technology as blessing. They also span the range of our understanding of 'technology', with Rudnick using the term to include structured, behavioral therapeutic modalities, Kaplan using it to include research methodologies, and Kruger, Iseminger, and Theobald using it to refer to concrete technological instruments.

In 'Psychiatric rehabilitation and the notion of technology in psychiatry', Abraham Rudnick invokes the 'technology' of psychiatric rehabilitation to defend the use of technology in psychiatric treatment. He argues that psychiatric technologies are often viewed as 'tools' used to 'fix problems' and that this technological language—and perspective—of tools and fixing is inherently dehumanizing. Rudnick challenges this point of view as too narrow and invokes psychiatric rehabilitation to illustrate how a technology can be viewed as in fact humanizing. That is, the technology—in this case the technical methods of rehabilitation—can be viewed as a set of tools that help individuals achieve their goals. Rudnick's analysis readily brings to mind the wide range of behavioral therapies and the way in which they are at times seen as mechanical and thereby dehumanized.

Stuart Kaplan's 'Drugs, not hugs: clinical psychopathology trials in children—A case history in the philosophy of science as an argument for the need for improved technology in psychiatry,' shares features with the chapters of the second section. He critiques the primitive technology in place for the assessment of psychopharmacological agents in children, the need for a more sophisticated methodology, and the multitude of difficulties in developing such an improved methodology. While recognizing the double-blind study as the indispensable technological instrument for the evaluation of pharmacological agents, he addresses the multiplicity of problems in the implementation of this methodology and the need for further refinement of the 'instrument'.

The last two papers in this section demonstrate the use of concrete instruments in research and practice. Iseminger and Theobald provide an example of a technological instrument, an Internet-enabled, computer-automated telephone and computer psychiatric symptom monitoring system. In 'Philosophical considerations of an Internet-enabled telephone and computer psychiatric symptom monitoring system: maintaining the balance between subjectivity and objectivity in research,' they discuss the use of such technology for symptom-reporting and communication with home-bound cancer patients. They evaluate the philosophical implications of such technology, whether the technology impedes or promotes the desired human communication between patient and treater. Finally, in 'The assessment of emotional awareness: can technology make a contribution?', Robert Kruger shows how the use of a simple piece of technology, the video recorder, can be of great assistance in dealing with a complex clinical phenomenon, the assessment of emotional awareness. The ability to identify the emotional states of others (even that they have emotions) has been an active topic in our understanding of conditions like autism. Kruger shows how the assessment tools using videotaping can assist in the assessment of this capacity (and possibly be useful in the treatment of individuals who are deficient in the capacity).

4.5 Ethical issues in technology and psychiatry

We complete this volume with chapters on ethical issues in technology and psychiatry. Jennifer Radden's 'Thinking about the repair manual: technique and technology in psychiatry' takes us back to John Sadler's chapter on the generic clinician. Her approach to the overly technical psychiatrist, however, moves in a more directly ethical direction. She questions whether the good psychiatrist must possess not only technical skills but also moral virtues. She addresses issue in terms of the psychiatrist's character. That is, being a good psychiatrist requires having a 'good character'. Radden argues that the current emphasis on technical expertise has led us to forget and neglect the time-honored recognition of moral virtue in the good doctor.

In 'Beyond repugnance: human enhancement and The President's Council on Bioethics,' Michael Cerullo addresses a different ethical issue, that of the use of putative enhancement medications in psychiatry. He centers his discussion around the recent report of the President's Council on Bioethics, entitled 'Beyond therapy: a report of the President's Council on Bioethics.' He argues that this report is the product of neo-conservative ideology and misrepresents both the nature of current antidepressants and the issue of cosmetic psychopharmacology. He offers a defense of so-called cosmetic psychopharmacology that is directed not just to the President's Council but at any extreme, conservative critique of such pharmacological technology.

The use of antidepressant medication makes another appearance in the final chapter of this volume. In 'The reflectively anxious and depressed: psychotropics and lives worth living,' Mark Jenkins questions whether there are situations in which the use of antidepressants is counterproductive, that is, whether for some individuals they impede the process of reflection. In this chapter Jenkins addresses the ethical ambiguity of using antidepressants to foreclose a confrontation of ordinary human existential dilemmas.

Endnotes

1 Writing from a continental perspective, Gadamer (1975 [1960]) relates Aristotelian practical knowledge to the hermeneutic tradition. See also Dunne (1993) and Phillips (2002*a*, 2002*b*). For an account of instrumental reason from the perspective of the Frankfurt school see Marcuse (1964) and Adorno (1966). For further discussion of technical reason in medicine and psychiatry, see: Agich 1981; Beresford 1996; Clouser 1977; Gadamer 1996; Hunter 1989; Leder 1990; McWhinney 1978; Munson 1981; Pellegrino and Thomasma 1981; Sadler 2005; Toulimn 1976; Zaner 1990.

References

Achterhuis H. (ed.) (1999). *American Philosophy of Technology: The Empirical Turn* (Bloomington: Indiana University Press).

Adorno T. W. (1966). *Negative Dialectics* (New York: Continuum).

Agich, G. (1981). 'The question of technology in medicine' in S. Skousgaard (ed.) *Phenomenology and the Understanding of Human Destiny* (New York: The Center for Advanced Research in Phenomenology and The University Press of America), 81–92.

Beresford E. (1996). Can phronesis save the life of medical ethics? *Theoretical Medicine* **17**, 209–223.

Borgmann A. (1984). *Technology and the Character of Contemporary Life: A philosophical inquiry* (Chicago: The University of Chicago Press).

Bunge M. (1972). 'Toward a philosophy of technology' in C. Mitcham and R. Mackey (eds.) *Philosophy and Technology: Readings in the philosophical problems of technology* (New York: The Free Press), 62–76.

Clouser K. (1977). Clinical medicine as science: editorial. *Journal of Medicine and Philosophy*, **2**, 1–7.

Descartes R. 1955 [1644]. 'The principles of philosophy' in *Philosophical Works of Descartes* (Cambridge: Dover Publications).

Dreyfus H. (1972). *What Computers Can't Do: A critique of artificial reason* (Cambridge: MIT Press).

Drefus H. (1992). *What Computers Still Can't Do: A critique of artificial reason* (Cambridge, MIT Press).

Dunne J. (1993). *Back to the Rough Ground: 'Phronesis' and 'techne' in modern philosophy and in Aristotle* (Notre Dame: University of Notre Dame Press).

Dusek V. (2005). *Philosophy of Technology: An introduction* (Indianapolis, Wiley and Sons).

Ellul J. (1964). *The Technological Society* (New York: Vintage Books).

Feenberg A. (1981). *Lukacs, Marx, and the Sources of Critical Theory* (New York: Oxford University Press).

Feenberg A. (1991). *Critical Theory of Technology* (New York: Oxford University Press).

Feenberg A. (1995). *Alternative Modernity* (Berkeley: University of California Press).

Feenberg A. (1999). *Questioning Technology* (New York: Routledge).

Feibleman J. (1972). 'Pure science, applied science, and technology: An attempt at definitions' in C. Mitcham and R. Mackey (eds.) *Philosophy and Technology: Readings in the philosophical problems of technology* (New York: The Free Press), 33–41.

Gadamer H.-G. (1975) [1960]. *Truth and Method.* (New York: Continuum Press).

Gadamer H.-G. (1996) [1993]. *The Enigma of Health: The art of healing in a scientific age* (Stanford: Stanford University Press).

Heidegger, M. 1976.'The question concerning technology' in D. Krell (ed.) *Martin Heidegger: Basic writings* (New York: Harper & Row), 283–318.

Hunter K. (1989). A science of individuals: medicine and casuistry. *Journal of Medicine and Philosophy*, **14**, 193–212.

Ihde D. (1991). *Instrumental Reason: The interface between philosophy of science and philosophy of technology* (Bloomington, Indiana University Press).

Ihde D. (1998). *Expanding Hermeneutics: Visualism in science* (Evanston, IL: Northwestern University Press).

Jarvie I. C. (1972). 'Technology and the structure of knowledge' in C. Mitcham and R. Mackey (eds.) *Philosophy and Technology: Readings in the philosophical problems of technology* (NewYork: The Free Press), 54–61.

Jonas H. (1966). 'The practical uses of theory' in *The Phenomenon of Life* (Westport, CT: Greenwood Press), 188–210.

Jonas H. (1974). 'Seventeenth century and after: the meaning of the scientific and technological revolution' in *Philosophical Essays: From ancient creed to technological man* (Chicago: The University of Chicago Press), 45–80.

Kaplan D. M. (2004). *Readings in the Philosophy of Technology* (Lanham, MD: Rowman and Littlefield).

Leder D. (1990). *The Absent Body* (Chicago: The University of Chicago Press).

Marcuse H. (1964). *One Dimensional Man* (Boston: Beacon Press).

McWhinney I. (1978). Medical knowledge and the rise of technology. *Journal of Medicine and Philosophy*, **3**, 293–304.

Mitcham C. and Mackey R. (eds.) (1972). *Philosophy and technology: Readings in the philosophical problems of technology* (New York: The Free Press).

Mumford L. (1963). *Technics and Civilization* (New York: Harcourt, Brace & World, Inc.).

Mumford L. (1972). 'Technics and the nature of man' in C. Mitcham and R. Mackey (eds.) *Philosophy and Technology: Readings in the philosophical problems of technology* (London, The Free Press), 77–85.

Mumford L. (1973). *The Condition of Man* (New York: Harcourt Brace Jovanovich, Inc.).

Munson R. (1981). Why medicine cannot be a science. *Journal of Medicine and Philosophy*, **2**, 183–208.

Olsen J.-K. and Selinger E. (2007). *Philosophy of Technology* (Copenhagen: Automatic Press).

Pellegrino E. and Thomasma D. (1981). *A Philosophical Basis of Medical Practice: Toward a philosophy and ethic of the healing professions* (New York: Oxford University Press).

Phillips J. (2002*a*). 'Technical reason in the DSM-IV: An unacknowledged value' in J. Z. Sadler (ed.) *Descriptions & Prescriptions: Values, mental disorders, and the DSMs* (Baltimore: The Johns Hopkins University Press), 76–95.

Phillips J. (2002*b*). Managed care's reconstruction of human existence: the triumph of technical reason. *Theoretical Medicine*, **23**, 339–358.

Sadler J. Z. (2005). *Values and Psychiatric Diagnosis* (Oxford: Oxford University Press).

Scharff R. D. and Dusek V. (eds.) (2003). *Philosophy of Technology: The technological condition* (Oxford: Blackwell).

Sharfstein S. S. (2005). President's column. *Psychiatric News*, **40** (5 August), 3.

Skolimowski H. (1972). 'The structure of thinking in technology' in C. Mitcham and R. Mackey (eds.) *Philosophy and Technology: Readings in the philosophical problems of technology* (New York: The Free Press), 42–49.

Toulmin S. (1976). On the nature of the physician's understanding. *Journal of Medicine and Philosophy*, **1**, 32–50.

Toulmin S. (1990). *Cosmopolis: The hidden agenda of modernity* (Chicago: The University of Chicago Press).

Toulmin S. (2001). *Return to Reason* (Cambridge, MA: Harvard University Press).

Widdershoven-Heerding I. (1987). Medicine as a form of practical understanding. *Theoretical Medicine*, **8**, 1179–1185.

Winner L. (1977). *Autonomous Technology: Technics-out-of-control as a theme in political thought* (Cambridge, MA: MIT Press).

Winner L. (1986). *The Whale and the Reactor: A search for limits in an age of high technology* (Chicago: The University of Chicago Press).

Zaner R. (1990). Medicine and dialogue. *Journal of Medicine and Philosophy*, **15**, 303–325.

Part 1

Technical reason in psychiatry

Chapter 1

The instrument metaphor, hyponarrativity, and the generic clinician

John Z. Sadler

1.1 Introduction

Each day we encounter people in our lives whom we treat (to put it bluntly) as resources to be exploited. Any of us, given time and a notepad, could come up with hundreds of examples of this banal truth. My assistant is a resource who answers the phone for me, writes down progress notes, prepares manuscripts to journal specifications, maintains and files correspondence for me, and so forth. The 230 medical students I face in the lecture hall expect me to present a lecture on delirium that is informed, entertaining, and stimulating, not caring or even knowing my car is in the shop and that I had to hustle to show up on time. When the taxi driver en route to the airport starts to tell me about his problems, I am annoyed because I am not interested in his problems, but in getting to the airport on time. The CEO of the major corporation, despite its advertising campaign, is interested more in the stockholders' share values than in the public welfare. The politician is interested in her constituency as a means to re-election. And so on. In each of these very ordinary situations, people are treated not as ends in themselves, but, *contra* Kant, as means to ends. That is, people put themselves up, and are put up, to be used as resources in various projects, and we all, most of the time, accept this use of people as resources in everyday contemporary life.

I do not deny that there are many worthy ends to which these people-as-means are contributing: my work projects are important at least to me; the students' understanding of delirium may result in their saving many lives in years ahead; in another setting I might, as a psychiatrist, be very interested in helping the cab driver with his problems; and indeed the CEO's attention to profit-making contributes to economic growth and the creation of new jobs, which in turn make a substantial contribution to the public welfare.

So to recognize the idea that people are resources to be used is more a condition of being human rather than a moral failing, more of a moral–existential limitation than a uniform moral failing. From this existential context, so to speak, this essay will comment on this tension between people as means and as ends.

1.2 **Instrumentality**

Having pointed out this instrumental character of everyday life, for this chapter I would like to explore the manner in which 'instrumentality' has increasingly saturated mental health work. My thesis can be simply stated: instrumentalist thinking has subtly, yet inexorably transformed the practice of mental health care and even the self-experience of clinicians and patients. Acknowledging the value of instrumentalist thinking, I claim that the balance between instrumentalist, and (what I shall call for the time being) 'non-instrumentalist' thinking has profoundly shifted to the former. Just as with the fact of our existential use of other people, so does this transformation generate ambivalence in our thinking about utility.

What do I mean by instrumentalist thinking? For my purposes here, instrumentalism is a style of thinking dominated by the values of efficiency, efficacy, production, and outcome (over process). Within the instrumentalist mode, we evaluate ourselves, our projects, and our lives in terms of outcomes and production. Indeed, the very notion of an 'evaluation' in everyday talk has come to mean assessment in terms of productivity or accomplishment. For some, thinking of how to evaluate ourselves and our projects outside this value system may be difficult to imagine—but this chapter will indicate other, alternative values that could characterize our thinking and our self-evaluations.

The inspiration for this idea comes from Martin Heidegger's *The Question Concerning Technology* (1976), though Heidegger does not cast his version of instrumentalist thinking in terms of characteristic, concrete values as I do here (this treatment is given a more thorough account in my 'Technology' chapter in *Values and Psychiatric Diagnosis* (Sadler 2005)). What worried Heidegger about technological ways of thinking was the framing of our experiences and projects as problems and solutions—a frame that results in an ever-expanding network of technological fixes which limit our potential as humans. We can recognize this network through picking any example of a technological artifact and then consider its history and practical interconnections in the social world. Take a light bulb for example—a solution to the problem of darkness. A solution that is interconnected to the problems of adequate glass production, adequate energy production, adequate refinement of metals, the development of standards of function and design, the regulation and control of waste materials, and indeed to a veritable cascade of such things as child labor laws, where electric light boosted the potential for meaningful nighttime labor, and the problem of night labor by children became 'illuminated'. The examples could go on. Each example would have its own layers of social–functional interconnections, and indeed would link intimately with the broad notions of economic production and the link between technology and capitalism (Feenberg 1991), though the latter is a discussion for another time. Although we can easily recognize this 'enframing' of our human experience, how it limits our potential may be less obvious. Let me turn to an illuminating example from Hubert Dreyfus, an example of which I am quite fond.

1.3 Technological and poietic values

Dreyfus (1991, 1995) contrasts the artifacts of the Styrofoam cup and Japanese teacup. The former, he shows, is deeply technological in character, the latter, less so. The Styrofoam cup exemplifies the technological artifact embodying the values of efficiency, efficacy, thrift, and disposability. The Styrofoam cup keeps my beverage warm or cold, it is inexpensive, and when I am finished with it, I simply toss it away (in a designated trash receptacle, preferably for recycling, of course). The Japanese teacup, however, as Dreyfus points out, is situated in a rich history and tradition, drawing together families, shared memories, spiritual themes, and the like. Moreover, the Japanese teacup is anything but efficient or disposable: it is fragile, expensive, it requires washing, careful storage, and protection. Yet Japanese families cherish the teacup in ways barely conceivable when considering a cup of plastic foam.

Through his example Dreyfus contrasts the ways the vessels are 'evaluated'—the values that are built into and embodied by them—values that are in marked contrast to each other. The Styrofoam cup embodies the values of efficiency, efficacy, economy, productivity—the values consonant with technology. The teacup embodies another set of values—tradition, family ties, emotional bonds, spirituality, a connectedness with Nature and art. When we live by and think under the metaphor of the Styrofoam cup, I (again inspired by Heidegger) call this way of living and thinking the 'technological mode of being' and the latter, under the metaphor of the Japanese teacup, the 'poietic mode of being'.

Restating my thesis against this background, mental health care has increasingly found itself operating in the technological mode rather than the poietic mode. I shall now present some cultural 'artifacts' that provide evidence of the dominance of the technological mode in mental health care.

Consider this clinical case: Ms Y, a middle-aged clerk with a bachelor's degree in math, presented for individual therapy because of chronic pelvic pain, marital problems, and diffuse anxiety. Her initial presentation could be characterized as a hodgepodge of somatic symptoms—'chronic pelvic pain', 'headache', 'tired all the time', 'nervous', along with externalizing complaints about others—'annoyed with Joe (her husband)', 'the kids never listen to me', 'employers are unreasonable', 'people take advantage of me', etc. She presented herself and to others almost entirely through strings of evaluations: 'The doctors can't control my pains, I've had three operations that were no good...my children don't listen to me because I'm so controlling...Joe is so hung up on religion that I can't talk to him...I can't work because things are bothering me all the time...'. She was a complainer.

When asked about more detailed examples of these problems, she made noble efforts but could not couch her life in terms of a narrative. She could not identify her own emotions, only could identify pain as 'feelings'. She could not place herself into a narrative line in which she was an actor among an interplay of other actors with their own motivations, beliefs, concerns, and histories. I believe this difficulty partly explains her sense of being lost amid a crowd of seemingly exploiting others. She had little in the way of an 'observing ego', or 'self-reflection', at least at first.

Her therapy consisted in my teaching her how to cast her life in terms of stories, including her own emotional reactions to life events and how she handled them. Her chronic pelvic pain disappeared very quickly, but her anxiety became more pronounced as she came to see her own role in her misery—as a powerful actor in her life. Assuming this 'role' proved to be the most challenging aspect of her treatment and for herself.

Ms Y, I would contend, lived within, and was consumed by, the technological mode of being—her identity and selfhood was wrapped up with being a good wife, mother, and employee, and saw herself as planted in a network (framework) of functionary people serving goals that only partly overlap with her own—as coworkers, as husband/provider, as kids– products of child-rearing. What was remarkable in her talk was the absence of meaningful family traditions, recognition of individuality, or connectedness apart from performing/producing/generating outcomes around school, finances, housekeeping. She was exceptional in not recognizing traditional holidays and (material) gift-giving (she gave no gifts for birthdays and holidays), as disengaged as she was from people and 'poietic values'.

As a second example, consider this (modified, anonymized) medical record template from a respected colleague:

PATIENT:
ID#
DATE
TYPE OF SERVICE:

☐ medication management	☐ individual	☐ family	
☐ psychotherapy 30 min.	☐ individual	☐ family	☐ group
☐ psychotherapy 45 min.	☐ individual	☐ family	☐ group
☐ psychotherapy 90 min.	☐ individual	☐ family	☐ group
☐ diagnostic evaluation			

DIAGNOSIS:
Axis I:
Axis II:
Axis III:
Axis IV: ☐ economic ☐ occupational ☐ primary support group ☐ social environment ☐ educational
☐ housing ☐ access to health care ☐ legal ☐ other____
Axis V: current highest past year
CURRENT SYMPTOMS:
SIGNIFICANT LIFE EVENTS:
MEDICATION CHANGES:
CONTINUED MEDICATIONS:
MEDICAL CONCERNS:
ADVERSE EFFECTS:

SUICIDAL IDEATION:	☐ none currently	☐ nihilism	☐ thoughts	☐ plans ☐ indent
HOMICIDAL IDEATION:	☐ none currently	☐ thoughts	☐ plans	☐ intent ☐ means
PSYCHOTIC SYMPTOMS:	☐ none currently	☐ chronic baseline		☐ exacerbation

PSYCHOSOCIAL INTERVENTIONS:
THEME OF THERAPY:
PROBLEM/PLAN:

1.
2.
3.
4. ***Patient education/informed consent:***
5. ***Need for continuing care:***

This standard document is her primary means to document her clinical care in the medical record. Designed to be compliant with Medicare billing requirements, it is a model of efficiency, efficacy, brevity, and productivity. The template serves to shorten, systematize, organize, and satisfy all the requisite billing requirements. It conveniently systematizes the clinical data required for fair billing of Medicare. Moreover, it embraces the values of the technological mode of being. Interestingly, like Ms Y's discourse, the template leaves little room for story-telling—as if the patient's story is irrelevant, much less the doctor's interpretation of that story, the practical and moral considerations of clinical problem-solving, or even the macroscopic 'trajectory'of the treatment process. What will happen to the narrative thread of the patient's life and therapy as this 'chart' develops? How will an idiographic understanding of the patient be retained?

A third example of the expansion of the technological mode within psychiatric practice comes from psychiatric residency training accreditation requirements.

> 2. The program must demonstrate that residents have achieved competency in at least the following forms of treatment:

a. brief therapy
b. cognitive–behavioral therapy
c. combined psychotherapy and psychopharmacology
d. psychodynamic therapy, and
e. supportive therapy

(Accreditation Council for Graduate Medical Education (ACGME), Program requirements for residency training in psychiatry, February 2000, effective January 2001: 31)

What is remarkable about these requirements is what they presuppose or imply: (1) that psychiatrists practice each of these therapies routinely, and as Nassir Ghaemi has pointed out, by pure patient 'indication' (Ghaemi 2003); (2) that all psychiatry residents should have the capability of achieving competency in all of these therapies; and (3) that a three- to four-year psychiatric postgraduate training period is adequate to prepare, in principle, all residents for *competency* in these therapies. I have noted elsewhere (Sadler 2007) that these requirements imply that each of these therapies can be applied to any suitable patient, with the homogeneity of administration and effect comparable to the administration of a medication. I have called this phenomenon the 'psychotherapy pill' because it, like the administration of a pill, assumes an anonymous, competent administrator, whose personal character, history, and selfhood are irrelevant to the treatment effects (other than placebo effects, of course!). The delivery of a pill requires competency, but once launched, the mode of action takes place independently of the agent of delivery. The implied rendering of psychotherapy as a treatment independent from the agent–deliverer makes up the 'psychotherapy pill' metaphor. As might be inferred, I would question all three of these assumptions, as well as the idea that psychotherapy can be administered like a pill.

Over the past 25 years, standardization procedures have increasingly characterized mental health and medical practice. Standardization has made mental health care more accountable, fairer in many ways, and has probably spared many patients the adversities of incompetent care. Indeed, the success of standardization has prompted its proliferation. To mention several prominent examples: (1) the development of explicit diagnostic criteria for diagnosis in the Diagnostic and Statistical Manuals of Mental Disorders (DSMs; American Psychiatric Association 1994, 2000); (2) pre-certification, review, case management in managed care settings; (3) treatment guidelines for particular conditions or disorders; (4) psychopharmacology treatment algorithms; (5) instruction manuals for psychotherapy; and (6) structured diagnostic interviews. These procedures have the laudable, even crucial goal of promoting consistent, competent, and effective care (Sadler 2007). Indeed, standardization, efficiency, and efficacy are crucial values that these procedures have aspired to promote and respect, and in so doing have allowed psychiatry and mental health to offer more certain scientific knowledge and the development of more effective therapies. But life is full of trade-offs, and although there are many praises to be sung for the DSMs, treatment guidelines, and the like, my focus here is 'What do we lose by promoting these values in our treatment paradigms?'.

The literature on computer-assisted or -provided psychotherapy is growing. Indeed, at least one specialized journal, *CyberPsychology and Behavior*, has appeared, prominently featuring empirical studies of computer psychotherapy or 'robotherapy' (Libin and Libin 2003). What could be more efficient than eliminating the therapist altogether, especially if there is no loss in efficacy? Moreover, mechanized therapeutic tools potentially expand the ability to treat more people (Gega *et al.* 2004; Krija *et al.* 2004; Tate and Zabinski 2004). The metaphor of doctors as machines then becomes a concrete reality, and automated therapy brings a similar set of assets and problems as Henry Ford's assembly-line did.

In 2004, philosopher Louis Charland reported on internet phenomena concerning mental health and illness. Charland, after 'lurking' in internet chat rooms about mental health and illness issues, found substantial numbers of participants debating the significance, meaning, and importance of their diagnostic categories or 'labels'. The reified categories seemed to determine the person's identity, rather than the reverse. Some participants were threatened by proposed revisions to DSM diagnostic categories; as if changing the name somehow changed their self:

> The relative independence and persistence of psychiatric diagnostic labels despite their abolishment by institutional psychiatry raises several novel ethical problems. First, because persons often identify with their label, to remove a label is to threaten a person's identity. Saying the label is no longer legitimate, or was a mistake in the first place, can therefore cause serious harm, particularly to persons already suffering from disorders that implicate identity. Second, the retention of psychiatric labels by consumer forces that operate independently of the psychiatric establishment can possibly cause further harm to patients of the labels are truly empirically invalid. New more scientifically appropriate labels may not be adopted and more effective treatments may not be sought.
>
> (Charland 2004: 347)

What do these seemingly discrepant cultural phenomena have in common? I would claim at least three things, which I will call the 'instrument metaphor,' 'hyponarrativity' and the 'generic clinician'. Let me discuss each in turn.

1.4 The instrument metaphor

When people are used and regarded primarily as instruments in larger social projects, and these larger social projects are evaluated in the language of production and utility, I call this existential condition the 'instrument metaphor.' The metaphor is the 'as if' character, and 'instrument' refers to the instrumental character of our condition.

I would contend that the regarding of people in terms of the instrument metaphor is unavoidable, tied to the existential truths of everyday social life, but it is not the way we should always or perhaps even predominantly regard people, as Kant claimed. As with the Styrofoam cup of Dreyfus' example, the life according to the instrument metaphor is bereft of spiritual depth, of emotional connection. Life under a predominating instrument metaphor is artless and joyless (but perhaps depressionless!). We become concerned with the acquisition of material possessions because these things help us meet our 'objectives.' We become alienated from others because they slow us down from our quest for efficiency and productivity. Like Ms Y, we consume and produce, but are not satisfied, content, or gratified. Like Charland's chat participants, we are nominalized by others' objectives and purposes. Our compliance with Medicare billing requirements makes us an instrument of a larger healthcare system, along with our residents whose individuality is irrelevant to their clinical competence.

1.5 Hyponarrativity

In *Values and Psychiatric Diagnosis* (2005), I coined the awkward locution 'hyponarrativity' to describe what appeared to be a guiding assumption of the DSM:

> What I mean by 'hyponarrativity' in the case of the DSMs has to do with the choosing of the descriptive or categorical route to diagnosis, rather than seeing 'the patient as a subject responding to a set of circumstances and understand[ing] the distressing symptoms as reactions to the misfortune.
>
> (Sadler 2005: 177)

Hyponarrativity is the marginalizing of the narrative, 'storied' dimension of human existence. In the DSM, hyponarrativity is formalized into the very concept of mental disorder through the emphasis on 'social and occupational functioning'. My colleague Jim Phillips sees the symptom concept in mental health as 'emblematic' of the technological mode (J. Phillips, personal communication 2007). I tend to agree, but as will be clarified later, what counts is not emblems but the uses of concepts in practice. (Whether symptoms are technological-mode depends on their practical use.) What this means is psychopathology is assessed in large part on whether the patient succeeds in fulfilling the technological values of productivity, efficacy, and efficiency. Under this criterion of qualifying for a mental disorder, the narrativizing of the poietic mode is existential background and irrelevant. The DSM does not so much ignore the patient's interpersonal relationships as a measure of pathology: rather, it overlooks the poetic aspects of human life, for instance, the *attachments* people have to each other. Ms Y's compulsion to evaluate herself and others makes her both the embodiment of the DSM ontology and a hyponarrativity. Her self-talk appears to be tailored for DSM diagnostic criteria. Her talk about her family sounds more corporate than familial.

We can readily recognize the hyponarrativity in the Medicare template, algorithms and treatment guidelines, Charland's chatroom participants, and ACGME requirements—and the efficiency value embodied by these artifacts is also obvious. Surely mental health involves some sort of engagement of the self as a participant in the world of others, but these artifacts obscure this truism.

1.6 **The generic clinician**

In the ACGME guidelines, the point of training appears to be to produce generically capable clinicians—anonymous because their individual predilections, talents, and faults do not count, capable through the administration of homogeneous, predictable, uniform modes of therapy, be they medications or psychotherapy interventions. The generic clinician responds to collective, corporate, uniform requirements and adheres to managed care requirements, Medicare billing requirements, treatment algorithms, and psychotherapy manuals. The 'pill' becomes the central metaphor for treatment: administration yields a standard, uniform effect; the administrator may be anonymous with no effect on outcome. When we consider 'robotherapy', the perfection of the faceless clinician has reached its apotheosis and the clinician can literally be replaced by a literally anonymous, compliant, and consistent machine. Will the patients respond and comply? Can clinicians provide the uniformity, predictability, and utility of intervention that machines can provide? Will psychiatrists become programmers for robotherapists?

1.7 **Re-engagement and reform**

The philosopher Albert Borgmann describes many of these societal ills in his *Technology and the Character of Everyday Life* (Borgmann 1984).

Sympathetic readers of this chapter might well be rewarded by reading Borgmann's prescriptions for altering our relationship to technology. Meaningful reform of our relationship to technology and the technological mode don't involve the rejection of technology, no more than reform necessarily involves the rejection of Medicare billing standards, the DSM, and treatment algorithms. Instead, reform involves altering our attitude and conduct regarding technology, and reorienting ourselves toward what is truly important. We might say reform involves a balance between the technological and poietic modes of being—though I think Borgmann's emphasis on the relationship between the two modes is more to the point.

The reform of our relationship to technology for Borgmann involves three key concepts: awareness, engagement, and a focus on 'ultimate concerns.' Awareness involves the recognition of these distinctions between the technological and poietic mode. Engagement involves investing the self in worthwhile, meaningful activities, which in turn depend on our ultimate concerns—our highest aspirations, ego-ideals, and guiding values. In my view, the reform of our relationship to technology involves both a redirection toward others and the external world, as well as an inward-directed element. From this standpoint, the question of 'balance' between technological and poietic mode is off the mark: if we are guided by the right values, technological tools are only means, and 'balance' is not an apt metaphor. Our values or 'the right way to live' arise within, or are embodied within, the poietic mode: the technological mode is secondary, a means to the poietic ends.

Some examples may be in order. From the 'external' perspective, reorienting toward ultimate concerns might redirect us toward shaping our psychiatric–professional lives toward the ultimate concern of 'patient welfare'. Technology and the technological mode are subserved to those goals. Medical records are to ensure quality care, and so engaging in the making-room for those considerations would be a reform. Instead of the DSM's highest priority being a 'helpful guide to clinical practice'(American Psychiatric Association 1994: xv), perhaps it should be 'the improvement of, or excellence in, the care of the mentally ill' (Sadler 2005: 349). Crucial to the reform would be to ensure that the reorienting toward ultimate concerns is not just a motto, but a commitment or engagement to work towards those ultimate concerns. A key virtue for the poietically engaged clinician might be *discipline*. Achievements through discipline seem to be irreplaceable compared with purchased achievements.

In terms of internal, self-directed 'reforms', one might think of office assistance, checklists, and algorithm efficiencies not as tools to 'save time' but as tools that offer opportunities for a more intimate doctor–patient relationship. These tools are the place where treatment considerations begin with patients, not end. Indeed, if there is substance to the idea that mental health involves an engagement with people and the world, then patients should be assisted in securing that engagement with ultimate concerns as well.

References

American Psychiatric Association (1994). *Diagnostic and Statistical Manual of Mental Disorders*, 4th edn. (Washington, DC: American Psychiatric Press).

American Psychiatric Association (2000). *Diagnostic and Statistical Manual of Mental Disorders*, 4th edn., text revision (Washington, DC: American Psychiatric Association).

Borgmann A. (1984). *Technology and the Character of Contemporary Life: A philosophical inquiry* (Chicago: University of Chicago Press).

Charland L. (2004). A madness for identity: psychiatric labels, consumer autonomy, and the perils of the internet. *Philosophy, Psychiatry, and Psychology*, **11**, 335–349.

Dreyfus H. (1991). *Being-in-the-World: A commentary on Heidegger's Being and Time, Division 1* (Cambridge, MA: MIT Press).

Dreyfus H. L. (1995). 'Heidegger on gaining a free relation to technology' in A. Feenberg and A. Hannay (eds.) *Technology & The Politics of Knowledge* (Indianapolis: Indiana University Press) 97–107.

Feenberg A. (1991). *Critical Theory of Technology* (Oxford: Oxford University Press).

Gega L., Marks I., and Mataix-Cols D. (2004). Computer-aided CBT self-help for anxiety and depressive disorders: experience of a London clinic and future directions. *Journal of Clinical Psychology*, **60**, 147–157.

Ghaemi S. N. (2003). *The Concepts of Psychiatry* (Baltimore: The Johns Hopkins University Press).

Heidegger M. (1976). 'The question concerning technology' in D. F. Krell (ed.) *Basic Writings* (New York: Harper and Row), 283–317.

Krijn M., Emmelkamp P. M. G., Olafsson R. P., and Biemond R. (2004). Virtual reality exposure therapy of anxiety disorders: a review. *Clinical Psychology Review*, **24**, 259–281.

Libin E. and Libin A. (2003). New diagnostic tool for robotic psychology and robotherapy studies. *Cyberpsychology and Behavior*, **6**, 369–374.

Sadler J. Z. (2005). *Values and Psychiatric Diagnosis* (Oxford: Oxford University Press).

Sadler J. Z. (2007). The psychiatric significance of the personal self. *Psychiatry: Biological and Interpersonal Processes*, **70**, 113–129.

Tate D. F. and Zabinski M. F. (2004). Computer and internet applications for psychological treatment: update for clinicians. *Journal of Clinical Psychology*, **60**, 209–220.

Chapter 2

Technological rationality in psychiatry: immanent critique, critical theory, and a pragmatist alternative

Peter Zachar and Scott Bartlett

2.1 Introduction

The purpose of this chapter is to acknowledge the importance of a critical analysis of technological and algorithmic approaches to problem solving in psychiatry without rejecting the progressive contributions of technology. We argue that there are negative consequences to relying on technological approaches, but technology is not fundamentally alien to our nature. Among the most articulate and insightful opponents of technological rationality were the members of the Frankfurt school of critical social theory. We claim that the critical theorists offered important insights, but they also adopted an overly hostile attitude toward technological reasoning. A less dystopian alternative is found in the pragmatism of Dewey. We describe the advantages of a reflective use of technology in which 'ends' are open to renegotiation as situations evolve, and also propose that many important shortcomings of technological approaches are discovered only by users of technology. Examples from the domains of statistical prediction, psychiatric taxonomy, and evidence-based medicine are explored.

2.2 Clinical psychology and technical methodology

In the middle of the twentieth century, Paul Meehl (1954) initiated a controversy within psychology over the value of statistical versus clinical prediction. Meehl asked whether it is better to make predictions about patients using expert judgment or using actuarial methods. Meehl's argument in support of actuarial methods challenged traditional assumptions regarding the value of expert opinion and experience in the healthcare professions. These arguments anticipated the conceptual basis of both the *Diagnostic and Statistical Manual of Mental Disorders, Third Edition* (DSM-III) revolution and evidence-based medicine. The field of psychological measurement is also the primary source of the various proposals for dimensional models in psychiatry.

Let us introduce Meehl's argument using a non-clinical example. The question is whether an applicant will be a successful college student. According to Meehl, admissions committees should give all applicants a normed test that assesses academic skills. Norms allow one to decide how capable an individual applicant is relative to everyone else. If we can also show that scores on the skills test are correlated with academic performance in college, we can create a formula for predicting future college grade point average from the score any subsequent applicant earns on the academic skills test. Such a formula can be used to not only predict success, but to predict who could benefit from remedial work—the latter goal being closer to the original purpose of IQ testing as introduced by Binet in 1905.

Meehl claimed that technical formulas, on the whole, consistently lead to equal or better predictions than expert evaluations. The statistical methods are better at assessing what variables are actually related to the criterion of interest and also better at weighing the variables in terms of relative importance (i.e., aggregation). Furthermore, individual differences between raters in skill level, cognitive biases, motivation, and fatigue are eliminated when using formulae. Every applicant is treated the same.

Since Meehl made his initial claims, statistical prediction has been found to be superior to clinical prediction in many domains, including the assessment of personality traits, malingering, and the denial of psychiatric problems. Statistical formulas can also distinguish neurotic from psychotic disorders, identify likely candidates for criminal recidivism and predict the length of psychotherapy (Dawes *et al.* 1989; Garb 1998; Morey 1996;).

2.3 The advantages of technological understanding

We are a technology-dependent species. Some technologies predated the development of *Homo sapiens* and may have served as selection pressures during evolution, such as the use of stone axes and fire by our ancestor *Homo erectus* (Futuyma 1998). Skills that potentiate the discovery and refinement of technology are arguably a part of our design.

In this chapter, technology refers not only to the use of physical tools, but also to acquired methods and procedures for solving problems so that the probability of a successful solution is enhanced. Technological procedures are *rules for action*. For example, if you want to begin your day with a cup of espresso, you cannot open a can of Folgers, throw a scoop of coffee in some hot water, and wait for it to turn into espresso. For espresso you need a specific kind of coffee bean, it has to be ground in a particular way, and then water at a certain temperature has to be forced through the grounds for a determinate amount of time.

Espresso, fine wine, supermarket doors that open themselves, endoscopic surgery, and magnetic resonance imaging renderings of internal organs are wonderful things. We don't need magic to make them, although without knowledge of the relevant techniques and their development, the final products can seem like magic. If such techniques are efficient and easy to use, their application can become habitual. Habitual use is reinforced by robust efficacy. For example, antibiotics work whether the patient believes in Western medicine, indigenous and holistic approaches, faith-healing, or miracles. For these reasons, they are widely used.

2.4 **Technological rationality**

Technological rationality refers to methodological approaches becoming norms of rationality so that thinking and acting in conformity with technology comes to define what it means to be rational. An endemic problem associated with increased technical prowess is that when we discover methods that successfully allow us to deal with particular kinds of problems, we can become so reliant on them that we rarely think about those problems outside of what is prescribed by our methods. Similar to the negative consequences associated with Cacioppo and Petty's (1982) concept of *low need for cognition*, a reliance on technological rationality encourages a preference for easy answers and magic bullets rather than thinking through a problem. This is potentially undesirable. As the singer Tom Waits (1993) writes:

> The more of them magics you use, the more bad days you have without them. So it comes down finally to all your days being bad without the bullets. It's magics or nothing.

John Sadler (2005) points out that we also rarely question the values enshrined in our methods, if we even notice values at all. For example, the belief that technology is value neutral is exemplified by claims such as 'Guns don't kill people, people do!'

Technological rationality is a form of instrumental reasoning, or reasoning with goals-in-mind. If you think it is important to own a Saab, then it is rational to take an extra job on the weekend. If you think it is important to develop close relationships with your family, then taking an extra job may be irrational.

In technological rationality, the *means* often dictate the *ends*. In other words, we sometimes choose to work on problems because the tools are available. In a memorable phrase conventionally attributed to Abraham Maslow, if the only tool you have is a hammer, then everything becomes a nail. Seeking and then pounding 'nails' becomes the rational thing to do.

An example of this process in the mental health professions would be picking goals for treatment based only on what goals a therapy manual prescribes. To illustrate, the solution focused therapy manual says the goal for therapy is to help clients imagine a better future and decide what behaviors they need to practice in order to make that future a reality (Miller and Berg 1996). The manual offers a host of techniques for doing this, for example, 'asking the miracle question'. For many users, 'focusing on solutions' is considered a good treatment goal because the manual claims it can be achieved efficiently and economically (in fewer than ten sessions!). In philosophical terms, this goal is the end because there is a means to achieve it. When following the dictates of technological rationality, the need to be *productive* and *efficient* can result in working on problems because we can, without always considering whether we should.

A more penetrating explication of the relationship between technological progress and norms of rationality is found in Ian Hacking's (2002*a*, 2002*b*) work on styles of scientific reasoning. Two scientific styles of reasoning that are important in psychiatry include *Ordering Diversity by Taxonomy* and *Statistically Analyzing Regularities Using Probability.*

According to Hacking, each style of reasoning engenders philosophical debates about realism versus antirealism. Examples include:

Is schizophrenia a natural kind?

Does the 'average' person exist?

Styles of reasoning also introduce new kinds of statements that are candidates for truth or falsity such as:

Does schizoaffective disorder belong on the schizophrenic spectrum?

Is the sample representative?

With the introduction of a style, new perceptions about how the world is structured emerge.

In the tradition of Foucault, Hacking (1990) points out that with the introduction of statistical reasoning, not only did *populations*, *normalcy* (versus deviancy) and *deviancy* (as quantitative variation) become things we observed, but the scientific determinism advocated by Enlightenment thinkers such as Laplace was downgraded in favor of chance. For determinists, outcomes are fated to be as a function of causal necessity and the concept of 'probability' refers to the subjective degree of confidence we have in predicting the eventual result. In a universe of chance the concept of 'probability' refers to the odds that a certain outcome will result from a series of event/actions. The difference between the two concepts of probability is important. With the second kind of probability, as with evolution, specific outcomes are not necessarily fated to be.

As the statistical style was being developed, a diverse set of technologies ensued for counting, summarizing, comparing, predicting and, eventually, explaining phenomena such as diseases and crime. The work of Marx (economic and historical laws), Durkheim (social science), and Darwin (populations of organisms) were each, in their own way, connected with statistical reasoning.

An important quality of a scientific style of reasoning is that it is self-authenticating. As noted, a style of reasoning nominates new candidates for truth or falsity, for example, 'Are the treatment and control groups significantly different?' The style is authenticated by subsequently being used to determine if any of the new candidate statements actually are true or false. For example, if we ask, 'Are the mean differences between the treatment group, the control, group and the placebo control group significant?', having a way to answer that question (i.e., formulating a null hypothesis, computing an *F* ratio and deciding to reject the null hypothesis) serves to authenticate statistical reasoning.

A subtle implication of Hacking's argument is that the presence of significant differences between groups is an objective fact, if you use the statistical style of reasoning. The style of reasoning provides a systematic way to answer a question which would not be asked if the style didn't exist. It constitutes a *norm of rationality*—a shared cognitive-methodological resource on which people can subsequently draw. Once the norms are established, doing something like merely eyeballing two means (e.g., treatment group = 8, control group = 10) and claiming one is larger than another violates the canons of rationality. Without a test of statistical significance, one cannot rationally rule out the possibility that the observed difference between the two means is due to random variation.

As stated earlier, the styles of reasoning or norms of rationality that are especially relevant to psychiatry are the statistical and the taxonomic styles. Each style prescribes different sets of methodological strategies. Learning how to think in these ways helps define what it means to be rational in psychiatry and clinical psychology. They also play a role in determining the goals that psychiatric nosologists seek to achieve.

2.5 Technological domination

The critical social theorists such as Horkheimer and Adorno (1944/2001) and Marcuse (1964) explored our dependency on technology in the form of technological domination. Marcuse also claimed that since instrumental reasoning operates according to its own relentless logic, technology tends to become autonomous and thus less subject to our control.

Exploring the role of the automobile in contemporary society offers an easily accessible example of technological domination. Automobiles allow us to get from one place to another efficiently. With the introduction of the automobile, people are able to live long distances from work, and cities are planned so that schools, stores, offices, and neighborhoods are placed with driving distance of each other; that is, cities are designed to require automobiles.

In the past seventy-five years, social norms regulating what is possible to accomplish in a single day have been recalibrated to take into account rapid travel on demand. Over time, an uncountable number of livelihoods have come to depend on making, selling, repairing, and insuring cars, building and maintaining roads, providing fuel, and regulating traffic.

One of the most penetrating insights of the critical social theorists is that new technologies also mold us personally by creating desires—we want sun roofs, quiet rides, more airbags, and GPS systems, and will work to get them. Humans also become a particular kind of object, *consumers*, and 'rational choice' itself is just another variable to be algorithmically manipulated. The cost of being freed from the limits of walking is a robust psychological and societal dependence on automobiles. Culture evolves both to accommodate and require the technology, and the ensuing social structure seems *natural* to those who never experienced anything different.

2.6 **Critical theory and 'identity thinking'**

Horkheimer and Adorno (1944/2001) argue that when it was developed in the seventeenth century, scientific reasoning was an advance over mythical and superstitious views of the world, for example, theories of demonic possession and a belief in divine punishment as explanations for what are currently identified as psychiatric disorders. Science abandoned supernatural explanations in favor of impersonal laws of nature. By explaining all of nature with respect to universal laws, however, Horkheimer and Adorno claim that scientific reasoning engendered its own kind of myth.

Adorno (1966/1973) refers to this myth as 'identity thinking' or believing that general concepts accurately represent the world in its particularity. According to the critical theorists, the real objects that exist out there in the world are always more complex and particular than the all-encompassing universal concepts and technological solutions acknowledge. For example the general concept of major depression articulated in the DSM-IV does not capture the complexities of depression as it is instanciated in distinct individuals.

Although written in a different philosophical tradition, the non-essentialist and nominalistic spirit of Adorno's critique of identity thinking has a close cousin in the domain of psychiatric classification, such as Zachar's (in press) claim that every good classification both reveals and conceals things about the objects being classified.

2.7 The critical theorist's response: immanent critique

The solution offered by the critical theorists to the problem of an all encompassing technological rationality was called immanent critique. Immanent critique takes existing norms as standards of measurement and examines failures to realize these norms. An example of an immanent critique would be pointing out that the Declaration of Independence stated that all men are created equal, but the subsequently created United States of America allowed slavery. Immanent critique works from within a system of thought, uncovering both its problems and its unrecognized possibilities.

By using immanent critique, the critical theorists believed that the tensions between the merely existent present and the possible future could be heightened. The goal would be, in some sense, to overcome the reified present. We note that the concept of the reified present can be applied not only to social systems, but also to institutionally approved technologies such as diagnostic manuals and treatment protocols.

Engaging in an immanent critique requires a sympathetic attitude with respect to the object of critique. One must be willing to validate what is legitimate in the target of the critique rather than merely discrediting or exposing what is invalid. To reveal the tensions existing internal to a particular way of seeing and acting in the world, the critical theorists attempted to trace out the full range of problems contained within that perspective.

Walter Benjamin (1936/1969) probably exhibited the 'sympathetic' dimension of the immanent critique of technology more thoroughly than the other critical theorists, especially in his essay 'The Work of Art in the Age of Its Technological Reproducibility.' After reviewing some of Benjamin's ideas on art and technology, the remainder of the chapter will advocate for the adoption of a likewise sympathetic attitude as a context for critical reflections in psychiatry.

In this essay, Benjamin examined the impact of mass-produced art, for example, the thousands of copies of Matisse paintings hung on walls throughout the world. He acknowledged that with mass reproduction there is a loss of the 'aura'; that is, the unique, irreplaceable, original object that has its own history. Aura is what is valued both in the Sistine chapel as a thing physically made by Michelangelo or in the patina on an old piece of furniture. The unique is precious and rare, not pedestrian and mass produced.

On the whole, Benjamin shared the critical theorists' view that art is a redemptive force in the face of relentless technological advancement. In this particular essay, however, he was less content to mourn what is lost or to adopt disdain for what is new. Photography and film, he noted, are also arts. They are a kind of art that would not exist without technology. As a matter of fact, there is no such thing as the original work in film or photography—the presence of multiple copies are inherent to these media. With the proliferation of director's cuts and other kinds of 'special editions', Benjamin's observations are even more perceptive today.

In line with the concept of technological rationality described earlier, Benajmin suggests that in film, the very norms of acting change. For example, a stage performance of *To Kill a Mockingbird* is given in two hours from beginning to end. In film, the performance may occur over a period of six months, and is not shot in sequence. More importantly, with close-ups, shadows, angles, and repeated viewings, film offers us something new—the perception of the artwork is configured in a totally unique way and a different reality is revealed. According to Benjamin, film is also accessible to more people than the elitist art forms of the past, save architecture, could possibly manage.

One of the important lessons we take from this essay is that technological products can have unique and progressive value. If this is true in art, it may also be true in science.

2.8 **A different species of immanent critique**

To their credit, the critical theorists provided important warnings that we should be vigilant to the ways in which we become blind to the institutional and technological forces that shape us. Their thoroughgoing rejection of instrumental reasoning, however, had the consequence of dampening their sympathy for technology. This limits their relevance to both psychiatry and psychology, which are each committed to accentuating the progressive nature of scientific understanding. As Wolin (2006) suggests, given their dystopian sensibilities related to their personal experience of the technological horror that was Nazi Germany, in the criticial theorists' hands, immanent critique came to function as a species of external critique of the Enlightnement project itself.

It is possible that the philosophical umbilical cord with the generation of Heidegger could not be cut and, as a result, the critical theorists tended to see technology as something alien and inhumane, exemplified in a reliance on philosophical distinctions such as natural versus artificial, authentic versus false and humanistic versus scientific. This led them to sometimes overstate the ways in which technology controls us and miss the myriad ways that we work creatively with technology.

John Dewey (1925/1981) offers an interesting contrast with the critical theorists. He referred to his philosophical method as *instrumentalism*, but what Dewey meant by the term 'instrumental' cannot be reduced to the instrumental reasoning that the critical theorists so vehemently criticized. For the critical theorists, instrumentalism is limited to finding means to secure already existent ends. It operates like a recipe, a decision procedure that if followed to the letter will yield the desired end. For Dewey, instrumental reasoning is dynamic. It demands constant readjustment between ends and means. Ends, for Dewey, should not be taken as given, but as ends-in-view.

We recommend Dewey's more flexible concept of ends. This concept potentially offers a way out of the either/or dichotomy of human values on the one side and scientific or technological imperatives on the other, especially in psychiatry. As with pragmatism generally, Dewey's concept is also consistent with both Darwinian theory and the likelihood that technology predated human evolution.

Dewey argues that human existence is a mixture of the precarious and stable, so there is no guarantee that our methods or techniques will always be suitable for our present problems. Often, our methods cease to be properly instrumental to the ends we have previously chosen. Problems in application and outcome represent the need for further inquiry. An important purpose of intelligence itself is the ability to see problematic situations *as* problematic, and to realize that methods may have to be reflectively reconstructed as the circumstances change. Doing so requires us to also reason about values. In this process of adaptation, ends too can be renegotiated.

More concretely, if manuals/cookbooks/algorithms summarize well-founded knowledge in a way that can be beneficially applied, then they are valuable tools. They are, like beliefs themselves, rules for action. Examples include psychotherapy manuals and decision-making algorithms for diagnosis. Uncritical adherence to manuals and decision rules, however, may foster stagnation. Progress, a key Enlightenment value, occurs when we have the gumption to confront the unknown (by preference or by necessity) and find better ways to do things than we were taught. The skeptical and self-correcting process of scientific reasoning is itself, a critical theory.

Technology is something that we use. As Hacking's concept of scientific styles of reasoning suggests, we have to work hard to learn to use 'technology.' For an immanent critique to be more than a methodological strategy for engaging in an external critique, it has to arise of its own accord from the users of technology, often from experienced users who have a degree of expertise. Some limitations become evident only in use. The flaws of identity thinking become evident in practice, or as Adorno says—the object inevitably eludes the concept. Although this different species of immanent critique is only one form of critique and should not be all-encompassing, it uncovers important value considerations that are invisible not only to unreflective users, but to external critics as well.

2.9 **Criticism from the inside out**

Let us return to the non-clinical example of predicting college grade point average to illustrate what we are proposing. The principle that will be emphasized in this section is the notion that technology can be used to make better decisions, but these decisions are not necessarily made in a value-free manner. With a reflective use, technological solutions can make values issues explicit, and their use is defended and rejected with respect to those goals and values.

Using a valid standardized test, the grade point averages of students entering college can be predicted with a formula better than they can with expert judgment. This means not that the formula will predict everyone's specific grade point average accurately; rather, it means that, on the whole, the average errors in prediction will be smaller using the formula than they will be by using professional judgment.

It is not that formulas provide the 'correct' answer to the question (i.e., will a given student graduate or not graduate); rather, they accurately identify more cases than intuitive approaches. They also mistakenly classify cases and the extent to which they do so can be quantified. A technique borrowed from epidemiology, hit rate analysis, tells us how many correct predictions and incorrect predictions are made when using the formula in combination with a cut score. An examination of costs and benefits using a hit rate analysis and the values issues they make subject to consideration, particularly as used in epidemiology, is the primary methodological strategy of evidence-based medicine. Hit rate analysis was also used to evaluate individual diagnostic criteria during the DSM-IV revision process.

Returning to the non-clinical example, with a very low ACT score, we may find that 80% of those who the formula-based decision rule says will fail actually do fail. That means that 20% of the time, the formula leads us to predict that someone will fail when they will actually succeed. A complicated series of value judgments can now be made about the costs and benefits of certain kinds of errors of prediction. Being able to obtain information about hits and misses, and consequently being able to engage in new kinds of value judgments, is an advantage of the formulas.

As a psychologist and chairperson of the academic standards committee at his university, one of us (P.Z.) was responsible for assessing the success and failure rates of students relative to their performance on a standardized aptitude test, namely the ACT. His analysis indicated that that, even with intensive remediation and academic advising, students with very low scores (ACT $\leq$ 15, or SAT $\leq$ 730) were unlikely to successfully earn an undergraduate degree at that institution. Students with slightly higher scores also had variable success rates, but benefited more from remedial education than those with low scores.

As we suggested earlier in this chapter, technology is used by humans for their purposes. With a reflective use of technology, values are not merely imposed. Values issues are also revealed and made subject to consideration. For example, the values issues that were made subject to consideration in this instance involved passionate debates about (a) the meaning and limits of *opportunity* at comprehensive institutions, (b) whether or not to take money from students who had a small chance of success, (c) whether the institution had a responsibility to avoid burdening such students with loan debt only to see them fail out in three years, and (d) the possibility re-allocating resources to those students who might succeed with additional help; that is, students with ACT 17 who were not eligible for more intensive services. The re-allocation of resources as a way to increase success rates for students who might not otherwise succeed was an important factor in the university's board of trustees agreeing to raise admissions standards.

What was interesting about this process was that the faculty were quite pleased with the changed policy, believing that raising the standards was going to eliminate the poorer-performing students from their classes. This was a notion that had to be repeatedly disputed. The number of students who would no longer be admitted was minuscule relative to the total number of students, and more importantly, most of the failing grades were being earned by students who had average scores on the ACT. The occasional Ds and Fs earned by the students with average ACTs dwarfed the number of consistent poor grades earned by those the very low ACTs. In this case, those having more experience with the relevant technology had to educate others about its limits.

It is the responsibility of the insider or the person schooled in the technology not only to implement the technology, but when the time comes, to explain to those who want the easy answers, all reasons why it is not as easy as it seems from the outside. Doing so is a matter of professional honesty and conscientiousness.

2.10 **Expertise—qualified**

Another issue in this example worth exploring is the notion of an 'expert'. In some cases considerable expertise is required to use a manual. For example, most scientific psychologists are not statisticians proper. They understand statistical logic and know how to use computer programs to answer specific kinds of research question. One computer program, called SPSS, is a manualized approach to statistics that is popular in the social sciences and is designed to be used by those who are not mathematicians.

Users of technology have graded ranges of expertise, and therefore, graded abilities to engage in an immanent critique. No individual can master all aspects of any technology. As such, a thorough immanent critique is the responsibility of the community of users. This principle applies not only to statistical reasoning, but also to psychiatric diagnosis, psychiatric consultation, pharmacology, and psychotherapy.

Qualified users have a professional responsibility to be reflective users. They should be 'thinkers'. Reflective use means being able to step back and become more conscious of one's professional activity. In this respect, the two sins of expertise are fooling yourself and fooling others. Fooling yourself represents a lack of critical reflection. To some extent, everyone is ignorant of the limits of their own methods and techniques. Many of us are also trained to accentuate the positive in the service of career advancement. A consistent lack of doubt, however, represents a failing. Another important failing is fooling others—to recognize the problems/limits but to offer what Leo Strauss (1964/1978) referred to as the *noble lie*; that is, playing politics and engaging in positive spin when you know it is not true. Both fooling yourself and noble lies undermine the intellectual honesty, skeptical analysis and the community's ongoing correction of error that defines the kind of scientific reasoning that inspired the better part of the Enlightenment, and also spawned most of the technologies that we use today.

2.11 **Examples from psychiatry**

In our terms, an immanent critique of technology requires an insider's critical awareness of the limitations of a field's methods-in-application. This kind of internal critique has also emerged in psychiatry, especially in the development and promulgation of the DSM-IV. For example, the introduction to the manual specifically cautions mental health professionals from using the diagnostic criteria in a cookbook fashion. The introduction also states that use of the manual requires appropriate training and experience, and should not be applied in a mechanical fashion by untrained individuals. Many an author of the manual has lamented that this introduction is rarely read, or applied (First *et al.* 1999; Williams *et al.* 1985).

The mechanistic or cookbook approach to diagnosis, where the goal is to find out which DSM diagnosis a patient has by merely checking whether criteria are met, is a kind of technological rationality. When using the mechanistic approach, if a patient meets criteria for any diagnosis in the manual, then he or she is considered to be both mentally ill and qualitatively distinct from everyone else. This represents an insidious variety of diagnostic literalism where issues of relative severity, compensating mechanisms, situational influences, and developmental issues are not considered.

The DSM was not written by merely discovering what disorders are really out there. The DSM revision process involved an extended period of evaluating evidence and engaging in debates about its meaning. Many of these debates began where the evidence ended, and involved considering the purposes of the DSM (communication, treatment, experimental research, correlational research, epidemiology, etc.) and the values it tends to express (personal flexibility, accurate self-assessment, social relatedness, etc.).

Many of those who participated in these debates are acutely aware of the extent to which these manuals are cobbled together based on available evidence and theory. As Michael First (2006) has written, the DSM is not a bible. Or, more precisely, unlike a bible, it is not canonical. It is subject to revision. Borrowing a concept used by Giere (1999), we suggest that the DSM diagnoses are analogous to maps. Like maps, they are not supposed to contain all the information about a landscape. In psychiatry, that additional information should be taken from clinical training and experience, plus scientific evidence that became available after the current edition of the manual was published. Non-professionals may not always grasp these complexities; or if they do, they sometimes flip the error of diagnostic literalism upside down and conclude that because they are imperfectly cobbled together, psychiatric disorders and the criteria used to assess them are just made up.

Another example of an immanent or insider's critique is in the work of Kenneth Kendler (1990), a prominent scientific psychiatrist who was involved in the development of both the DSM-III-R and the DSM-IV. After sitting through multiple committee meetings and listening to passionate debates about picking appropriate diagnoses and diagnostic criteria, Kendler became aware that choosing criteria and 'validating' a particular DSM diagnostic category could not proceed independently of choosing a construct for the disorder in question. For example, deciding to *prioritize* the classification of major mental illnesses might lead a committee to define a diagnostic category narrowly and validate it with poor prognosis indicators; for example, diagnosing schizophrenia means normalcy is unlikely to be recovered. Deciding that mental disorders are biological conditions individuated by means of genetic causes might lead to the development of broader diagnostic categories; for example, awkward, odd and suspicious personality styles are also part of the schizophrenia family.

This means that validators are good, partly, in relation to constructs. Deciding what disorders are out there is not only a matter of conducting more research. In addition to research, developing a scientifically valid nosology involves emphasizing scientific values such as homogeneity, confirmability, inter-rater reliability, and sensitivity. Kendler's reflections on psychiatric taxonomy call attention to a range of issues that extend beyond the conventional empirical ones, and more importantly, brings them into awareness and makes them more subject to rational consideration.

One example of needing to think through the choice of validators more carefully rather than just selecting them from the pre-printed validator menu can be seen in schizophrenia. One of the contributions of the Feighner criteria in the early 1970s was to offer a narrower definition of schizophrenia that made the diagnosed conditions more obviously mental illnesses. Proposing more narrow criteria was related to standardizing diagnostic practices in the United States and Britain—which earlier had shown that the different prevalence rate of schizophrenia between New York and London was actually an artifact of each country using different diagnostic criteria.

Kendler's essay helps us to see that the Feighner criteria and its offspring, the Research Diagnostic Criteria (RDC) and the DSM-III, did not represent a scientific discovery of what schizophrenia really was, but a rational decision about where to draw classificatory boundaries. In effect, it was considered more important to recognize poor outcome and/or psychotic symptomatology. About this same time, research in genetics showed that familial validators are also important, leading to the development of the schizophrenic spectrum concept, which echoes the broader Bleulerian criteria once used in the USA.

2.12 A Note on evidence-based medicine

As noted in the opening paragraphs of this chapter, the debate in psychology about clinical versus statistical prediction foreshadowed current controversies regarding *empirically-validated treatments*, *evidence-based medicine*, and the role of clinical expertise. The proponents of empirically validated treatments believe that clinical judgment is fraught with error and, as a result, harmful. They transform Meehl's skepticism about clinical decision-making into an axiom that reliance on clinical expertise is inherently antiscientific. For them, statistical evidence that a particular treatment protocol is effective for a specific type of disorder is a *sine qua non* of practice. If a type of disorder is present, the actuarial approach says a validated treatment protocol should be applied because the chances of having a positive effect with that population are good.

They also believe that practice outside the scope of empirical validation (i.e., treatment manuals) should not be allowed (McFall 1991).

Such an approach raises concerns. One concern is that the wisdom gained through clinical experience will be marginalized in favor of assembly-line approaches to practice based on a relatively narrow list of research studies (Norcross 1999). Another concern is that assembly line approaches will appeal to bureaucrats whether or not they provide better care and whether or not the demonstrated effects are practically significant (Charlton and Miles 1998). A third concern is that practice in conformity with treatment manuals and mechanically applied decision algorithms makes every mental health professional the same: specifically, well-educated clerks (Phillips 2002).

In contrast to the advocates of empirically validated treatments, however, proponents of evidence-based medicine are not exclusively disorder-focused, they are also patient-focused. As such, they are more likely to value clinical expertise as a way to address individual differences between clinical cases (Sackett *et al.* 1996; Sackett 1998). Although they also seek to identify empirically supported treatment strategies, proponents of evidence-based medicine are less willing to reduce every clinical problem to a 'one size fits all' solution. Patients in the real world with multifaceted problems represent populations not sampled in the carefully screened participant groups used to validate treatment manuals.

The proposals made by proponents of evidence-based medicine are more reflective and, in principle, congruent with a pragmatist attitude. For example, Haynes *et al.* (2002) define three sources of information that need to be considered in formulating treatment decisions. These are (1) research evidence, (2) clinical state and circumstances of the patient, and (3) patient preferences, actions and values. These three spheres are integrated in practice; that is, means and ends are readjusted relative to each other on a continual basis. According to Haynes and his colleagues, *clinical expertise* emerges as an overarching, integrative sphere. This fits Giere's map metaphor quite well—the research evidence provides only partial information and cannot exclusively guide action.

Fundamental to evidence-based medicine is the view that each sphere of information deserves consideration, but each is not weighted equally. Randomized controlled trials are given a higher weight than other kinds of evidence, but research evidence by itself, proponents of evidence-based medicine claim, is incomplete. To illustrate, the research evidence may suggest prescribing clozapine for a particular psychiatric patient. However, it transpires that she has epilepsy and also lives over 150 miles from a medical center where the blood tests can be performed. Clozapine therefore probably is not the best choice. In evidence-based medicine, clinicians systematically consider general principles, available formalized techniques and their knowledge of the patient as a guide to developing treatment recommendations.

One of the important insights of the EBM proponents is their awareness that researchers cannot merely expect clinicians to read journal articles and formulaically apply the results to practice. Understanding that results have to be translated into a clinically usable form represents an acknowledgement of empirical reality constraints. For example, Zachar and Leong's (2000) study of scientist and practitioner differences among psychologists showed that practitioners are interested in research, but not interested in statistics and design, which makes them less likely to seek information from journal articles. Similar findings were reported by Beutler *et al.* (1995). Translation from science to practice is necessary.

For the issue of evidence, expertise, and clinical decision-making, pragmatists would be uncomfortable with romantic approaches to problem solving that consist primarily in emotional appeals combined with strident views of what counts as relevant evidence. Romantic approaches come in both traditional and technological forms.

Romanticism is traditionally associated with a more conservative, resentful hostility to technology, dreams of simpler times, and a longing to return to some primordial authentic state where life was meaningful and myth was alive. The conservatism of Heidegger is one example of this tendency. In contrast to such backward-looking philosophies, evolutionary theory suggests that the use and continual refinement of technology is part of our species' design.

Equally unpalatable is the romantic advocacy of technological approaches, where *emotional appeals* are made about the worthiness of clinical scientists relative to the 'pseuodoscientific' illogic of practitioners. Like their counterparts in the arts, these thinkers write manifestos and dream of revolutions that will be managed by the wise few who know the truth.

Romantic inclinations of all stripes and their associated feelings of certainty lend themselves to tyrannical approaches. In the end, traditional romantics reject statistically supported treatment protocols as dehumanizing and alienating. In doing so they fail to see their tangible benefits or what pragmatists call cash value. On the other hand, the romanticized advocacy of technological methodology eventuates in a demand that practice occur according to the dictates of treatment manuals and operationalized decision-making algorithms, or not at all. Such demands transform science into shallow ideology.

2.13 **The role of trenchant external criticism**

Technical approaches favor specialization. It is beneficial to have experts in statistical prediction, the pharmacology of psychotic disorders and marital therapy.

The more intensive the training, the more a professional learns to see things that others miss. Unfortunately they may learn to see only those things. As social psychologists discovered several years ago, actively practicing a particular set of beliefs or system of thought also leads to acquiring convictions about their purported truth–value (Nisbett and Ross 1980).

The development and promulgation of scientific approaches to problem solving, be they statistical algorithms or psychiatric diagnostic manuals, are a function of communities rather than single individuals. Both Hacking (2002*b*) and Davidson (2001) discuss the self-stabilization of scientific styles of reasoning in which the meaning of the concepts, the relationships between them and how they are to be applied are continually negotiated within the community in such a way that meanings and proper uses become stable. Norms become regimented. Hacking refers to this as *philosophical technology*. For example, in psychiatric taxonomy proposing observable criteria that can be shown to distinguish cases from non-cases with some fidelity contributes to the perceived objectivity of categories. Redefining a heteregeneous category as a higher-level spectrum that includes distinct kinds which share underlying properties plays a similar role. Philosophical technology can be considered a set of tools for iteratively sculpting objective categories and true generalizations.

One virtue of this process is that the members of the community who participate in this stabilization process are, in a sense, each authors/owners of the style. Learning to adopt a sense of ownership in this way is an important aspect of doctoral-level education. The same is true of the development of therapy and diagnostic manuals. In theory, because they should not place the manual on a pedestal or see it is as magically handed down by the psychiatry gods, those who adopt an ownership attitude should be less likely to buy into literalism. Of course, the process of advocating for what they helped produce may also lead professionals to adopt undue conviction.

For various reasons, external critiques are also valuable, especially when technological approaches become dominant. Shaking insiders loose from a complacent trust their groups' internal norms of rationality was one of the purposes of immanent critique in critical theory. What we refer to as trenchant external criticism is a hostile critique, where the technological approach being examined is considered more harmful than helpful. Examples in psychiatry include Szasz's (1961) critique of the concept of mental illness, Kirk and Kutchins' (1992) claims about the guild interests underlying the DSM, Murphy's (2006) complaints about descriptive psychopathology, and Bracken and Thomas's (2006) postmodernist reinterpretation of scientific psychiatry. One does not have to agree with an external criticism to benefit from it, particularly if it initiates some honest doubt and leads to another cycle of reflective analysis and adjustment.

2.14 **Conclusions**

Consistent with the Darwinian emphasis of pragmatism, we do not believe that technological approaches are inherently alien to human nature, and believe that they play an important role in progress. Philosophical analysis clearly demonstrates the various ways in which technological rationality can have negative consequences. We have suggested that some of those consequences can be compensated for by adopting a more philosophical or contemplative attitude toward the use of technology and related procedures. We advocated the virtue of intellectual honesty about the limits of our methods that is akin to the intellectual honesty enshrined in idealized scientific practice, but also realize that both a community of expert users and external critics are required for such honesty. A thorough consensus should not be expected, or even desired.

References

Adorno T. W. (1966/1973). *Negative Dialectics* (New York: Continuum Publishing).

Benjamin W. (1936/1969). 'The work of art in the age of mechanical reproduction' in H. Arendt (ed.) *Illuminations* (trans. H. Zohn). (New York: Schocken Books) 217–252.

Beutler L. E., Williams R. E., Wakefield P. J., and Entwistle S. R. (1995). Bridging scientist and practitioner perspectives in clinical psychology. *American Psychologist*, **50**, 984–994.

Bracken P. and Thomas P. (2006). *Postpsychiatry: Mental health in a postmodern world.* (Oxford, UK: Oxford University Press).

Cacioppo J. T. and Petty R. E. (1982). The need for cognition. *Journal of Personality and Social Psychology*, **42**, 116–131.

Charlton B. G. and Miles A. (1998). The rise and fall of EBM. *Quarterly Journal of Medicine*, **91**, 371–374.

Davidson A. (2001). *The Emergence of Sexuality* (Cambridge, MA: Harvard University Press).

Dawes R. M., Faust D., and Meehl P. E. (1989). Clinical versus actuarial judgment. *Science*, **243**, 1668–1674.

Dewey J. (1925/1981). 'Experience and nature' in J. A. Boydston (ed.) *The Collected Works of John Dewey, The Later Works, Vol. 1* (Carbondale, IL: Southern Illinois University Press).

First M. B., Pincus H. A., and Frances A. (1999). Another perspective on 'Putting the DSM-IV in perspective'. *American Journal of Psychiatry*, **156**, 499–500.

First M. B. (2006). Beyond clinical utility: broadening the DSM-V research appendix to include alternative diagnostic constructs. *American Journal of Psychiatry*, **163**, 1679–1681.

Futuyma G. J. (1998). *Evolutionary Biology*, third ed (Sunderland, MA: Sinauer Associates).

Garb H. N. (1998). *Studying the Clinician: Judgment research and psychological assessment.* (Washington, DC: American Psychological Association).

Giere R. (1999). *Science without Laws* (Chicago: University of Chicago Press).

Hacking I. (1990). *The Taming of Chance* (Cambridge, UK: Cambridge University Press).

Hacking I. (2002*a*). Inaugural lecture: Chair of philosophy and history of scientific concepts at the Collège de France, 16 January 2001. *Economy and Society*, **31**, 1–14.

Hacking I. (2002*b*). *Historical Ontology* (Cambridge, MA: Harvard University Press).

Haynes B. R., Deveraux P. J., and Guyatt G. H. (2002). Clinical expertise in the era of evidence-based medicine and patient choice. *Evidence Based Medicine*, **7**, 36–38.

Horkheimer M. and Adorno T. W. (1944/2001). *The Dialectic of Enlightenment* (New York: Continuum Publishing).

Kendler K. S. (1990). Toward a scientific psychiatric nosology: strengths and limitations. *Archives of General Psychiatry*, **47**, 969–973.

Kirk S. A. and Kutchins H. (1992). *The Selling of DSM* (New York: Aldine De Gruyter).

Marcuse H. (1964). *One Dimensional Man* (Boston, MA: Beacon Press).

McFall R. M. (1991). Manifesto for a science of clinical psychology. *The Clinical Psychologist*, **44**, 75–88.

Meehl P. E. (1954). *Clinical versus Statistical Prediction: A theoretical analysis and a review of the evidence* (Minneapolis: University of Minnesota Press).

Miller S. D. and Berg I. K. (1996). *The Miracle Method* (New York: Norton).

Morey L. C. (1996). *An Interpretive Guide to the Personality Assessment Inventory (PAI)* (Lutz, FL: Psychological Assessment Resources).

Murphy D. (2006). *Psychiatry in the Scientific Image* (Cambridge, MA: The MIT Press).

Nisbett R. E. and Ross L. (1980). *Human Inference: Strategy and shortcomings* (Englewood Cliffs, NJ: Prentice Hall).

Norcross J. (1999). Collegially validated limitations of empirically validated treatments. *Clinical Psychology: Science & Practice*, **6**, 472–476.

Phillips J. (2002). 'Technical reason in the DSM-IV: an unacknowledged value' in J. Sadler (ed.) *Descriptions and Prescriptions: Values, mental disorders, and the DSMs* (Baltimore: The Johns Hopkins Press), 76–94.

Sackett D. L., Rosenberg, W. M. C., Muir Gray J. A., Haynes R. B., and Richardson W. S. (1996). Evidence-based medicine: what it is and what it isn't. *British Medical Journal*, **312**, 71–72.

Sackett D. (1998). Evidence-based medicine. *Spine*, **23**, 1085–1086.

Sadler J. Z. (2005). *Values and Psychiatric Diagnosis* (Oxford, UK: Oxford University Press).

Strauss L. (1964/1978). *The City and Man* (Chicago, IL: The University of Chicago Press).

Szas T. (1961). *The Myth of Mental Illness* (New York: Harper and Row).

Waits T. (1993). 'Crossroads' on *The Black Rider* [CD] (New York: Island Records).

Williams J. B., Spitzer R. L., and Skodol A. E. (1985). DSM-III in residency training: results of a national survey. *American Journal of Psychiatry*, **142**, 755–758.

Wolin R. (2006). *The Frankfurt School Revisited* (New York: Routledge).

Zachar P. (in press). 'Real kinds but no true taxonomy: An essay in psychiatric systematics,' in K. S. Kendler and J. Parnas, (eds.) *Philosophical Issues in Psychiatry: Explanation, phenomenology and nosology* (Baltimore: The Johns Hopkins University Press).

Zachar P. and Leong F. T. L. (2000). A 10-year longitudinal study of scientist and practitioner interests in psychology: assessing the boulder model. *Professional Psychology: Research and Practice*, **31**, 575–580.

Chapter 3

Technological reason and the regulation of emotion

Louis C. Charland

Treatment is not a matter of coming to the truth but of restoring flexibility.
(David Healy 1990: 201)

3.1 New technologies of emotion regulation

The regulation of 'emotion' is a popular topic in contemporary psychology and psychiatry. However, the concern is certainly not new. From antiquity to the present, numerous figures in the history of Western thought have worried about how to manage the influence of affective states like anger, fear, and love in our lives. However, there are two major differences between these earlier efforts and those of today. One is that we now speak of regulating the 'emotions' rather than regulating the 'passions'. The other is the nature of the means used to achieve the ends of regulation. The two developments are connected. Because the chief posits involved in regulation—passions, emotions—are vastly different, so, therefore, are the means used to regulate them.

There are now accepted technologies for regulating the emotions. These consist mostly of scientifically validated psychotherapeutic techniques (Beck 1976; Goleman 1995; Klerman *et al.*; 1984; Linehan 1993; Salovey and Mayer 1990). The *Merriam-Webster Online Dictionary* (2006) identifies one meaning of the word 'technology' as 'a manner of accomplishing a task especially using technical processes, methods, or knowledge'. Technical processes, in turn, are defined as 'of or relating to a practical subject organized on scientific principles'. It is in this sense that current techniques for emotion regulation can be called 'technological'. They are all developed and organized according to scientific principles. Of course, there are a wide array of pharmaceutical products for the regulation of affective states available today. These, too, can be called 'technological', because their development and application are based on scientific principles. However, the present discussion will be limited to the regulation of affective states using psychotherapeutic techniques only, leaving pharmaceutical regulation for another occasion.

In what follows, I try to cast doubt on the possibility of regulating the emotions using scientific psychotherapeutic techniques alone. I do not deny that such techniques are sometimes practically effective and valuable. Nor do I suggest that we should dispense with them. Instead, I scrutinize and evaluate their philosophical credentials to get a clearer idea of their promise and limitations. My conclusion, which is tentative and an invitation to further discussion, is that current technological approaches to emotion regulation are not sufficient for their stated tasks. Indeed, there are even limitations at the level of how the tasks are defined. My argument is that emotion regulation requires an ethical and moral component that cannot be avoided or dispensed with. Current scientific efforts in the domain of emotion regulation either omit or deny this. They pretend to be scientific, ethically neutral, and self-sufficient, but they are not. There is an empirical dimension to this criticism. At some point, it needs to be empirically demonstrated that regulation without ethical assumptions is incomplete, or maybe even impossible. However, before we can empirically test such a hypothesis, it is first necessary to formulate it and understand its underlying motivation. It is this prior task that I propose to address. My strategy will be to turn to history for clarification of what the hypothesis means and what motivates it.

There are already some precedents for the view that, when dealing in matters of emotional regulation, psychotherapy cannot brazenly ignore questions of morality and ends of life as it currently does. For example, psychoanalyst Peter Lomas notes that 'our contemporary model of psychotherapeutic endeavor omits the moral dimension of living' (Lomas 1999: 4–6). In addition, recent philosophical attempts to revive interest in early Stoic therapies of emotion also bear directly on our topic, although their ethical presuppositions vary and can be hard to interpret (Nussbaum 2001; Sorabji 2000). The ensuing discussion will add to these initiatives, but take a slightly different historical route.

We start with Descartes' pioneering theory of the passions, and then proceed to the rise of psychiatric 'moral treatment' in the late eighteenth century. These developments will be set against the background of a wider set of historical transitions in which ethical 'passions' are said to have ceded their place to modern secular 'emotions' (Dixon 2003). This alternate historical analysis should provide further impetus for questioning the disingenuous secular aspirations and professed neutral self-image of modern psychotherapy.

The example of moral treatment is a fitting note on which to end, because it should remind us of just how far we have strayed from the premise that hope and judicious kindness are not simply adjuncts or prerequisites for psychotherapy, but rather part of what psychotherapy essentially is and must aspire to. The example of moral treatment also has the merit of having been clinically tested and evaluated in its own day, something that is notably absent from the more speculative hypothetical status of the early stoic emotional therapies and their modernized counterparts. Indeed, historians concur that moral treatment was an extremely effective therapy in its own day (Charland 2007). This is good reason for taking it seriously today, as we consider the ethical shortcomings of our current technological therapies of emotional regulation.

3.2 **Regulating the passions**

To illustrate the nature of the ethical considerations that are being omitted and denied in modern scientific theories of the regulation of emotion, it is helpful to revisit the regulation of the passions in earlier times. A pivotal figure here is Descartes. His commitment to rigorous scientific explanation in this domain is unparalleled. However, his commitment to remaining true to the phenomena proved to be even stronger. Descartes, the arch scientist, thought that there were principled limits to the scientific attempt to understand and regulate the passions. Studying his views should help us discover what those limits are.

Towards the end of his life, Descartes published a treatise on the passions entitled *Les Passions de l'Âme* [*The Passions of the Soul*] (Descartes 1650/1990). It represents a milestone in the history of physiological thinking about the emotions. What is seldom noted is that it also represents an important contribution to ethics. It is this peculiar methodological alliance between science and ethics in Descartes' work on the passions that will especially concern us here.

According to Descartes, the passions are embodied and their study requires that we consider the mind and body as an *indissoluble organic unity* (James 1997: 94–96, 106–107). Dualism here is sharply constrained, because it is impossible to consider the mental aspects of the passions in isolation from their union with the body. Thus we are told that the passions cannot be referred 'either to the mind alone, or to the body alone' (Cottingham *et al.* 1984: 336–339). They arise, instead, 'from the close and intimate union of our mind with our body' (ibid., 339, 341). It follows that the explanatory vocabulary we use to explain the workings of the passions will require both mental and physical terms and both mental and physical posits. This is decidedly not a reductionist account. Nor is it really a dualist account. It is, in fact, misleading to accuse Descartes of dualism where his work on the passions is concerned (Damasio 1994). He committed no such 'error'. On the contrary, in the case of the passions, he was keenly aware of the need to transcend dualism and treat the relation of mind and body as an organic unity.

So, for Descartes, the passions are mental phenomena but they are also embodied. To the extent that they are embodied, the explanation of the passions falls within the purview of science and their operations can be explained mechanistically. However, as a scientist, Descartes must also tell us what the passions are for. We need to know this to understand and regulate their operations. Before we can regulate the passions, we must know what regulation is for; its ends. Otherwise, we do not know what we are trying to achieve. What then are the passions for?

Descartes tells us that '...l'usage de toutes les passions consiste en cela seul, qu'elles disposent l'âme a vouloir les choses que la nature dicte nous être utiles, est a persister en cette volonté...'(Art. LII) ['The customary use or function of the passions consists only in this, that they dispose the soul to will only those things which nature tells us are useful to us, and to persist in this volition' (Cottingham *et al.* 1984: 349)]. The passions, then, present options to the will; they suggest what we should strive for and avoid. But which options and why? We need to disentangle descriptive and normative questions here. The passions may in fact dispose the soul to will certain things. But should we will those things? The problem is that the passions often lead us astray. Many of them implicate or lead to immoral forms of behavior. We must accordingly learn how to regulate our passions, not only to survive biologically, but to live ethically. This requires employing our will along with the insights of reason. Although Descartes is optimistic about the power of the will to rule over and control the passions, he also recognizes that this involves a moral struggle. It is simply a fact that we have unhealthy passional inclinations. Against these, we must struggle; the exercise of such passions must be regulated.

There can be no doubt that in his treatise Descartes set out to understand and explain the passions and their operations scientifically. However, at the same time he firmly demonstrates that the passions are inextricably ethical in nature. Although they have a physical dimension and are therefore amenable to scientific scrutiny, one cannot completely strip away or ignore their ethical aspects without falsifying their nature as a whole. Thus, in explaining the workings of the passions there is a point where scientific reasoning and mechanistic explanation must be supplemented by ethical reflection and the normative influence of morals. Regulation must ultimately be guided by 'knowledge of good and evil, which the soul has resolved to follow in guiding its conduct' (Cottingham *et al.* 1984: 347). Consequently, in matters of emotional regulation, we must move from instrumentalist technological reasoning associated with how to realize certain specified passional ends, to the moral appropriateness and selection of those passional ends themselves. In addition, we must also consider how those ends conform with the dictates of morality and wider questions about the ends of life.

In his treatise, Descartes tried to walk the fine line between the normative and descriptive dimensions of the passions; between a scientific account of the passions that stresses their physiological basis as natural phenomena, and an ethical account that focuses on their characteristics as felt experiences reported in a normative mentalistic vocabulary used to guide and explain behavior. He insisted on charting the descriptive natural terrain of the passions as far as he could go as a 'natural philosopher', a scientist. However, at the same time, he also maintained that a theory of the passions was invariably a practical normative affair. Somewhat paradoxically, working as a natural scientist, he nonetheless delivered an ethical treatise (Levi 1964: 248). There is an irony to this conclusion, because at one point he indicates that his intention was 'to explain the passions only as a natural philosopher, and not as a rhetorician or even as a moral philosopher' (Cottingham *et al.* 1984: 327).

Descartes' integrity and unfailing commitment to the explanatory exigencies of his topic is impressive. One suspects that he knew that the normative and descriptive requirements of his theory of the passions would be difficult to reconcile. Yet he laid them down side-by-side anyway. This being his last major work, the problems were left to posterity. Evidently, they are still with us today. However, although in Descartes' work the problems are clearly exposed for all to see, in modern theories of emotion regulation they remain hidden under the rhetoric of technological scientism.

3.3 From ethical passions to secular emotions

Like many writers of his time—especially the so-called 'French Moralists'—Descartes simply assumes that there is an ethical dimension to the regulation of the passions (Levi 1964). This general tendency to tie the regulation of the passions to ethics has a long history in the West. Starting with the ancient Greeks, concepts of the passions have often been intimately tied to ethical and religious notions of right and wrong (Knuuttila 2006; Nussbaum 2001; Sorabji 2000). Yet nowadays we speak more commonly of 'emotions', and ethics appears to have vanished from discussions of emotion regulation. What has happened? To answer this question, we must examine the history of affective terms and notions.

During the nineteenth century, the ethical passions of ancient and medieval times were superseded by the secular emotions of today (Dixon 2003; Rorty 1982). Psychiatry and psychology have yet to come to terms with this profound change in Western concepts of affectivity. The episode contains important clues why some experts have claimed the psychopathology of affectivity is so impoverished compared with other areas of psychopathology (Berrios 1985). This is especially true in descriptive psychopathology, the study of the signs and symptoms of mental disorder (Berrios 1996). Lack of progress in the psychopathology of affectivity is also largely responsible for the failure of modern psychotherapy to live up to its early scientific ideals; a hiatus that has been dubbed a 'suspended revolution' (Healy 1990). It is easy to overlook and downplay the significance of these differences in the attempt to compare early efforts to regulate the passions with modern psychotherapies of the emotions.

Historically, the passions were suffused with ethical connotations. However, once freed from those normative shackles, they started to appear in secular guise only; as emotions. Historian Thomas Dixon locates the culmination of this trend in the middle of the nineteenth century (Dixon 2003). There are remarkable transformations leading up to this conceptual transformation. Pride, the cardinal sin for Augustine, becomes the psychological foundation of the self in Hume (Rorty 1990). Avarice, another deadly sin, is converted into merchantile self-interest by Adam Smith (Hirshman 1977).

To capture the enormity of these developments, we might compare Augustine's passions with Darwin's emotions. It is not just the terminology and the labels that have changed. The underlying concepts and their associated forms of life have also changed. In Augustine, the passions are inextricably ethical and tied to spiritual salvation in another world. This is *The City of God*, a world reserved for human souls and other spiritual entities (Augustine 1972). In Darwin, the emotions are fundamentally biological and tied to corporeal survival in this world. This is the evolutionary milieu of *The Origin of Species*, a world humans share with animals. Darwin called his major work on emotion *The Expression of Emotion in Man and Animals*, thus explicitly emphasizing his thesis of a shared evolutionary heritage and biological continuity between human and animal emotions (Darwin 1872/1998). For Augustine, this probably would have been considered blasphemy. Obviously, in the Augustinian and Darwinian worlds, passions and emotions are associated with widely different forms of life.

So there appears to have been a conceptual revolution in which the ethical passions of the past have ceded their place to the secular emotions of today. However, careful analysis also reveals that the transition has been neither consistent nor complete. It is not so much that one map of the soul has replaced another. Rather, what we have is a 'palimpsest' (Berrios 1985: 745). As a result, culturally we find ourselves with an affective vocabulary that is historically staggered, somewhat incoherent, and in a general state of disarray. The situation is reminiscent of present-day moral philosophy, where we continue to use the language of virtue, even though most of its original supporting forms of life disappeared long ago (MacIntyre 1981). Of course, at any given time, there have been exceptions and objections to these trends in the evolution of affectivity. At various times, including the present, there have been debates over competing maps of the soul and its powers; disagreements over the nature of the mind and its division into natural faculties, and controversies over which faculties exercise control over the others. Still today, we have choices. We can choose to retain the ethical substance of the ancient passions in our theories of affective regulation, or we can try to jettison questions of ethics and the ends of life and opt for purely secular emotions.

3.4 **Regulating the emotions**

The response by modern psychiatry and psychology to the transition from ethical passions to secular emotions has been to embrace the change and choose to regulate the emotions scientifically. That 'thin' neutral explanatory vocabulary is thought to be better suited to the aims of an objective science of mental health and disorder. It is chosen because it promises to provide a simple and succinct description of emotional states and operations in terms that are fixed, frugal, and precise, requiring no metaphorical or other literary devices, and especially no 'thick' contextual narrative embellishments or elaboration (Williams 1986). Such a thin vocabulary allegedly makes operational definitions of emotional signs and symptoms more robust and reliable. And it nicely meets the exigencies of generalization and explanation across persons and cultures.

As a result of this choice to follow the lure of science and attempt to regulate the 'emotions' technologically, there is now a wide variety of promising scientific projects in the area. Indeed, it is now widely assumed that it is possible to speak of emotional disorders and their therapy without encroaching on questions of ethics and morals (Beck 1976; Goleman 1995; Klerman *et al.* 1984; Linehan 1993; Salovey and Mayer 1990). At least, it is possible to pretend (Charland and Zachar 2008). With a quick swipe of Ockham's razor, questions of ethics and fundamental life questions associated with the more normative dimensions of emotions have simply been excised from psychotherapy. On the whole, contemporary scientific efforts at emotion regulation assume it is possible to divorce normative ethical questions associated with emotional means and ends from the more 'mechanical' aspects of emotion. This for example is the position taken by psychiatrist David Healy, who has eloquently argued that contemporary psychotherapy is in a suspended state of scientific development because of its failure to fully banish ethics and associated questions of 'authenticity' from its practice and theory. His argument is that psychotherapy ought to avoid matters of *authenticity* if it wishes to be scientific (Healy 1990: 199–121). According to him, restoring *flexibility* to the psyche is the proper goal of a scientific psychotherapy, not authenticity.

The distinction between flexibility and authenticity is derived from another set of distinctions which Healy supports with a complex set of arguments taken from the philosophy of science. This is the distinction between the *psyche*, *mind*, and *brain* (ibid., 25, Table 1). Very roughly, the psyche is the domain of psychological operations, properly speaking, whereas the mind is the domain of mental operations. Both of these two levels of functioning differ from the brain, which represents a third level of organization. On this model, each explanatory level is relatively autonomous and independent with respect to the others. Levels are related to each other by a 'principle of emergence' (ibid., 8). The relationship between the levels is hierarchical, with lower brain operations supporting psychological operations, which in turn support mental operations. Mental operations arise out of the psyche, which consists of psychological capacities for 'intelligent behavior', 'perception', 'memory', 'learning', 'imagination', 'emotion', 'motivation', and 'habit' (ibid., 12-20). On its side, the psyche arises from possibilities inherent in the nervous system' (ibid., 12). In sum, 'there is something called the mind that differs distinctly from the psyche and the brain, but has emerged from them' (ibid., 27).

Now, unlike flexibility, which is a property of psychological operations and the psyche's special level of organization, authenticity is a property of mental processes and the mind's own special mode of organization. Inspired by ancient Greek concepts of the mind, Healy characterizes authenticity as a kind of striving; a 'yearning for order and personal coherence' (ibid., 5). It is 'something acquired by an individual subject only after a struggle to heed the call of reason' (ibid., 29). Authenticity, he says, involves a 'search for meaning' (ibid., 31). It involves 'creation' and 'self-definition' (ibid., 202). This makes authenticity inseparable from fundamental life choices (ibid., 202). Many of those choices will be moral; they have to do with the kind of persons we wish to be, with moral character (ibid., 28–29). They also have to do with the emotional ends we choose, as well as the means to those ends.

Healy states that authenticity is a peculiarly human concern, something we do not share with animals: Unlike an animal which can simply get on with life if particular problems remain unsolved, for humans a programme of action crucially revolves around the act of self-creation. As the correct answer to this problem is shrouded in mystery, human life, although free from many natural dangers, will nevertheless be fraught with moral concern (ibid., 32).

Animals then have psyches and share many of their psychological capacities with humans to some degree. However, they do not have minds, and therefore differ from humans on that point. In one instance, Healy appears to suggest that authenticity 'and its world of meaning is radically human in a way that *emotions* and personality are not...' (ibid., 28; emphasis added). The exact meaning of this last passage is hard to interpret. But it seems to suggest that, as a psychological capacity we share with animals, emotion can be squeezed within the envelope of science, without encroaching on issues of morals or the ends of life. Strictly 'psychological' problems in the area of emotion regulation would then involve restoring 'flexibility' to the relevant psychological processes and operations, and accordingly they would be amenable to psychotherapy, scientifically understood. However, of course human emotional problems go beyond the range of basic psychological processes and operations we share with animals. Invariably, human emotional problems implicate mental operations at the level of the mind and raise issues of authenticity that no amount of flexibility in psychological operations can solve. At this point, scientific psychotherapy has reached its limits.

It appears, then, that Healy wishes to divide problems associated with emotions and their regulation into two sorts. Some revolve around problems in functioning at the level of psychological operations and can be resolved by restoring flexibility. Others occur at the level of mental operations and involve ethical and normative issues that no amount of flexibility can solve. These latter problems fall within the boundaries of the quest for authenticity and require selecting goals and making fundamental life choices, many of them moral. However, can the domain of emotion really be divided up so neatly? Our historical example of Descartes and the French moralists suggests probably not. It shows that emotion regulation requires adverting to the normative evaluative dimensions of emotion, which cannot adequately be captured using a purely secular technological scientific explanatory framework.

A strategy very similar to Healy's can be discerned in the modern theory of 'emotional intelligence' and its concept of the regulation of emotion (Salovey and Mayer 1990; Goleman 1995). The theory starts with the assumption that 'there is a set of conceptually related mental processes involving emotional information'. The main aims and components of emotional intelligence are: (1) expression of emotion (goal: improving accuracy in self and others); 2. regulation of emotion (goal: channeling emotions appropriately to promote goals); 3.utilization of emotion (goal: harnessing emotions effectively to solve problems)

(Salovey and Mayer 1990: 189–200). It is interesting that no mention is made of the ultimate *ends* of emotion in this scheme. Everything revolves around emotions in that they function as *means* to unstated ends. Because the nature of and selection of emotional ends is not considered, it is relatively easy for the theory to avoid questions of morals and ethics. Moreover, when emotional means are considered, it is solely mechanistically; that is, from the point of view of whether they are effective relative to certain ends, which remain unstated and unquestioned.

It appears that questions of morals and the ends of life do not form any part of the theory of emotional intelligence. These aspects of emotion are summarily excluded, leaving the impression that it is possible to talk about emotional intelligence and emotional regulation without mentioning them. The exclusion is deliberate. This is because the theory and concepts of emotional intelligence are supposed to be scientific, and mental health and psychological science must avoid normative ethical questions. Problems in emotional intelligence on this view are mechanistic; they have to do with obstacles to effective emotional processing and with the instrumental success of the emotional means used to attain certain ends. Professionals in the area of emotional intelligence would probably bristle at the suggestion that it involves or requires ethical training for themselves, or ethical indoctrination for their patients. They see themselves as clinical scientists and practioners, not priests or judges or moralists. In the theory of emotional intelligence, the normative and evaluative aspects of emotion are considered descriptively, in the form of codified social norms and standards of acceptable behavior. However, genuine normative considerations are absent. They certainly do not recommend that you ought morally to live one way rather than another.

There is, in fact, an important normative ethical sense in which the theory of emotional intelligence is affectively empty. Its thin scientific vocabulary and descriptive methods render it unable to address the thick, sensually drenched, normative ethical questions emotions raise in daily life. It does not ask, and therefore does not answer, how morally we ought to use and regulate our emotions, and which emotions we ought morally to pursue or avoid as ends. In embracing this and other like secular concepts of affective life, psychology and psychiatry have stepped squarely into the domain of science. However, at the same time, they have lost their foothold in the terrain of ethics. It is tempting to talk of scientific advances and revolutions here, but let us not forget the paradigms that have been lost or overrun. In the present case, what has been lost is how affective states like passions and emotions actually function in daily life, where they are invariably associated with normative ethical questions and assumptions.

What has been lost is the content, the living color, the evaluative force, of affectivity. Stripped of its normative dimension, affective experience is now largely meaningless and empty. Therapists talk to their patients about their emotions using words devoid of any evaluative content or normative force; patients usually respond accordingly, using the same hollow shells. This is now a domain where it is important to be clinical and objective; where the decisions of the patient must be respected as a fundamental right of autonomy; and where the psychotherapist is neither trained nor sanctioned to give moral advice or criticism. No wonder it often feels so pointless; there neither is nor can be any real goal, ethically. How you ultimately should live does not enter into such discussions. That would violate professional and scientific neutrality. Anyway, the medium of discussion does not allow it. The thin explanatory currency and typology of affective states involved has been normatively devalued so many times that it is now almost worthless and is devoid of any substantial affective meaning. Clinical symptoms are so thinly described that they have no grip on the real circumstances of our lives. To adapt a dictum of Wittgenstein's, modern affective psychopathology is slipping and sliding on a frictionless plane. It is time to step back onto the rough ground; into history, culture, and literature, and the ethical import of affectivity in our lives.

3.5 **Moral treatment**

At this point it is appropriate to ask what exactly an attempt to regulate the emotions ethically might look like. We already have the theoretical example of Descartes. However, we need a more practical and clinical example. There is such an example of this sort in the history of psychiatry. It is called moral treatment.

Moral treatment arose simultaneously in different parts of Europe towards the end of the eighteenth century. It is associated with the work of the French physician Philippe Pinel (1745–1826) and the Italian physician Vincenzo Chiarugi (1759–1820). However, perhaps the most famous name in the history of moral treatment is William Tuke (1732–1822), a lay Quaker and wealthy tea merchant who opened a special Retreat for the Insane in York in 1796. Samuel Tuke, William's grandson, later characterized the Retreat as 'an Institution near York, for the reception of persons afflicted with disorders of the mind, among the Society of Friends' (Tuke 1813). The Retreat figures importantly in the annals of psychiatry, where it is noted for its innovative humanitarian reforms in the treatment of the mentally ill. Invariably, it is also cited as a focal point in the history of 'moral treatment'. Contemporary historians generally define this as the attempt to treat mental illness by psychological means. However, as shall become evident, the word 'moral' is sometimes used ambiguously in these contexts and often it means 'ethical' in addition to 'psychological'.

The main therapeutic objective of the Retreat was 'to assist nature in her own cure' (Tuke 1813: 216–217). For that reason, William often preferred to speak of promoting recovery rather than effecting a cure. It was recognized that simply following the Hippocratic injunction to 'do no harm' was already an important contribution to recovery. Early observations of patient care at the Retreat proved to be supportive of William's assumption that providing a friendly and intimate familial environment helped to assure patient comfort and promote recovery. Location and healthy activities were important ingredients of the healing environment, and much attention was paid to the geographical location and layout of the Retreat. To this day, the Retreat's buildings and grounds still constitute a splendid country estate.

Moral treatment at the Retreat was premised on the observation that core benevolent affections in humans remain mostly untouched by madness. Samuel notes that, even in madness, 'the existence of the benevolent affections, is often strongly evidenced' (Tuke 1813: 134). So despite their madness, the mad are apparently still capable of experiencing and expressing basic social affection and passions. Moral treatment at the Retreat capitalized on this premise, which was increasingly confirmed by observation. In fact, it is not an exaggeration to say that moral treatment at the Retreat was a therapy *of* the passions that worked *through* the passions. Reason had little to do with it. This was not primarily a 'talking' therapy like our modern cognitive psychotherapies. It was a primitive form of affective conditioning with benevolence at its core (Charland 2007).

In his *Description of the Retreat*, Samuel explicitly remarks that 'the influence of religious principles over the mind of the insane, is considered of great consequence, as a means of cure' (Tuke 1813:161). Indeed, analysis of the rules and regulations of the Retreat and its regime of moral management reveal five Quaker values that clearly have an ethical character: benevolence, charity, discipline, self-restraint, and temperance. This 'moralistic element' was pervasive in the early days of the Retreat (Digby 1985: 85). It was considered advisable to 'promote in the patient, an attention to his accustomed modes of paying homage to his creator' (Tuke 1813:, 161). This was done by nurturing and appealing to the 'inner light' which, through the grace of God, was thought to lead to salvation (Digby 1985: 28, 31). The ethical and religious goals of moral treatment at the Retreat explain why attendants were expected exemplify the Quaker way of life and its values (Digby 1985: 140–141, 155). Today they would be referred to as ethical role models. On the whole, this is a view of life and health where ethical passions and healthy passions are inextricably linked.

It is a model of the self where a healthy 'moral' life in a general *psychological* sense, requires a balanced 'moral' life in the *social* sense, which in turn requires an upright 'moral' life in the *ethical* sense.

Referring to the early, more religious, phase of moral treatment at the Retreat, historian Ann Digby states that, 'the ethos of these early years did include a disciplinary and moralistic element' (Digby 1985: 85). The Quaker religion and its values were the origin of that moral code. However, note that it was not simply a 'moral' code in the sense of defining socially appropriate conduct, such as when and whom to marry, and so on. Instead, it was that plus an ethical code in the strict sense. Thus the ultimate aim of 'moral' treatment in these early days of the Retreat was 'moral good' and the 'preservation of moral character' in this ethical sense (Digby 1985: 97). The 'moral feelings' that moral treatment was supposed to awaken were not only affectively tied to related passions and feelings; they were also ethical (Digby 1985: 96). Therefore, 'moral' treatment at the Retreat was not simply mental and psychological, though it was that. It was also 'moral' in a specific ethical sense that derived from Quaker values and morality.

3.6. Truth and authenticity

What our historical philosophical investigation suggests is that beyond a certain point you cannot explain and regulate the passions and emotions from a neutral interpretive and merely descriptive standpoint. Psychotherapy in the emotional domain must involve ethical evaluation as well as interpretation. What is at stake in this proposed expansion from interpretation to evaluation is both radical and profound. To be sure, restoring flexibility to emotional processes and operations remains an important goal of psychotherapy and much of that can perhaps be done scientifically, within a mechanistic paradigm. However, matters of authenticity, of truth and self creation, cannot be jettisoned entirely. The reason is that in matters of emotion regulation it is ultimately impossible to disentangle the descriptive and normative elements of affective life, with the former neatly housed in the domain of science and the latter reserved for ethics.

On this last question, Descartes was again a pioneer. As a natural scientist, he understood the importance of restoring flexibility and functionality to the passions. Yet at the same time, he was also on the side of truth and authenticity when it came to regulating them. This last point is clearly stated in Article 49 of *Les Passions de l'Âme*: 'Que la force de l'âme ne suffit pas sans la connaissance de la vérité' (Descartes 1650/1990: 73). ['The strength of the soul is inadequate without knowledge of the truth' (Cottingham *et al.* 1984: 347).] The passage is reminiscent of the powerful influence of Augustine, who argues that 'only truth and virtue can offer a centre of resistance against turbulent and degraded passions' (Augustine 1972: 345).

What Descartes saw was that regulating the passions was impossible without some overriding notion of truth, which he believed to be partly ethical in nature. He saw that in order to organize and regulate the passions it was necessary to appeal to some overarching normative ideal. He called it truth, but it can also be called authenticity—the personal call to truth; to self-creation; to re-making the self in the light of some normative ideal that gives life meaning. William Tuke intuitively reached the same conclusion as Descartes, although he did not state or defend it philosophically. He saw that restoring flexibility to the psyche was impossible without some normative direction and organization in the passions as a whole. His moral treatment endeavored to combine flexibility and personal authenticity as goals for therapy.

It is time that we rethink the meaning of the lessons of Descartes and Tuke for the theory and practice of emotion regulation today. The historical material reviewed here suggests that it may be wrong and inadvisable to try to rid psychotherapy of truth and authenticity entirely, as Healy suggests. At least in matters of emotion regulation. The question therefore is not whether psychotherapy can be either exclusively scientific or not. This appears to be a false dichotomy when it comes to emotion regulation. There is no purely scientific road for us to seek or follow here, although science may partly illuminate the way.

References

Augustine (1972). *The City of God* (D. Knowles, ed.) (Harmondsworth, UK: Penguin).

Beck A. (1976). *Cognitive Therapy of Depression* (New York: Guilford Press).

Berrios G. E. (1985). The psychopathology of affectivity: conceptual and historical aspects. *Psychological Medicine*, **15**, 745–758.

Berrios G. E. (1996). *The History of Mental Symptoms: Descriptive psychopathology since the 19th century* (Cambridge: Cambridge University Press).

Charland L. C. (2007). Benevolent theory: moral treatment at the York Retreat. *History of Psychiatry* **18**, 61–80.

Charland L. C. and Zachar P. (eds.) (2008). *Fact and Value in Emotion* (Amsterdam: John Benjamin Press).

Cottingham J., Stoothhof R., and Murdoch D. (eds. and tr.) (1984). *The Philosophical Writings of Descartes*, vol. II (Cambridge: Cambridge University Press).

Damasio A. (1994). *Descartes' Error* (New York: Putnam).

Darwin C. (1872/1998). *The Expression of Emotion in Man and Animal* (Oxford: Oxford University Press).

Descartes R. (1650/1990). *Les Passions de L'Âme* (Paris: Librarie General Française).

Digby A. (1985). *Madness, Morality, and Medicine* (Cambridge: Cambridge University Press).

Dixon T. (2003). *From Passions to Emotions: The creation of a secular category* (Cambridge: Cambridge University Press).

Goleman D. (1995). *Emotional Intelligence* (New York: Basic Books).

Healy D. (1990). *The Suspended Revolution* (London: Faber & Faber).

Hirshman A. (1977). *The Passions and the Interests* (Princeton: Princeton University Press).

James S. (1997). *Passion and Action: The emotions in seventeenth-century philosophy* (Oxford: Oxford University Press).

Klerman G. L., Weissman M., Rounsaville B., and Chevron E. (1984). *Interpersonal Therapy of Depression* (New York: Basic Books).

Knuuttila S. (2006). *Emotions in Ancient and Medieval Philosophy* (Oxford: Oxford University Press).

Levi A. (1964). *French Moralists: The theory of the passions 1585 to 1649* (Oxford: Clarendon Press).

Linehan M. (1993). *Cognitive Behavioral Treatment of Borderline Personality Disorder* (New York: The Guilford Press).

Lomas P. (1999). *Doing Good: Psychotherapy out of its depth* (Oxford: Oxford University Press).

MacIntyre A. (1981). *After Virtue.* (South Bend, IN: Notre-Dame University Press).

Merriam-Webster (2006). *Merriam-Webster Online Dictionary*, http://www.merriam-webster.com, accessed 17 September 2006.

Nussbaum M. (2001). *Upheavals of Thought: The intelligence of the emotions* (Cambridge: Cambridge University Press).

Rorty A. (1982). From passions to emotions and sentiments. *Philosophy*, **57**, 175–188.

Rorty A. (1990). Pride produces the idea of the self: Hume on moral agency. *Australian Journal of Philosophy*, **68**, 255.

Salovey P. and Mayer J. D. (1990). Emotional intelligence. *Imagination, Cognition, and Personality*, **9**, 185–211.

Sorabji R. (2000). *Emotion and Peace of Mind* (Oxford: Oxford University Press).

Tuke S. (1813). *Description of the Retreat* (reprinted, London: Process Press, 1996).

Williams B. (1986). *Ethics and the Limits of Philosophy* (Cambridge, MA: Harvard University Press).

Part 2

Critical approaches to technology in psychiatry

Chapter 4

Technology, aesthetic explanation, and psychoanalysis

Miguel Uribe

4.1 Introduction

Technology poses particular challenges to psychiatry, which can be faced through the study of the types of question we try to answer in our discipline. In psychiatry and psychoanalysis, the object of study, the human mind, cannot be explored and understood from a single perspective. We can obtain further clarity about these perspectives by differentiating the classes of explanation we are working with. Not all explanations are of the same nature. In psychoanalysis, the answers we find are our interpretations; however, some interpretations take the form of a causal explanation whereas others are similar to aesthetic explanations. To develop these ideas further, I will elaborate on Wittgenstein's views on aesthetics and psychoanalysis, and on Cioffi's (1998) work on Wittgenstein. The main contrast will be between causal and aesthetic explanations.

The use of different kinds of explanation has important consequences for psychiatry. In the first place, we would have to abandon the idea of having a single method for our discipline. Various ways of inquiry and explanation will necessarily stand side by side. Secondly, limits to the application of empirical investigations, many of which rely on technological applications, will become more evident. Psychiatry would have to pursue inquiries that might seem even contradictory; our many theoretical disputes illustrate this situation. The conceptual clarity that psychiatry needs requires acknowledging this multiplicity, beginning with a clear differentiation of the sort of questions we are dealing with, and the type of explanations required. Clarity, however, might be elusive, as many of the questions posed belong to a muddled territory.

It is well known that in mental health, patients may be bewildered by the fact that there are too many available treatments. Each school offers its own theory, therapy, and approach towards patients. Psychoanalysis and biological psychiatry differ in their understanding of the mind and treatment of mental disorders.

Placing psychoanalysis side by side with technology probably represents the opposite ends of our field, in that biological psychiatry greatly benefits from technology, whereas psychoanalysis seems to avoid technological applications. One of the most interesting aspects of psychoanalysis is the simplicity of its setting: nothing more than talking and listening. Now, in this ascetic setting, the questions asked can be rather compelling, urgent, and complex.

Technical reasoning occupies an important place in contemporary psychiatry, as shown by Phillips (2002). Technical rationality means 'that for any problem area there is a systematic body of generalized knowledge, with specific rules for application, that can define the handling of a particular case and thus minimize or eliminate the need for real judgement on the part of the individual practitioner' (Phillips 2002). As a therapy, psychoanalysis uses technical reasoning, trying to find generalities which will guide the therapist as he or she applies it to a patient. The therapist uses a general theory of technique such as Freud's technical papers, and applies it to particular cases. However, the practice of psychoanalytic psychotherapy remains largely a craft, and every individual therapy has such a degree of uncertainty and so many variables that it will inevitable remain unique. Complexity is part of the reason for its singularity: I want to suggest, however, that the use of aesthetic explanations is also an important ingredient.

Rather than engaging a confrontation between psychoanalysis and technology, however, I explore the following questions:

Is it useful, or clarifying, to hold a clear distinction concerning the use and application of aesthetic explanations versus causal explanations?

Is there a place for aesthetic explanation in clinical work, and specifically in psychoanalysis?

The rest of this chapter is organized as follows. I will begin by presenting some of Wittgenstein's ideas to approach the previous questions. Then I will expose different types of explanation and the characteristics of aesthetic answers, as well as the origin of questions and their relation with the object of study. Finally, I will study the process of validation of explanations and the presence of aesthetic explanations in therapeutic endeavors.

4.2 **Wittgenstein**

Wittgenstein's work tries to dissolve certain conceptual confusions arising from the fascination language exerts on us. These confusions, according to Wittgenstein, are found not only in the core of some of the most traditional philosophical problems, but also in psychology. Such was the case in Freud's work, an 'abominable mess' in Wittgenstein's words, resulting from confusing causes and reasons.

According to Wittgenstein, one of the biggest problems in philosophy is the confusion between empirical propositions and philosophical pseudo-propositions. Wittgenstein's method for philosophy proceeds through conceptual clarification, with a close attention to the way we use language, and it avoids trying to explain phenomena as if it were using hypotheses (Holguín 2001). Another mistake is seeing the scientific model as the only paradigm, as in philosophy's aspiration of becoming a science of sciences. If we apply the same reasoning to psychiatry and psychology, we could say that some of the problems we face cannot be solved through empirical investigation. The difference with philosophy is obviously the relevance of the scientific method in a broad area of clinical work. Nevertheless, if we see our work as dealing only with empirical propositions, we risk reductionism on the one side, or confusion on the other, when applying the same method to all questions. This would imply, among other perils, thinking that technology is the only, or the optimal, way to find answers to our problems. This risk arises from considering our problems exclusively as empirical questions needing scientific exploration and causal explanations. That does not mean technology has no place in psychiatry; it just means we should be careful in deciding to what extent and in which cases it can help us in our inquiries.

4.2.1 Types of explanation

Every explanation arises from a question, a 'Why?' 'Why did John suddenly begin to act in a strange way after having a stroke?' and 'Why does John feel touched by a passage in Borges?' may be alike in form. But it is clear that they are different questions: in the first case, we are looking for a causal explanation, and we may proceed with the methods of science; whereas in the second we are looking for a reason, or for a more complete description of the situation, and causal explanations find no place in it.

Another example, the words of a patient:

> I don't know if I can explain myself. The thing is: you say that if I take Lamictal I shall be less anxious; that might be so, but then, if I am less anxious I shall be optimistic and try to do again things like going to college, starting a relationship, trying to get out of myself, things in which I always fail, and that will be too painful.

The patient is looking for a very specific kind of explanation, something that will help her understand more clearly her way of relating to other people, and the painful confrontation between her ideals and the reality of her achievements, moving between the stillness brought about by severe symptoms and the disenchantment in life's limitations. On the other hand, the effects of lamotrigine on anxiety and affective symptoms in the patient would certainly be clarified by means of causal explanations.

Cioffi (1998) states the risk of offering a causal explanation of a phenomenon when we are really looking for a different explanation: 'When is it a mistake to take our interest in a phenomenon in the direction of an enquiry into its causes and conditions rather than towards an enhanced grasp of the impression it produces, or the ruminations it incites?'

In the first direction, we may proceed through an empirical inquiry, in which case technology is surely an important ally. However, we may also proceed along a different path, one more similar to an aesthetic explanation, a path that leads us to self-clarification, or to the 'untroubled contemplation' of our object of study. This second direction is the one we take when confronted with a work of art, for example. Is these cases, according to Wittgenstein, we try to understand our feelings or thoughts, to gain an 'enhanced grasp' of our reactions. The answer takes the form of an aesthetic explanation. We obtain a 'perspicuous view' (*Ubersicht*) when we just 'see the connections,' not the causes.

> This is connected, I believe, with our wrongly expecting an explanation, whereas the solution of the difficulty is a description, if we give it the right place in our considerations. If we dwell upon it, and do not try to get beyond it. The difficulty here is: to stop. (Wittgenstein 1967: 314)

Recently, in a clinical case, a neurologist argued that any kind of injury or malfunction could be detected by our current diagnostic methods. Technology has advanced to such a degree of precision, he argued, that if nothing is detected there is no neuropathology whatsoever. How different from other ways of investigating the mind. If we cannot find an answer, maybe we are not looking in the right place, or we are not asking the questions properly, or we are not looking from the appropriate perspective.

Therefore, our first task is defining what type of explanation we need for a specific problem, and the second is knowing when to stop searching for one. Putting an end to explanations cuts across both causal and aesthetic answers. It may even be more difficult in explanations such as those offered in psychoanalysis, where an endless pursuit of interpretations lies open for both the therapist and the patient.

Wittgenstein's work showing that aesthetic explanations are not causal hypotheses is illustrated in the following quotes from *Lectures and Conversations*, selected by Cioffi (1998):

> There is a 'why' to aesthetic discomfort, not a cause to it (Wittgenstein 1966: 14)
>
> The sort of explanation one is looking for when one is puzzled by an aesthetic impression is not a causal explanation (ibid.: 20)
>
> ...an aesthetic explanation is not a causal explanation (ibid.: 12)
>
> The puzzles arising from the effects the arts have are not puzzles about how these things are causes (ibid.: 28)
>
> The criterion for its being the one that was in your mind is that...you agree (ibid.: 18)

> Here explanation is on the same level as utterance – where utterance is the only criterion (ibid.: 18)
>
> The answer in these cases is the one that satisfied you... (ibid.: 18)

The first set of aphorisms challenges the causal nature of the relation between our impression and the object related to it, whereas the second set of questions shows that the way of verifying the explanation differs. In the following table, I summarize the differences between causal and aesthetic explanations, to be further developed in the remaining of this chapter.

Explanation (science)	**Clarification (aesthetic)**
Hypothesis	Further description Perspicuous view
Causal	Formal
External	Internal
Inference meaning	Aspect meaning
Empirical investigation	Intersubjective
Verification	Placing side by side, agreement Persuasion

In causal explanations we make hypotheses and may continue on to experiments or apply statistical methods to verify or disprove our hypotheses, whereas those methods are fruitless in aesthetic explanations, if used at all. Wittgenstein also stressed the formal or internal relation characteristic of aesthetic descriptions: the explanation names the source of a feeling or an impression, its object, not the causes, and is therefore immune to experimental examination. A formal relation is what I can know with no need of a hypothesis, once again, the source of the feeling. The relation between my feeling or impression, and the object it refers to is also an identifying feature of the object. It should be noted that there are instances where it is not clear whether an aesthetic impression may not be explained through some kind of experimental revision, as Cioffi shows in his work.

4.2.2 'Where are wild questions from?'

Where do questions arise from, what is their territory? For example, reasons someone has for undertaking a psychoanalytic treatment: feelings of emptiness, solitude, difficulties in interpersonal relationships, knowing oneself better, or becoming a psychoanalyst. We want to gain a deeper understanding of ourselves: why we are the way we are, why we are unhappy, etc. This class of question is correctly placed by Cioffi under the category of self-understanding. Are these questions susceptible to causal explanations through hypotheses and empirical investigations, or should we explore them through further descriptions and clarifications? Or both ways?

Turning to dreams: 'What is intriguing about a dream is not its *causal* connection with events in my life, etc., but rather the impression it gives of being a fragment of a story – a very *vivid* fragment to be sure – the rest of which remains obscure.[...]The dream affects us as does an idea pregnant with possible developments' (Wittgenstein 1980: 68). This can be illustrated by another clinical example. A female patient has the following dream: 'I am alone in a room, and someone approaches me. I can see a neck tie, an elegant suit, but no face. I feel lost, and I try to see his face, but when I do so, he always turns away.' Simplifying, two different interpretations occurred to the therapist. In the first one, the patient is expressing her wish of seeing clearly the face of a man (her father), or as we say, confronting him face to face. Actually, the patient made a long trip to ask her father some urgent question she had about her history. In the second interpretation, the classical castration anxieties seem to be more important, as well as the anxiety about a sexual encounter.

That is to say, when interpreting a dream we can try do discover the causes of the dream (childhood sexual wish) and trace its mechanism (condensation, displacement, etc.) as Freud did. Or we can take the dream as a stimulating image that, linked with other aspects of the emotional life of the dreamer, may foster a more complete self-understanding. Freud was certainly looking for something more: something beyond the dream, its origin, a cause, and not just a good or pregnant idea.

If we move from dreams to symptoms the situation may not be so clear. Dreams are not usually taken as a problem as such, with some exceptions (e.g., nightmares), so the dreamer and listener may feel it has a peculiar attraction, something inviting further description, as Wittgenstein shows. However, in the case of a symptom we try to find its causes. Obviously, there are some symptoms inviting further descriptions, symptoms with some kind of charm. Delusional ideas may fit into this class: part of their difficulty is precisely that the patient is looking for a way to make them part of his own story, and he would be dissatisfied if we showed him that their cause is excessive dopaminergic activity.

The core of the problem might then be identifying which type of question we are dealing with, an aesthetic question or an empirical one. We can err both ways. Not undertaking the investigation of the origins of a symptom and offering only interpretations, or by an endless empirical pursuit trying to find the cause of some particular situation, for example through multiple diagnostic tests. However, many of the problems we deal with in clinical practice are what we may call limit cases or boundary problems, questions arising from a muddled territory, questions addressing us without the clarity of a name. Wittgenstein's metaphor of the lamp comes to mind: you find dark areas, lighted ones, and a gray zone where it is not possible to tell if there is light or not. Such cases abound in psychiatry. Some may well lie in a clear arena, for example, in the application of technology. Another way of trying to solve them is pragmatic: let us just proceed through an empirical inquiry, with the aid of available technological innovations, and wait to see how far we get. I believe this will be a commonly trodden path, even though Wittgenstein would tell us we were wrong from the start.

An additional source of tension between explanation and clarification arises from those cases in which after finding a causal explanation of a phenomenon through empirical enquiry, we nevertheless remain unsatisfied. Something is left out by the causal account. Take the case of depression; will it be enough for many of us to be told that our depression really is nothing else but the deregulation of such and such pathways and neurotransmitters in the brain? Many would feel the urge to find other explanations, without denying the correctness of the neurophysiologic description.

4.2.3 Relation to the object of study

An aesthetic view is different from other ways of looking at an object. For example, we may see the object as something to be explained and conquered. The aesthetic explanation does not try to possess the object, as much as trying to understand it. It does not intend to change or manipulate the object as a thing, but seeks to be moved and changed by the object. We are confronted with the other, or in Sartre's words, quoted by Cioffi (1998) 'the other who assaults our being'. Or we can fail to establish any kind of relationship with the object (patient, art work). In such cases we usually think: 'it says nothing to me', it fails to become 'a problem that troubles us'. According to Cioffi (1998), the 'natural form' of an aesthetic enquiry is 'What does this experience mean to me?' in opposition to 'what is its cause?' Clearly, as psychotherapists we are familiar with the 'natural form' of the first type of question. 'Every explanation is a hypothesis…But for someone worried by love, an explanatory hypothesis will not help much. It will not bring peace…the crush of thoughts that do not get out because they all press forward and are wedged in the door' (Cioffi 1998: 107).

We may ask: for someone troubled by love, what can technology offer? A thorough description of the positron emission tomography scan of the cerebral areas activated by his longings? Electron microscopic analysis of the oxytocin receptors involved in love at first sight? Thus formulated, the answer seems to be of no use. However, this should not prevent an empirical inquiry: the biological bases of attachment, for example, are important contributions to our field. Take the case of a similar phenomenon: grieving. Freud tried to offer a causal account (the shadow of the object falls upon the ego, identification being the main mechanism). He also acknowledged that something mysterious and difficult to understand remained when we tried to explain its painful quality. The important point is that we can explore grief in different ways: for example, looking at a functional magnetic resonance image. If someone wished to enroll in such investigation, he could be asking himself: 'well, it would be interesting to know how the brain is involved in this peculiar process' and at the same time go on with a different, more personal process of grieving, using further descriptions, struggling to find its place life's story.

In psychoanalysis or psychotherapy, the therapist is not only trying to understand the patient; he is also paying attention to his inner world, his own way of understanding, feeling, thinking, etc. Often we are in fact changed by our patients. In contrast, many of the insights gained through technological application do not affect the person who is applying it. He gains knowledge, no doubt; but this is knowledge about the object and not self-understanding.

Being touched or moved by a problem or a question is part of a feeling of wonder, a strong motivation for any kind of inquiry. Wittgenstein thought science was not a way of fostering wonder, but rather, of sending man to sleep. Wittgenstein's temperament shines through this saying, as many people feel they are 'awakened' by science. However, there is a contrast. In a more pragmatic way, we can just say that we are interested in a different set of questions. Aesthetic explanation will leave many persons completely unsatisfied; they will probably not choose to become therapists.

Turning to psychoanalysis, the case of Freud's development of his ideas shows a gradual but fundamental change in the type of questions he struggled with. How to explain the conversion symptoms seen in hysteria and how to understand the erotic and destructive forces hidden inside us seem to belong to territories far apart. However, not only Freud changed: the patients seeking psychoanalysis have also changed. They ask us different questions, less about symptoms and more about their life, such as 'Why do I feel empty, or why can't I find a deep connection with other persons?'.

In a sense, psychoanalysis begins as an aesthetic approach, asking what my reaction to this patient is, what do I imagine, my own floating associations. The patient has an 'aesthetic impact' on the analyst that sets in motion the process of mutual self-understanding or misunderstanding, or in other words, the movements of transference–countertransference. When we only try to find a cause, the patient can feel misunderstood, as if some of his own depth of singularity is being neglected. No wonder he or she may feel dehumanized and accuses psychiatry of being too reductionistic. The challenge lies in keeping the aesthetic dimension without excluding other types of exploration.

If we deny the relevance of empirical inquiries, we may fall into obscurantism. Indeed, Wittgenstein's limits to the adequacy of empirical enquiry on many subjects has been criticized as obscurantism (see Cioffi 1998). He could be charged on obscurantism of limits, for placing limits to the explanatory power of empirical enquiry; of an obscurantism of method, for giving reflection more explanatory potential than it has; and an obscurantism of sensibility, for preferring one method over the other.

4.2.4 **Validation**

'Here it occurs to me that in conversation on aesthetic matters we use the words: "You have to see it like *this*, this is how it is meant"..."When you see it like *this*, you see where it goes wrong"..."You have to hear this bar as an introduction"..."You must hear it in this key"..."You must phrase it like *this*" (which can refer to hearing as well as to playing)' (Wittgenstein 1953: 202). The role of persuasion in aesthetic explanation was underlined by Wittgenstein (Meléndez 2003). This means that the criteria for deciding whether an explanation is correct or not is going to be different: it is the one that leads to agreement and is accepted by the person who is trying to understand the impression or problem. Persuasion helps us view things in a new way, leading us to say, 'yes, I see it clearly now.' Once again, the parallel with psychotherapeutic work is apparent. Indeed, Wittgenstein criticized Freud on this account, for persuading patients without recognizing he was doing so, and the only evidence available for psychoanalysis would ultimately 'always be essentially the product of successful persuasion' (Bouveresse 1995).

> If you are led by psycho-analysis to say that really you thought so and so, or that really your motive was so and so, this is not a matter of discovery, but of persuasion. In a different way you could have been persuaded of something different. (Wittgenstein 1966)
>
> Now, I could imagine that someone seeing the unfolded picture might exclaim: 'Yes, that's the solution, that's what I dreamed, minus the gaps and distortions'. This would then be the solution precisely by virtue of his acknowledging it as such.
>
> (Wittgenstein 1980: 68)

It is indeed difficult to prove an interpretation in psychoanalysis; sometimes we can aspire only to make a good case, something convincing for the patient.

4.3 **Types of interpretation in psychoanalysis**

In this section I explore the different types of use of interpretation in Freud's work and in psychoanalysis. Interpretation may be understood as finding the cause of a symptom or a dream, as exemplified in Freud's earlier ideas. If we are looking for a cause, we are bound to use the scientific method. In other passages, however, Freud uses interpretation to give a new meaning to the patient's experience. This second use implies clarification, helping the patient see through a different perspective, placing the problem in a broader context, connecting it to other experiences; in short, something not that different from aesthetic explanations presented above.

Furthermore, there is no way of doing psychoanalysis without using both types of explanation. Some may argue this is not the case, and see psychoanalysis as working with only one kind of interpretation, for example, defending an exclusively hermeneutical approach.

As I have argued before (Uribe 2004), in their practice psychoanalysts frequently resort to several sorts of interpretation. Elias Mallet da Rocha Barros (2000) shows rich clinical material, including dream images of his patient. He discusses the case of a patient who consulted him because of mood oscillations and not being able to sustain stable intellectual output. Taking into account the patient's dreams of clams and oysters as well as his associations during the session, Rocha Barros concludes: 'I see the "clams" that turned into "oysters" as a condensed expression of several different emotional experiences... The tension produced by these emotional experiences in the internal world of the patient is an expression of the absent meaning with which they are linked. The resulting image has a great power to evoke experiences. Evocative language is characteristic of the process of dream work, which produces pictorial images, and is also present in painting, poetry and music.' (Rocha Barros 2000: 1091).

The 'absent meaning' and the evocative power of the images recall the above characterization of aesthetic explanations. The dream and our images from the emotional experiences are 'saying something' to both patient and analyst, and the tension derived from trying to understand them resembles 'what is in the back of the mind', leading hopefully to an assent like 'yes, that is what I was trying to say'. Note also the comparisons made with painting, poetry, and music. Finally, working with the 'absent meaning' belongs more to the domain of aesthetic explanation. The author also talks about potential significations, which I think are also frequently used in psychoanalysis in general, as there is plenty of room for expanding, completing, and wording through emotional experiences.[1]

However, we also find causal hypotheses: for example, Rocha Barros (2000) suggests that his patient's intellectual inhibition is due to repression and competitiveness with his father and other male figures. I believe the presence of different types of interpretation can be found in many clinical examples: this task, however, exceeds the limits of this chapter.

4.4 **Aesthetics in therapeutics**

The study of the relation to the object characteristic of aesthetic explanations opens the way for a deeper understanding of the therapeutic effects in psychoanalysis. Clarification and self-understanding are essential aspects of psychotherapeutic work; the analogy, however, runs deeper, as has been discussed by Edwards (1982). In effect, Wittgenstein's method of doing philosophy has been compared to a therapeutic enterprise (see also Baker 2003). For Edwards, the reason for a therapeutic aspect in Wittgenstein's work resides precisely in his view of aesthetics. He even suggests that Wittgenstein's work can be understood as an 'aesthetic model of philosophy'. He looks at the way aesthetic disputes end according to Wittgenstein.

> For the clarity we are aiming at is indeed *complete* clarity. But this simply means that the philosophical problems should *completely* disappear. The real discovery is the one that makes me capable of stopping doing philosophy when I want to. The one that gives philosophy peace, so that it is no longer tormented by questions which bring itself in question.
>
> (Wittgenstein 1953, sec. 133)

What Edwards is trying to rescue is the value of a comparison between Wittgenstein's method and a therapeutic method. In the first place, for philosophy the problem (disease or question) arises from a perplexity, which is a symptom of confusion, whereas in psychiatry the problem is the disease, the symptom, or a vague sense of uneasiness. Secondly, in the case of an aesthetic relation one is changed by the object. Following a similar line, Edwards argues that when we apply the aesthetic method in philosophy, there should be a 'fundamental change in the philosopher'. This change is brought by a 'change in sensibility' in the patient or the philosopher, a change in 'some of those deep perspectives in terms of which experience is appropriated, ordered, understood' (Edwards 1982: 134). In aesthetic reasoning, finally, a dispute or a problem is also solved through a change in sensibility.

The way therapeutic effects have been depicted in psychoanalysis has not so far mentioned explicitly a change in sensibility. However, other ways of describing therapeutic changes are congenial with sensibility, as those mentioned above, like seeing things in a different way, a more complete or coherent view; in short, a new understanding. Central in this method is comparing an object or situation with another, typical in Wittgenstein's use of 'intermediate cases'. As he wrote in *Zettel*: 'I wanted to put this picture before your eyes, and your *acceptance* of this picture consists in your being inclined to regard a given case differently; that is, to compare it with this series of pictures. I have changed your *way of seeing*' (1967: 461).

Finally, it is important to underline the individuality common to a psychotherapeutic work and an aesthetic impression. The object of study in both areas almost always involve a specific reaction or perspective on a single object of study, no matter how useful a comparison with many other cases can be.

4.5 Conclusions

Psychiatry as a discipline cannot expect to find a single theoretical approach as the basis for its practice. The difference in the nature of questions it explores and the type of answers pertinent for each inquiry is one of the reasons we need multiple perspectives. In this chapter, I have explored the contrast between empirical inquiries with their own explanations, and a clarification that takes the form of aesthetic explorations.

The distinction between explanation and clarification runs close to Jaspers' (1946/1993) well-known distinction between explaining and understanding. For Jaspers, we use psychological explanations to understand psychic manifestations when we see them 'from the inside', whereas we explain them causally when we use an objective approach, 'from the outside'. Both approaches are needed and useful, but they are completely different sources of knowledge. Aesthetic explanations in the sense presented here would be but a very specific way of understanding among others. Jaspers also thought both methods were part of science, whereas Wittgenstein considers aesthetic explanation as belonging to a field quite apart from science.

The need to include various modes of explanations also coincides with Ghaemi's (2003) recent formulation of the plurality in psychiatry. He relies mainly on the methods used in multiple approaches rather than studying the contrast between aesthetic and causal explanations. Ghaemi takes psychoanalysis as an example of one perspective to be included in the plurality, whereas this chapter argues for the existing plurality within psychoanalysis itself. It is also important to keep in mind the risk of eclecticism, severely criticized by Ghaemi. As I have argued above, taking aesthetic and causal explanations to be equally valid as forms of inquiry is a mistake. Not every problem or question is suitable for both kinds of exploration. In that sense, eclecticism is nothing other than treating all questions and answers alike. If psychoanalysis wishes to avoid being called an 'abominable mess', it should state clearly what type of explanation is being used, acknowledging the need for various perspectives without running into confusion.

The relation to the object marks an interesting difference that might open the path for a further discussion of the technological impact in psychiatry. As shown by Ihde (2003), technology can be not only a means to an end but also a way of disclosure and revealing. The relation with this activity could even be liberating, if we are able to stand in a free relation with technology. The problem with technology might be its tendency to elicit a sense of possession and domination of objects; that is, standing to the object as something to be conquered, changed, and most important, something that will not change me. An aesthetic approach, as has been underlined here, always opens more clearly the possibility of being changed by the object. Technological applications in psychiatry could well be revealing, disclosing, even liberating; however, they are easily transformed into a mere tool leading to an estrangement from the object.

An empirical enquiry into the causes and conditions of a phenomenon might be supported by technology, whereas it is useless for certain kinds of problem. The role of technology in self-understanding (as an auxiliary tool) is misplaced. When formulated this way, it seems clear. So where lies the difficulty, if there is any? For psychiatry, the difficulty lies in the clinical situation; what is expected and demanded from psychiatry or psychoanalysis is not just self-understanding: the patient constantly expects some kind of explanation. As long as psychotherapy uses aesthetic explanations, our field will never be just an instance of techne.

Finally: the presence of aesthetic explanations in psychoanalysis seems to confirm Wittgenstein's criticism of mixing causes and reasons. However, as has been argued above, part of the solution is precisely in accepting different types of explanation without mixing them. The philosophical cure for the psychoanalytic dimension of psychiatric theory would be to offer clarity, not oversimplification.

Endnote

1 It should be mentioned that Rocha Barros quotes Wittgenstein saying that images can be recognized as forms of something, 'whose meaning can be understood only in terms of their relationship with other things' (p. 1092).

References

Baker G. (2003). 'Wittgenstein's method and psychoanalysis' in B. Fulford, K. Morris, J. Sadler and G. Stanghellini (eds.) *Nature and Narrative: An introduction to the new philosophy of psychiatry* (Oxford: Oxford University Press), 57–63.

Bouveresse, J. (1995). *Wittgenstein Reads Freud. The myth of the unconscious* (Princeton, NJ: Princeton University Press).

Cioffi F. (1998). *Wittgenstein on Freud and Frazer* (Cambridge, UK: Cambridge University Press).

Edwards J. (1982). *Ethics without Philosophy: Wittgenstein and the moral life* (University Presses of Florida).

Ghaemi S. N. (2003). *The Concepts of Psychiatry. A pluralistic approach to the mind and mental illness* (Baltimore and London: The Johns Hopkins University Press).

Holguín M. (2001). 'Wittgenstein: la lógica de una ilusión' in J. Botero (ed.) *El Pensamiento de L. Wittgenstein* (Bogotá: Universidad Nacional de Colombia), 93–109.

Ihde D. (2003). 'Heidegger's philosophy of technology' in R. Scharff and V. Dusek (eds.) *Philosophy of Technology. The technological condition. An anthology* (Oxford, UK: Blackwell), 277–292.

Jaspers K. (1946/1993). *Psicopatología General* (México:, Fondo de Cultura Económica).

Meléndez R. (2003). 'Persuasión en el pensamiento tardío de Wittgenstein' in A. Flórez, M. Holguín, and R. Meléndez (eds.) *Del Espejo a las Herramientas. Ensayos sobre el pensamiento de Wittgenstein* (Bogotá: Universidad Nacional de Colombia), 183–198.

Phillips J. (2002). 'Technical reason in DSM-IV: an unacknowledged value' in J. Sadler (ed.) *Descriptions and Prescriptions: Values, mental disorders, and the DSMs* (Baltimore, MD: The Johns Hopkins Press).

Rocha Barros E. M. da (2000). Affect and pictographic image: meaning in mental life. *International Journal of Psychoanalysis*, **81**, 1087–1099.

Uribe M. (2004). Determinismo, explicación e interpretación en psicoanálisis. *Revista Sociedad Colombiana Psicoanálisis*, **29**, 489–510.

Wittgenstein L. (1953). *Philosophical Investigations* (Oxford, UK: Blackwell).

Wittgenstein L. (1966). *Lectures and Conversations on Aesthetics, Psychology and Religious Belief* (C. Barrett, ed.) (Oxford, UK: Blackwell).

Wittgenstein L. (1967). *Zettel* (G. E. M. Anscombe and G. H. von Wright, eds.) (Berkeley and Los Angeles: University of California Press).

Wittgenstein L. (1980). *Culture and Value* (G. H. von Wright, ed.) (Chicago: The University of Chicago Press).

Chapter 5

Focusing the lenses of feminist theories to reflect on technology and psychiatry

Sue V. Rosser

5.1 Introduction

On 14 January 2005, I was an invited speaker at the National Bureau of Economic Research at Harvard University where President Larry Summers delivered his now infamous speech. When he resigned as President of Harvard on 21 February 2006, most of the news articles covering the projected second vote of no confidence and his resignation cited the 'dispute over women in science' as a factor that led to his failed presidency (Finder *et al.* 2006). As the transcript is now available on the Harvard website, www.president.harvard.edu/speeches/2005/nber.html, here I will not recount the faulty logic and absence of research that he used to support his three primary hypotheses for the paucity of women scientists and engineers: (1) women are unwilling or unable to work the 80-hour weeks required for success in science at top-flight academic institutions; (2) innate or biological factors, rather than socialization, probably account for sex differences in mathematical aptitude and in adult preferences for choice of academic study and occupational field; (3) discrimination, which he defined as a 'taste' for hiring people like oneself, does not exist in academia because that would be eliminated through market forces by lesser institutions hiring highly qualified women and minorities, thereby gaining a competitive advantage.

Rather than rehashing the arguments and research for Summers' discussion of why women are not in science, here I will examine another aspect of the topic: What differences have or can women make in science and engineering? Specifically, can the lenses of feminist theories provide reflections useful for the topic of technology and psychiatry?

Most researchers in the behavioral, biomedical, and physical sciences are trained in the scientific method and believe in its power. Few, however, are aware of its historical and philosophical roots in logical positivism and objectivity. Positivism implies that 'all knowledge is constructed by inference from immediate sensory experiences' (Jaggar 1983: 355–356). It is premised on the assumption that human beings are highly individualistic and obtain knowledge in a rational manner that may be separated from their social conditions. This leads to the belief in the possibilities of obtaining knowledge that is both objective and value-free, the cornerstone of the scientific method.

Longino (1990) has explored the extent to which methods used by scientists can be objective and lead to repeatable, verifiable results while contributing to hypotheses or theories that are congruent with non-objective institutions and ideologies of the society. 'Background assumptions are the means by which contextual values and ideology are incorporated into scientific inquiry' (Longino 1990: 216). The institutions and beliefs of our society reflect the fact that the society is patriarchal. Even female scientists have only recently become aware of the influence of patriarchal bias in the paradigms of science.

A first step for feminist scientists was recognizing the possibility that androcentric bias would result from having virtually all theoretical and decision-making positions in science held by men (Keller 1983). Not until a substantial number of women had entered the profession (Rosser 1986) could this androcentrism be exposed. As long as only a few women were scientists, they had to demonstrate or conform to the male view of the world to be successful and to have their research meet the criteria for 'objectivity.'

In the past two decades, feminist historians and philosophers of science (Fee 1982, 1983; Haraway 1978, 1989, 1997; Harding 1986, 1993, 1998; Longino 1990) and feminist scientists (Birke 1986; Bleier 1984, 1986; Fausto-Sterling 1992; Keller 1983, 1985, 1992; Rosser, 1988, 1994, 1997; Spanier 1995) have pointed out the bias and absence of value neutrality in science, particularly biology. By excluding females as experimental subjects, focusing on problems of primary interest to males, using faulty experimental designs, and interpreting data based in language or ideas constricted by patriarchal parameters, scientists have introduced bias or flaws into their experimental results in several areas. These flaws and biases were allowed to become part of the mainstream of scientific thought and were perpetuated in the scientific literature for decades. Because most scientists were men, values held by them as males were not distinguished as biasing; rather, they were congruent with the values of all scientists and thus became synonymous with the 'objective' view of the world (Keller 1982, 1985) and what aspects of it were studied.

The demonstration that contextual values, including gender, bias not only the scientific research of individuals but also what is accepted as valid science by the entire scientific community represents one of the major contributions that feminism has made to science. In this chapter, I use different feminist theories to explore feminist impact in choice and definition of problems chosen, approaches used, and theories and conclusions drawn from the research. To approach these questions, I shall use the lenses of feminist theories to focus on examples from biology and technology to reveal why women bringing new, significant perspectives serve as a crucial link between science and society. I choose examples from biology and technology because these are the areas in which I have some expertise. I shall then suggest, from a position of non-expertise, how it appears that each feminist theory might apply in psychiatry to somewhat parallel situations, those of selective serotonin reuptake inhibitors (SSRIs) and functional magnetic resonance imaging (fMRI). I hope this theoretical framework stimulates new thoughts on the inter-relationships among gender, technology, and psychiatry.

5.2 Liberal feminism

A general definition of liberal feminism is the belief that women are suppressed in contemporary society because they suffer unjust discrimination (Jaggar 1983). Liberal feminists seek no special privileges for women and simply demand that everyone receive equal consideration without discrimination on the basis of sex.

5.2.1 Biology

Feminists have revealed a source of bias in many double-blind studies that were run using only male rats, human beings, or other primates as experimental subjects. In a double-blind study, neither the researcher nor the subjects know who among the subjects receives the true drug and who receives the placebo. This method is thought to ensure objectivity because neither party is biased by knowing who receives the drug. Perhaps the notion that the double-blind study ensures objectivity made the researchers overly confident of their results. In many cases, as demonstrated again by the study released in March 2005 documenting differential effects in men and women of aspirin in preventing heart attacks and strokes (Ridker *et al.* 2005), researchers universalized the results beyond what the data warranted (Steering Committee of the Physicians' Health Study Group 1989; MRFIT 1990). Because the studies were done on males only and because the differing levels of hormones in males and females frequently cause significantly different interactions with drugs in the two sexes, their extrapolation from the study population of males only to the entire human species is inaccurate and inappropriate. A liberal feminist would argue that adding women to the original research design would correct this bias.

A 2000 Government Accountability Office Report concluded that the National Institutes of Health (NIH) 'has made less progress in implementing the requirement that certain clinical trials be designated and carried out to permit valid analysis by sex, which could reveal whether intervention affects women differently from men' (U.S. Department of Health and Human Services 2000). The NIH then put into effect new guidelines for phase III clinical trials covering both the inclusion of women and sex-based analysis for reviewers and scientific review administrators. Is this, including the direction to publish data including gender-based analyses, being applied to SSRIs?

Applications of liberal feminism to current research agendas and their translation into practice and products might lead to the following sorts of changes. Equal numbers of women would be involved in setting the research agenda for the Human Genome Initiative (HGI) or Project. Women scientists would have equal access to the grant moneys and sequencing equipment provided by the HGI, instead of the current male dominance of such resources. Because of their awareness of potential androcentric bias such as the possibility of increased interest in mapping genes for diseases causing increased mortality and morbidity in men, both men and women scientists would strive to eliminate such bias from research designs and interpretations of data. In April, 2001, the Institute of Medicine published *Exploring the Biological Contributions to Human Health: Does Sex Matter?* This grew out of the 1999 proposal from the Society for Women's Health Research to the Institute of Medicine to review the available research on basic biology of sex differences and to set a research agenda. The agenda validated the study of basic biologic and molecular bases for sex and gender differences in disease, including 'sex-based biology as an integral part' of research conducted by the institutes involved in the initiative on brain research.

5.2.2 **Technology**

Male dominance in engineering and the creative decision-making sectors of the information technology workforce may result in similar gender bias, particularly design and user bias. Shirley Malcom suggested that the air bag fiasco suffered by the US auto industry serves as an excellent example of gender bias reflected in design; this fiasco would have been much less likely had a woman engineer been on the design team. Because on the average, women tend to be smaller than men, women on the design team might have recognized that a bag which implicitly used the larger male body as a norm would be flawed when applied to smaller individuals, killing, rather than protecting, children and small women. Are as many women, as men, setting the research agendas that use fMRI? Do the diseases and topics of prevalence and importance for women have equal footing with those of men in studies using this technology?

In contrast to liberal feminism, all other feminist theories call into question the fundamental assumptions underlying the scientific method, its corollaries of objectivity and value neutrality, or its implications. They reject individualism for a social construction of knowledge and question positivism and the possibility of objectivity obtained by value neutrality. Many also imply that men and women may conduct scientific research differently, although each theory posits a different cause for the gender distinction.

5.3 Socialist feminism

Marxist critiques form the historical precursors and foundations for socialist feminist critiques and define all knowledge, including science, as socially constructed and emerging from practical human involvement in production. Because knowledge is a productive activity of human beings, it cannot be objective and value-free because the basic categories of knowledge are shaped by human purposes and values. In the early twenty-first century United States, capitalism, the prevailing mode of production, determines science and technology and favors the interests of the dominant class. This Marxist/socialist theory undergirds the work of numerous scholars of science and technology who have used this framework for their studies, producing a large body of research commonly known as 'the social shaping of science and technology' (MacKenzie and Wajcman 1985).

Feminist scholars rightly point out, that science and technology and the social shaping of technology (Wajcman 1991; Webster 1995) and science (Rose 1994) have often been conceptualized in terms of men, excluding women at all levels. Socialist feminist critiques include women and place gender on equal footing with class in shaping science and technology. In this dual systems approach (Eisenstein 1984; Hartmann 1981) capitalism and patriarchy function as mutually reinforcing parts of a system where the sexual division of labor stands with wage labor as a central feature of capitalism, and where gender differences in wages, along with failing to count contributions of women to reproduction and child rearing as 'productivity' in a capitalist economy, reinforce patriarchy and power differentials in the home.

5.3.1 Biology

The billions of dollars spent on the HGI would be interpreted as reflecting the interests of the dominant class. The focus on genes and the considerable publicity that surrounds the isolation and copying of 'disease genes' suggest to most laypeople not only that most disease is biologically determined but more specifically that it is genetically caused. This diverts valuable research dollars away from environmental causes of, and contributions to, disease, and away from public health, long demonstrated to be more effective in eradicating more communicable, and other, diseases than the high-tech solutions developed by medical research. Centering on genes also places responsibility on the individual and takes it away from the system and broader society. The obvious question for psychiatry that follows from this line of thinking revolves around the extent to which the current fascination with a reductionistic, biomedical model focused on drugs for treatment diverts resources and research from the more comprehensive biopsychosocial model for mental health and away from non-drug therapies and social services also shown to be effective in treatment. Does the research money from the pharmaceutical companies distort the approaches and types of research undertaken? Why did the experts involved with revising the Diagnostic and Statistical Manual (DSM) not reveal their monetary connections with drug companies to uncover actual or perceived conflicts of interest that might bias their descriptive categorizations (Vergano 2006)? Very specifically, are SSRIs the most effective treatments for all individuals at all times who suffer from depression?

The decisions about which products are developed from the numerous patented genes isolated and sequenced by the biotechnology industries fall more under the influence of capitalist interests in profit margins than the needs of people in developing countries for nutritious foods or the health and medical interests of the public as a whole. For example, Monsanto owns a patent covering all genetically engineered cotton seeds and plants, and genes governing Alzheimer's disease have been patented by Duke University (King and Stabinsky 1999). What other anti-depressants are not being developed because of patents for a very successful SSRI already held by powerful pharmaceutical companies? Are socioeconomically disadvantaged people steered to the generic drugs and denied access to more appropriate drugs because of the successful use of patents by the pharmaceutical companies to maintain high drug prices?

5.3.2 Technology

Understandings of class relations emerging under capitalism and gender relations under patriarchy help to explain the intertwining of military and masculinity (Enloe 1983,1989; MacKenzie and Wajcman 1999) which drives much technological innovation in this country and elsewhere. These understandings also explain the choices made to develop technologies in a certain way. This exemplifies engineering decisions that favor fewer rich people over relatively less expensive technologies such as devices for the home to aid many people, especially women.

Caro (1974) revealed that Robert Moses, the master builder of New York's roads, parks, bridges, and other public works from the 1920s to the 1970s, had overpasses built to specifications to discourage buses on parkways. White upper- and middle-class car owners could use the parkways, such as Wantagh Parkway, for commuting and for accessing recreation sites, including Jones Beach. Because the twelve-foot height of public transit buses prohibited their fitting under the overpass, blacks and poor people dependent upon public transit did not have access to Jones Beach (Winner 1980).

This example of bridges raises the issue of access quite directly. Specifically, who has access, both as researchers and as patients/clients, to the use of fMRI? The expense of the machines prohibits research by those not at well-funded institutions. Are studies flawed because people on Medicaid or who are uninsured are not participating in the research?

5.4 African-American/womanist and racial/ethnic feminism

Just as socialist feminist theory provided insights into the gender and class distributions of science experiments and technological innovation, African-American critiques uncover the place/role of race. Racism intertwines and reinforces differing aspects of capitalism and patriarchy. Like socialist-feminism, African-American/womanist feminism, based on African-American critiques of a Eurocentric approach to knowledge, also rejects individualism and positivism for social constructionist approaches and questions methods that distance the observer from the object of study.

5.4.1 Biology

Not surprisingly, some view the HGI as providing a further opportunity for genocide of ethnic populations. The Human Genome Diversity Project, which samples indigenous and other 'vanishing' tribal populations, may be viewed from an ethnic perspective as an attempt to preserve genes, while allowing the peoples themselves to become extinct. Some have questioned the motives of Axys Pharmaceuticals, with its application for patents on cells and genes of New Guinea tribes, to use in developing treatments against viruses to which the tribes may have developed immunities (King and Stabinsky 1999). A possible critique of the use of SSRIs centers on the use of medication to 'even-out' moods and control rage that, in some cases, may be an appropriate reaction to racism in our society. African-American women, in particular, experience significant racism, sexism, and social inequities; some would question the use of medications or even therapy to mediate anger and depression that may constitute appropriate responses to their social situation.

In contrast, Professor Georgia Dunston and Carole Broome have founded the Human Genome Center at Howard University. They wish to use the information from sequencing the human genome to focus study on diseases significant for the African-American population, recognizing that certain genetic frequencies are higher in black populations and that historically Black Howard University provides a good environment in which to study this. One can imagine that some individuals would actively seek race/ethnic-based clinical trials of SSRIs, other anti-depressants, and medications to understand differences in responses to these medications that might be racially/ethnically based.

5.4.2 Technology

Because technology involves practical application of more abstract, basic scientific research, the problem of the distance between engineer (researcher) and the technology (object of study) needs to be understood, discussed, and addressed to make technological research methodologies clearer to both developers and users. Unlike theoretical scientific projects, which do not necessarily have immediate practical outcomes, projects in computer science or engineering must accommodate the impact of the uses of technology with particular attention to the users of technology. When designing technologies, engineers, designers, and computer scientists should not only ask how and under what conditions the technology will be used, but also allow the potential consumer to shape the design of the product. Gender, class, race, and other factors such as age and ability status, should be considered in defining who the user will be. Technology historically reflected and reinforced race relations, and traditional Web programming has typically ignored minorities. For example, the Blacksburg Electronic Village, an on-line community network, 'routes around' race and relies on the 'digital default' of White, male, heterosexual, middle-aged, middle to upper class (Silver 2000: 143).

This raises the issue of the 'norm' for MRI and fMRI. Upon what population have these technologies been 'normed'? Is the White, middle-aged, middle class, mentally healthy (by whose definition?), heterosexual, right-handed male used as the norm against which MRI or fMRI of individuals are compared?

5.5 Essentialist feminism

African-American and socialist feminist critiques emphasize race and class as sources of oppression that combine with gender in shaping and being shaped by science and technology. In contrast, essentialist feminist theory posits that all women are united by their biology. Women are also different from men because of their biology, specifically their secondary sex characteristics and their reproductive systems. Frequently, essentialist feminism may extend to include gender differences in visuo-spatial and verbal ability, aggression and other behaviors, and other physical and mental traits based on pre-natal or pubertal hormone exposure. For example, some sociobiological research such as that by Wilson (1975), Trivers (1972), and Dawkins (1976) and some hormone and brain lateralization research seems to provide biological evidence for differences in mental and behavioral characteristics in males and females.

5.5.1 **Biology**

Some individuals who might be categorized as essentialist, and possibly as conservative, push for more research that would result in discoveries such as the *BRCA1* and *BRCA2* genes. This focus on genetic causes of cancer, which may result, in the case of these genes, in the testing of some families and in women who have the genes having radical mastectomies before any sign of cancer is detected, might be supported by conservative essentialist feminists. Essentialists, who might be seen as extreme biological determinists, would push for more women scientists to be involved in this research to ensure that more HGI dollars would be directed toward isolation of genetic diseases that are particularly problematic for women.

The era of the human genome has produced a particularly reductionistic version of a biodeterministic, biomedical model, in which extreme attention is drawn to genetic causes for diseases. This genetic focus became necessary to justify the huge amount of resources diverted from epidemiology and public health measures to prevent disease, and studies of other causes for disease, to pour them into the $3 billion HGI. For breast cancer research, this helps to explain the focus on the isolation of *BRCA1* and *BRCA2* genes. The media attention surrounding the isolation and copying of the breast cancer genes fueled the public perception that the overwhelming cause of breast cancer is hereditary and that a cure for the genetic cause would soon be found; the reality is that only five to ten per cent of breast cancer is inherited and that the *BRCA1* and *BRCA2* genes are responsible for only half of the inherited cases (King *et al.* 1993). This leaves ninety or ninety-five per cent of breast cancer cases unaccounted for by the *BRCA1* and *BRCA2* genes, and points to the role caused by social, behavioral, and environmental factors.

Essentialism might be interpreted as the basis for the emphasis on the extreme biomedical, in which all mental illness results from biochemical, physiological, or anatomical imbalances, to the almost complete exclusion of psychosocial elements in the model of psychiatry. The reliance on medications such as SSRIs only, without accompanying individual, group, or other therapies exemplifies this.

5.5.2 Technology

Essentialist feminism suggests that men, because of their biology and inability to conceive, also develop technologies to dominate, control and exploit the natural world, women, and other peoples (Easlea 1983). Women, in contrast, because of our biology, not only have less testosterone, but also have the ability to give birth. Giving birth gives us less direct control over our bodies and connects us more closely with nature, other animals, and life (King 1989; Merchant 1979). In its most simplistic extreme form, essentialism implies that men use technologies to bring death and control to other people, women, and the environment, whereas (or because) women give birth and nurture life in all its forms. In his study of the discovery and development of nuclear weapons and the atomic bomb, Easlea (1983) examines the language and behavior of the scientists. Analyzing the aggressive sexual and birth metaphors the scientists use to describe their work, he argues that men 'give birth' to science and weapons to compensate for their inability to give birth to babies.

Some have noted the current fascination of the fields of psychology and psychiatry with MRI and fMRI and the underlying assumptions that differences in brain images have significant meaning for behavior, intelligence, and/or mental health. Lack of understanding of causes or meaning of many currently observed differences often drives research agendas and questions. Others have noted the relatively high percentage of male researchers working in neuroscience, especially using the technologies of MRI and fMRI, relative to the percentage of male researchers in other areas of psychology and psychiatry.

5.6 Existentialist feminism

In contrast to essentialist feminism, existentialist feminism purports that it is not the biological differences themselves, but the value that society assigns to biological differences between males and females which has led woman to play the role of the Other (Tong 1989). The philosophical origins of existentialist feminism emphasize that it is man's concept of woman as 'other' that has led to his willingness to dominate and exploit her (de Beauvoir 1947).

The methodological implications arising out of existentialist feminism are that a society that emphasizes gender differences would produce a science that emphasizes sex differences. In such a society, men and women might be expected to create very different sciences because of the social construction of both gender and science. The possibility of a gender-free or gender-neutral (positivist) science evolving in such a society is virtually nil. Elizabeth Fee (1982) summed up the situation very well: She states that a sexist society should be expected to develop a sexist science. Conceptualizing a feminist science from within our society is 'like asking a medieval peasant to imagine the theory of genetics or the production of a space capsule' (p. 31).

5.6.1 Biology

Existentialist feminism provides a theoretical explanation for the significant gender differential in research and treatment in cardiovascular disease in men compared with women that existed in the twentieth century. Because this society defines women as 'other' in contrast to men, the fact that heart disease strikes men at an earlier age than women, served as sufficient reason to direct most research funds and treatment protocols toward men. The similar frequency of heart disease in women compared with men was ignored because difference in age rather than similarity of frequency was emphasized in keeping with the definition of women as 'other'. This emphasis on difference resulted in extreme bias in research, such as women's exclusion from eighty-two per cent of studies between 1960 and 1991 of clinical trials for medications to prevent myocardial infarctions (Gurwitz *et al.* 1992), and an in-hospital death rate for women ten times that of men after angioplasty when the procedure was first developed (Kelsey *et al.* 1993).

Several recent studies (Kornstein *et al.* 2000; Young 2001) have explored the gender differences in responses to SSIs and tricyclic antidepressants. Despite the fact that depression is approximately twice as common in women than men, were women of reproductive age initially included in clinical trials and basic research in this area? Has the research adequately explored appropriate dosage responses correlated with age and stage of the reproductive cycle? Although the reasons for the gender differences may be related to the effects of female sex hormones on serotonergic neurotransmission and in particular on the function of the 5-HT1A receptor (Young *et al.* 1993), the evidence for gender differences in treatment response to antidepressants is not definitive (Kornstein *et al.* 2001; Quitkin *et al.* 2001). Sorting out the biological, compared with social, effects on depression requires additional study.

5.6.2 Technology

In direct ways, the use of the male norm to design technology excludes women as users of these technologies. Military regulations often apply Military

Standard 1472 of anthropometric data so that systems dimensions use the ninety-fifth and fifth percentile of male dimensions in designing weapons systems. This led to the cockpits of airplanes being designed to fit the dimensions of 90% of male military recruits (Weber 1997). This worked relatively well as long as the military was entirely male. In the case of the Joint Primary Aircraft Training System, used by both the navy and air force to train its pilots, the application of the standard accommodated the fifth through ninety-fifth percentile (90%) of males, but only approximately the sixty-fifth through ninety-fifth percentile (30%) of females. The policy decision by Secretary of Defense Les Aspin (1993: 1) to increase the percentage of women pilots uncovered the gender bias in the cockpit design. Designed to exclude only 10% of male recruits by dimensions, the cockpit excluded 70% of women recruits. Exclusion of such large numbers of women by dimensions alone, made it extremely difficult to meet the military's policy goal of increasing women pilots. The officers initially reacted by assuming that the technology reflected the best or only design possible and that the goal for the percentage of women pilots would have to be lowered and/or the number of tall women recruits would have to be increased. This initial reaction, which represented the world viewpoint of men (de Beauvoir 1947) changed. When political coalitions, the Tailhook scandal, and feminist groups reinforced the policy goal, a new cockpit design emerged which reduced the minimum sitting height from 34 to 32.8 inches, thereby increasing the percentage of eligible women (Weber 1997: 379).

Studies correlating the results of fMRI with handedness, SAT scores, and sexual orientation imply or are interpreted by many to suggest that these have a biological or even genetic basis. However, because society and culture may also influence these characteristics, the exact contribution of genes or biology remains unclear. What do these sex differences in fMRIs really mean and are there alternative ways to interpret them?

5.7 **Psychoanalytic feminism**

Based on the Freudian prejudice that anatomy is destiny, psychoanalytic theory assumes that biological sex will lead to different ways for boys and girls to resolve the Oedipus and castration complexes which arise during the phallic stage of normal sexual development. Rejecting the biological determinism in Freud, Dinnerstein (1977) and Chodorow (1978) in particular have used an aspect of psychoanalytic theory known as object relations theory to examine the construction of gender and sexuality during the Oedipal stage of psychosexual development which usually results in male dominance. They conclude that the gender differences resulting in male dominance can be traced to the fact that in our society, women are the primary caretakers for most infants and children.

Keller (1982, 1985) in particular applied the work of Chodorow and Dinnerstein to suggest how science, populated mostly by men, has become a masculine province, in its choice of experimental topics, use of male subjects for experimentation, interpretation, and theorizing from data, as well as the practice and applications of science undertaken by the scientists. Keller (1982, 1985) suggests that because the scientific method stresses objectivity, rationality, distance, and autonomy of the observer from the object of study (i.e., the positivist neutral observer), individuals who feel comfortable with independence, autonomy, and distance will be most likely to become scientists. Feminists have suggested that the objectivity and rationality of science are synonymous with a male approach to the physical, natural world. Psychoanalytic feminists would view the current vogue of using medication and focus on neuroscience as a reflection of objective, distant, and autonomous models created to explain mental health and function.

5.7.1 Biology

The current medical/research model has led to the need for a group of professionals, the genetic counselors, who explain the results and implications of tests and technologies to 'consumers', who then must decide whether to have a mastectomy because they carry the mutant copies of the *BRCA1* and *BRCA2* genes, abort a child when amniocentesis suggests that it would have spina bifida, or elect not to have 'genetic' children at all because of the results of tests indicating a certain statistical probability that genes they carry may lead to the production of a 'defective' offspring. In a similar fashion, using psychoanalysis, talk therapy, and other therapeutic approaches in conjunction with SSRIs would be favored by psychoanalytic feminists as a way of shortening the distance between the psychiatrist and the patient. Although most research supports such combinations of therapeutic approaches, what is the practice, particularly in understaffed rural areas and inner cities?

5.7.2 Technology

Critiques of information technologies from a psychoanalytic feminist perspective raise the very interesting question of how systems design might change, if more feminine values and connection became priorities. Sorenson (1992) explored whether male and female computer scientists worked differently. He found that men tended to focus on mathematical models and computer programming whereas women spent more time running experiments, reading scientific literature, and plotting data. After studying the technological and political values of men and women engineering students, graduate students, and junior R&D scientists at the Norwegian Institute of Technology, Sorenson found that women brought 'caring values' to research in computer science. 'Caring values' included empathy and rationale of responsibility. 'In computer science, this means that women have a caring, other-oriented relationship to nature and to people, an integrated, more holistic and less hierarchical worldview, a less competitive way of relating to colleagues and a greater affinity to users' (Sorenson 1992: 10).

Computers and use of on-line programs have become extremely popular, especially on college campuses and in some rural areas, as a mechanism for diagnosis and therapy. While increasing access and lowering costs, does using computers for diagnosis and therapy provide the caring values exhibited by many therapists and needed by many clients?

Understanding the importance of relationships and power, some women computer scientist designers (Microsysters 1988; Suchman 1994) have attempted to link users with systems design as an explicit attempt to empower women. Although some might view this as an example of Harding's 'strong objectivity', this shortening of distance between the user and the system design mimics Keller's (1983) description of McClintock's work in 'A Feeling for the Organism'. In the shortening of the distance between the observer and the object of study, Keller describes less autonomy, independence, and separation as classic hallmarks of psychoanalytic feminism when applied to the work of women scientists.

Researchers using fMRI might formulate research questions and agendas based less on what the technology can DO/SHOW. Issues of importance to both researchers and patients would set the agenda and drive the research questions.

5.8 Radical feminism

Radical feminism maintains that women's oppression is the first, most widespread, and deepest oppression (Jaggar and Rothenberg 1992). Scientific institutions, practice, and knowledge are particularly male-dominated and have been documented by many feminists (Bleier 1984; Fee 1983; Griffin 1978; Haraway 1978; 1989; Hubbard 1990; Keller 1985; Merchant 1979; Rosser 1990) to be especially effective patriarchal tools to control and harm women. Radical feminism rejects most scientific theories, data, and experiments precisely because they not only exclude women but also because they are not women-centered.

5.8.1 Biology

Because of the belief of radical feminists in connection and a concept of the world as an organic whole, they reject dualistic, hierarchical approaches, and dichotomies that fragment the organic whole of reality. Cyclicity as a concept of time and thinking as an upward spiral seem more appropriate ways to study a world in which everything is connected in a process of constant change (Daly 1978, 1984). Under radical feminism, the female body, with its cyclicity of menstruation, serves as the ideal model for other, non-reproductive hormones and continual biological change (Hoffman 1982); the static male body is a deviation from the female norm.

Several recent studies have revealed differences not only between men and women in response to SSRIs, but also among women depending upon the phase of the menstrual cycle and whether or not the woman is post-menopausal. For example a study (Kornstein *et al.* 2000) of responses to sertraline compared with imipramine in chronic depression revealed that pre-menopausal women responded significantly better to sertraline than to imipramine and that post-menopausal women had similar rates of response to the two medications. Radical feminism suggests that this cyclicity would have been anticipated and considered the norm had the research on antidepressants started initially with the female body.

5.8.2 Technology

Some might define the work of Bratteteig and her co-workers as radical feminism, because it originates from women's discourse on computer science problems and methods. Indeed, they insist on prioritizing applicability of systems and putting users and developers in the same plane as collaborators in systems development. This starting from the understanding of a woman worker and her abilities and then focusing on how her professional competence can be augmented by the use of a system, does begin with women's experience. This focus on women (Hacker 1989; Thoresen 1989) is consistent with feminist principles. Actually radical feminists would be likely to reject the use of fMRI, questioning what this technology really reveals, because we have ample evidence of poverty, sexism, and racism that lead to genuine differences and causes for depression in women's lives. However, if radical feminists did use fMRI they might start by developing research questions articulated by women themselves as significant for their lives, to be explored by fMRI.

In addition to the focus on women and seeking to empower women, MacKinnon (1987) adds a further criterion to radical feminism. She suggests that the consciousness-raising group provides a methodology for radical feminism. Because patriarchy pervades and dominates all institutions, ideologies, and technologies, women have difficulty placing their experiences, lives, and needs in central focus in everyday life and environments. A successful strategy that women use to obtain reliable knowledge and correct patriarchal ideology is the consciousness-raising group (Jaggar 1983). Using their personal experiences as a basis, women meet together in communal, non-hierarchical groups to examine their experiences to determine what counts as knowledge (MacKinnon 1987). Suchman in her work at Xerox PARC, uses this approach in her view that knowledge held by users is central to the design process. They are 'Taking computerization as an occasion to articulate unacknowledged forms of expertise and to take that knowledge seriously as a basis for design' (Suchman and Jordan 1989: 158). In recognizing the gap between technologies created by experts and their use in real working environments, they have produced a 'radical reconceptualisation of the computer systems development process which recognises the innovatory character of the implementation process and places the local expertise of users at the centre.' (Webster 1995: 165). Could computers be used to link women in their homes or other dispersed environments, particularly in rural areas, for group therapy?

The interplay between designing and use, or designer and user, described in the Suchman example, also might be seen to demonstrate the cyclicity, often associated with radical feminism: Because of the belief of radical feminists in connection and a concept of the world as an organic whole, they reject dualistic, hierarchical approaches, and dichotomies which fragment the organic whole of reality.

Radical feminists examining information technologies might interpret the binary 0,1 foundation of computers and computing, as based upon the primary dichotomy/dualism of male-female. The 'switchers', 'controls', and 'operations' language of computing fit the patriarchal mode of control. The dichotomy receives reinforcement by the domination of men and relative absence of women from the design process. 'So, the domination of men and the absence of women from the design process is *one* factor which creates technologies which are closely geared to the needs of men and which are inappropriate to women's requirements' (Webster 1995: 179). In a similar fashion, radical feminists would question the whole basis of what it means to say a part of the brain does or does not 'light up' in response to stimulation as depicted in fMRI. Is this not a binary, simplistic approach based on the initial male versus female dichotomy, likely to overlook more complex interactions?

5.9 **Postmodern feminism**

Liberal feminism suggests that women have a unified voice and can be universally addressed (Gunew 1990). In postmodernism, the self is no longer regarded as 'masterful, universal, integrated, autonomous, and self-constructed; rather it is socially constructed by ideology, discourse, the structure of the unconscious, and/or language' (Rothfield 1990: 132). Postmodernism dissolves the universal subject and postmodern feminism dissolves the possibility that women speak in a unified voice or that they can be universally addressed. Postmodern perspectives stress that due to her situatedness—the result of her specific national, class, and cultural identities—the category of woman can no longer be regarded as smooth, uniform, and homogeneous. Postmodern feminist theories imply that no universal research agenda or application of technologies will be appropriate and that various women will have different reactions to science and technologies depending upon their own class, race, sexuality, country, and other factors.

5.9.1 Biology

A limitation of the biomedical model with its cellular, hormonal, and genetic approaches becomes its tendency to center on the individual and her body, while bringing less attention to surrounding social, economic, and political factors that may contribute to disease and its progress. Breast cancer serves as a good example of how numerous factors including age, class, race, sexuality, and country impact its incidence. The incidence of breast cancer has increased one percent per year since 1940 (Harris *et al.* 1992). This fact, coupled with studies from the 1970s which documented a fivefold variation in breast cancer rates around the world (Armstrong and Doll 1975), and that the incidence of breast cancer in Japanese women who migrate from their low incidence home country to the USA becomes that of US women, suggests that factors apart from genetics, such as country, race, class, and sexuality, emphasized in postmodern theory, are significant for the disease.

In a similar fashion, postmodern feminism would see SSRIs as one of many possible effective treatments for depression, which may work for some women but not others. The effectiveness of SSRIs in treating any particular individual would depend upon her race, class, sexuality, nationality, and other issues, as well as her biochemistry.

5.9.2 Technology

As postmodern feminist theory recognizes limitations with perceiving women as a universal group, so have deeper, more complex studies of technology industries revealed limitations of simplistic assumptions in technology designs. For example, Webster suggests that critiquing the absence of understanding of women's needs is easier than identifying what women's needs and priorities really are.

> First of all, they are of course not uniform across all women or across all social classes, nationalities and cultures. Then, making the link between women's needs and the consequently desirable features of an IT system is a vexed question, and one that is too often dealt with in an essentialist manner by reference to the supposedly universal

> characteristics of women IT users (for example, as lacking in confidence with computers, as disinterested in computers except as tools, as caring and sociable rather than rational and technical). Feminist design initiatives have often encountered this difficulty. Most have addressed it by focusing away from the eventual characteristics of the IT *products* which they shape, and towards the *processes* of shaping which offer scope for permanently redefining the role of female users in systems design.
>
> (Webster 1995: 178)

Postmodern feminists would probably view fMRI as useful for providing some information, although not all would accept its dominance of neuroscience research today. fMRI constitutes one of many approaches with potential to provide insights into the brain and behavior.

5.10 **Post-colonial feminism**

Beginning in 1947, after various campaigns of anti-colonial resistance, often with an explicitly nationalist basis, many colonial empires formally dissolved and previously colonized countries gained independence (William and Crissman 1994). Although the end of colonial rule created high hope for a proper post-colonial era, the extent to which the West had not relinquished control became clear quickly. The continuing Western influence, particularly in the economic arena, but also in the political, ideological, and military sectors, became known as neo-colonialism by Marxists (William and Chrisman 1994). Feminists have suggested that patriarchy dominates post-colonial and neo-colonial, much as it dominated colonial, everyday life.

Not surprisingly, science and technology reflect the varying complex aspects of the inter-relationships among developed and developing countries in general and between the particular cultures of the colonized and colonizing country. General themes include the underdevelopment of the southern continents by Europe and other northern continents (Harding 1993); ignoring, obscuring, or misappropriating earlier scientific achievements and history of countries in southern continents; the fascination with so-called 'indigenous science' (Harding 1998); the idea that the culture, science, and technology of the colonizer or former colonizing country remains superior to that of the colony or post-colonial country; and the insistence that developing countries must restructure their local economies to become scientifically and technologically literate to join and compete in a global economy (Mohanty 1997). In northern, former colonizing countries, the concurrent restructuring effects of multi-national corporations and other forces of globalization are evidenced in downsizing, privatization, and widening economic gaps between the poor and very wealthy. The particular forms and ways that these general themes take shape and play out varies, depending upon the history, culture, geography, and length of colonization for both the colonized and colonizing countries.

5.10.1 Biology

The issues surrounding postcolonial science vary considerably between India and Kenya, for example. Although both India and Kenya were colonized by the British, the differences in indigenous cultures, geographies, and length of time since independence have led to remarkably different problems and uses of modern science and technology. In India, amniocentesis has been used for sex determination to abort undesired female fetuses. The particularities of Indian culture, economics, and religion, in which sons are highly valued, the elderly are cared for by sons, and dowry prices to find a good marriage partner for daughters can be very expensive, encourage this use of amniocentesis. In Kenya, in contrast, the indigenous culture, including polygamy, valuing of children in general, and agricultural production, discourages such sex selection and abortion.

Post-colonial feminism raises issues of culture and differences, particularly between developed and developing countries, with relevance for transnational psychiatry. Do diagnoses of depression for women in First World countries who respond well to SSRIs translate appropriately as diagnoses and elicit effective responses for women in developing countries with very different cultures and experiences? How different are the responses of women in the same, less developed country to antidepressants, depending upon whether they come from rural or urban parts of the country, their educational and marital status, and whether they have experienced war or other trauma?

5.10.2 Technology

Globalization, technology, and multinational corporations characterize and unite the northern, developed and the southern, developing countries at the beginning of the twenty-first century. Countries of the north serve as the headquarters for most of the technology and multinational corporations, whereas countries of the south provide raw materials, cheap labor, and markets for the products. Biotechnologies follow this pattern, with the developed countries purchasing the seeds from the varieties of plants women have cultivated over generations and genetically engineering them. After gene splicing or other technology has been used to produce monocultures of the crop, which has been made resistant to particular environmental parameters and adapted to agricultural methods in developed countries, the seeds are sold back to the people in the developing world at increased prices. The source of food and the labor of the people, especially of the women, in the developing countries have been devalued. They must pay more for the seeds and accompanying fertilizers and pesticides, and work the land without mechanized help.

The information technology industry uses subcontracted female labor in developing countries, particularly for software development. Western managements control the conduct of software development projects, relying on women from India, China, Mexico, Hungary, and Israel as programmers. Telecommunications technologies ease the transmission of specifications and completed work between the workers in developing countries and client companies in the West. Women from these developing countries are preferred as workers over those in developed countries because of their technical and English proficiency, relatively high roles of productivity, and relatively low costs of labor.

These examples clearly demonstrate aspects of post-colonialism in that control of the economy of developing countries remains in the hands of developed countries. They demonstrate patriarchal control because women, not men, in the developing countries become the sources of cheap labor. Language becomes an interesting feature which continues to tie former colony with colonizer. Theoretically, satellites and telecommunications transcend geographical barriers and allow any developed country to use labor in any developing country. Practically, the former ties developed between colony and colonizer, as well as the language of the colonizer learned by the colonized during the period of colonization, means that former relationships continue in the neo-colonial modern world. Does the conversion of some Indian universities to software factories exemplify this language connection in the information technology world where English dominates?

Postcolonial feminist perspectives raise questions about what differences in fMRI in individuals from very different countries and cultures really mean. Do they represent differential responses to subtleties of language, of culture, sex differences, or other differences in brain processing?

5.11 **Cyberfeminism**

Cyberfeminism stands not only as the most recent feminist theory but also as the theory that overtly fuses modern science and technology with gender. As the name suggests, cyberfeminism explores the ways that information technologies and the Internet provide avenues to liberate (or oppress) women. In the early 1990s the term 'cyberfeminism' first began to be used in various parts of the world (Hawthorne and Klein 1999), with VNS Matrix, an Australian-based group of media-based artists being one of the first groups originating the term.

The individuals who defined cyberfeminism (Millar 1998) saw the potential of the Internet and computer science as technologies to level the playing field and open new avenues for job opportunities and creativity for women. Absence of sexism, racism, and other oppression would serve as major contrasts between the virtual world and the real world:

> Cyberfeminism as a philosophy has the potential to create a poetic, passionate, political identity and unity without relying on a logic and language of exclusion. It offers a route for reconstructing feminist politics through theory and practice with a focus on the implications of new technology rather than on factors which are divisive.
>
> (Paterson 1994)

As Millar and other cyberfeminist critics point out, the existing elites have struggled to seize control and stabilize the commercial potential of digital technologies, as well as their research and development. Discontinuity, speed, symbolic and linguistic spectacle, and constant change characterize information technology and digital discourse. Although these characteristics of instability and indeterminacy, because of the changing technology, open the possibility for other changes in the social realm and power relations, it is very unclear that information technologies and cyberculture will result in such social changes.

Some critics suggest that the current information technology revolution has resulted in a rigidifying and reifying of current power relations along previously existing gender, race, and class lines. The Internet becomes a tool, making women more vulnerable to men using it for ordering brides from developing countries, prostitution, cybersex, assumption of false identities, and pornography (Hawthorne and Klein 1999).

5.11.1 Biology

Despite their postmodern veneer of fragmentation, shifting identities, and speed, information technologies rest upon the power of science and technology to emancipate humans and a faith in abstract reason. Millar (1998) defines this situation as 'hypermodern'. 'Hypermodern' describes the packaging of modernity power relations that are universally patriarchal, racist, and bourgeois in a postmodern discourse of discontinuity, spectacle, and speed. Do the computer programs used in diagnosis and therapy reflect these same power relations? More broadly, does the use of SSRIs to treat or modulate depression, diagnosed approximately twice as frequently in women as in men, represent patriarchal control and power exercised through the use of pharmaceutical means?

Biomedicine fuses technology with the biological human body in the forms of artificial hips, heart valves, pacemakers, and implants to deliver drugs, creating the cyborgs discussed by Donna Haraway (1997). Simultaneously, new media technologies explore the reciprocity between science and media, where in this age of genetics as the life code, culture may become biology. Analyses of metaphors in genome research suggest that because researchers transpose literature on to biology, it is not possible to critique science without critiquing culture.

5.11.2 Technology

Haraway moves beyond the use of computers to sequence the human genome to explore how the image of the cyborg embodies the extent to which technoscience interventions have become part of us as humans. She uses the image of the 'virtual speculum' in *Modest-witness@second-millennium.femaleman-meets-oncomouse: Feminism and technoscience* to 'open up observation into the orifices of the technoscientific body politic to address these kinds of questions about knowledge projects'. As the pioneer of feminist science studies, Haraway focuses on interdependencies and interrelationships among bodies, technologies, and cultures.

One of the many theories used to explain the increased incidence of autism centers on exacerbation or development of autistic tendencies resulting from excessive interaction patterns from computers, games, and other technologies and less emphasis upon personal, human interactions. Do technologies increase the incidence of certain types of mental illness?

Technologies, particularly visual or imaging technologies of science or medicine, allow mapping of the human body. These maps and images in the forms of X-rays, MRI, computer-aided tomography (CAT) scans, and ultrasound are now common parts of popular culture that appear not only in medical settings but also in the movies and on the nightly news. The media coverage of people's reaction to each not only entrenches it in popular culture, but also affects the evolution and use of the visual technology itself. What is the interaction between fMRI and mental health? If no difference is evident from comparing the fMRI of a mentally, behaviorally 'normal' individual with someone who has been diagnosed with a mental illness, what does it mean? Do negative or positive correlations between fMRI and particular behaviors or sex differences change DSM diagnoses?

5.12 Conclusion

This also raises the question of whether cyberfeminism is really a feminist theory. Could cyberfeminism merely represent an attempt to see information technology as the latest venue for women's liberation, much as Shulamith Firestone (1971) envisioned such liberation resulting from reproductive technologies?

Although reproductive technologies have resulted in significant feminist critiques, theorizing, and discussion, no one considers them a feminist theory or method.

Each one of the feminist perspectives discussed here might also be applied to aspects of cyberfeminism. Liberal feminism would raise issues of women's equal access to digital hardware and the digital world. Socialist feminism would raise the issues of class in terms of who profits from and who loses from cybertechnology. African-American feminism would focus on issues of race and the 'digital divide'. Existentialist feminism and psychoanalytic feminism raise gender difference based on women's role as caregiver and socialization to remain connected with friends, workers, and families. Radical feminists would point out the potential use of information technology to create alternative versions of reality and even to avoid interactions with men in the real world, whereas in contrast, queer and transgender theories would sever prescriptive links between sex, gender, and sexual orientation. Postmodern feminists would underline the fast, fragmented, and situation-dependence of information technologies and digital discourse, and the impossibility of universalizing its use, design, or impact for all women. Postcolonial feminists might highlight the widening gap between the software designers from one of the universities in developing countries now being converted to specialize in educating information technology workers, and those who do not even have electricity, let alone computers, in their homes, as the globalization of the information technology industry continues. Focusing the lens of varying feminist theories on cyberfeminism reflects multiple interactions among information technologies, women, and feminism. In a similar fashion, focusing these feminist theoretical lenses on technology and psychiatry may reveal some of the ways that these theories might be used to ask new questions, take new approaches, and/or draw different theories and conclusions from data gathered on SSRIs and fMRI.

References

Armstrong B. and Doll R. (1975). Environmental factors and cancer incidence and mortality in different countries, with special reference to dietary practice. *International Journal of Cancer*, **15**, 617–631.

Aspin L. (1993). *Policy on the Assignment of Women in the Armed Forces*, 28 April (Washington, DC: Department of Defense).

Birke L. (1986). *Women, Feminism, and Biology: The feminist challenge* (New York: Methuen).

Bleier R. (1984). *Science and Gender. A critique of biology and its theories on women* (New York: Pergamon Press).

Bleier R. (1986). 'Sex differences research: science or belief?' in R. Bleier (ed.) *Feminist Approaches to Science* (New York: Pergamon Press), 147–164.

Caro R. (1974). *The Power Broker: Robert Moses and the fall of New York* (New York: Random House).

Chodorow N. (1978). *The Reproduction of Mothering: Psychoanalysis and the sociology of gender* (Berkeley and Los Angeles: University of California Press).

Daly M. (1978). *Gyn/Ecology: The metaethics of radical feminism* (Boston: Beacon Press).

Daly M. (1984). *Pure Lust. Elemental feminist philosophy* (Boston: Beacon Press).

Dawkins R. (1976). *The Selfish Gene* (New York: Oxford University Press).

de Beauvoir S. (1947). *The Second Sex* (H. M. Parshley, tr. and ed.) (New York: Vintage Books).

Dinnerstein D. (1977). *The Mermaid and the Minotaur. Sexual arrangements and human malaise* (New York: Harper Colophon Books).

Easlea B. (1983). *Fathering the Unthinkable: Masculinity, scientists and the nuclear arms race* (London: Pluto Press).

Eisenstein H. (1984). *Contemporary Feminist Thought* (London: Allen and Unwin).

Enloe C. (1983). *Does Khaki Become You?: The militarisation of women's lives* (London: Pluto Press).

Enloe C. (1989). *Bananas, Beaches and Bases* (Berkeley, CA: University of California Press).

Fausto-Sterling A. (1992). *Myths of Gender* (New York: Basic Books).

Fee E. (1982). A feminist critique of scientific objectivity. *Science for the People*, **14**, 8.

Fee E. (1983). Women's nature and scientific objectivity' in M. Lowe and R. Hubbard (eds.) *Women's Nature: Rationalizations of inequality* (New York: Pergamon Press), 9–27.

Finder A., Healy P., and Zernike K. (2006). President of Harvard resigns, ending story 5-year tenure. www.nytimes.com/2006/02/22/education/22harvard.html. Retrieved 3 April 2006.

Firestone S. (1971). *The Dialectic of Sex* (New York: Bantam Books).

Griffin S. (1978). *The Death of Nature* (New York: Harper & Row).

Gunew S. (1990). *Feminist Knowledge: Critique and construct* (New York: Routledge).

Gurwitz J.H., Nananda F.C., and Avorn J. (1992). The exclusion of the elderly and women from clinical trials in acute myocardial infarction. *Journal of the American Medical Association*, **268**, 1417–1422.

Hacker S. (1989). *Pleasure, Power and Technology* (Boston, MA: Unwin Hyman).

Haraway D. (1978). Animal sociology and a natural economy of the body politic. *Signs*, **4**, 21–60.

Haraway D. (1989). *Primate Visions: Gender, race, and nature in the world of modern science* (New York: Routledge).

Haraway D. (1997). Modest witness @ second_millenium. female man ⊕ meets–oncomouse™ *Feminism and Technoscience* (New York: Routledge).

Harding S. (1986). *The Science Question in Feminism* (Ithaca, NY: Cornell University Press).

Harding S. (1993). 'Introduction' in S. Harding (ed.) *The Racial Economy of Science* (Bloomington: Indiana University Press), 1–22.

Harding S. (1998). *Is Science Multicultural? Postcolonialisms, feminisms, and epistemologies* (Bloomington: Indiana University Press).

Harris J. R., Lippman M. E., Veronesi U., and Willett W. (1992). Breast cancer. *New England Journal of Medicine*, **327**, 319–328.

Hartmann H. (1981). 'The unhappy marriage of Marxism and feminism: towards a more progressive union' in L. Sargent (ed.) *Women and Revolution: A discussion of the unhappy marriage of Marxism and feminism* (Boston: South End Press), 1–41.

Hawthorne S. and Klein R. (1999). *Cyberfeminism* (Melbourne, Australia: Spinifex).

Hoffman J. C. (1982). Biorhythms in human reproduction: the not-so-steady states. *Signs*, **7**, 829–844.

Hubbard R. (1990). *The Politics of Women's Biology* (New Brunswick, NJ: Rutgers University Press).

Jaggar A. (1983). *Feminist Politics and Human Nature* (Totowa, NJ: Rowman & Allanheld).

Jaggar A. and Rothenberg P. (eds.) (1992). *Feminist Frameworks* (New York: McGraw-Hill).

Keller E. F. (1982). Feminism and science. *Signs*, **7**, 589–602.

Keller E. F. (1983). *A Feeling for the Organism* (San Francisco: Freeman).

Keller E. F. (1985). *Reflections on Gender and Science* (New Haven: Yale University Press).

Keller E. F. (1992). *Secrets of Life, Secrets of Death* (New York: Routledge).

Kelsey S. F., *et al.*, and Investigators from the National Heart, Lung, and Blood Institute (1993). Percutaneous Transluminal Coronary Angioplasty Registry. Results of percutaneous transluminal coronary angioplasty in women: 1985–1986. *Circulation*, **87**, 720–727.

King Y. (1989). 'The ecology of feminism and the feminism of ecology' in J. Plant (ed.) *Healing the Wounds: The promise of ecofeminism* (Philadelphia: New Society), 18–28.

King M.-C., Rowell S., and Love S. M. (1993). Inherited breast and ovarian cancer: what are the risks? What are the choices? *Journal of the American Medical Association* **269**, 1975–1980.

King J. and Stabinsky D. (1999). Patents on cells, genes, and organisms undermine the exchange of scientific ideas. *Chronicle of Higher Education*, 5 February, B6–B7.

Kornstein, S. G., Schatzberg, A. F., Thase, M. E., *et al.* (2000). Gender differences in treatment response to sertraline versus imipramine in chronic depression. *American Journal of Psychiatry*, **157**, 1445–1452.

Kornstein, S. G., Schatzberg, A. F., Thase, M. E., *et al.* (2001). Dr Kornstein and colleagues reply. *American Journal of Psychiatry*, **158**, 1532–1533.

Longino H. (1990). *Science as Social Knowledge: Values and objectivity in scientific inquiry* (Princeton, NJ: Princeton University Press).

MacKenzie D. and Wajcman J. (1985). *The Social Shaping of Technology* (Milton Keynes, UK: Open University Press).

MacKenzie D. and Wajcman J. (1999). *The Social Shaping of Technology*, 2nd edn. (Milton Keynes, UK: Open University Press).

MacKinnon C. (1987). *Feminism Unmodified: Discourses on life and law* (Cambridge, MA: Harvard University Press).

Merchant C. (1979). *The Death of Nature* (New York: Harper & Row).

Microsysters (1988). *Not over our Heads: Women and computers in the office* (London: Microsyster).

Millar M. (1998). *Cracking the Gender Code: Who rules the wired world?* (Toronto: Second Story Press).

Mohanty C. T. (1997). 'Women workers and capitalist scripts: ideologies of domination, common interests, and the politics of solidarity' in M. Alexander and C. Mohanty (eds.) *Feminist Genealogies, Colonial Legacies, Democratic Futures* (New York: Routledge).

Multiple Risk Factor Intervention Trial Research Group (1990). Mortality rates after 10.5 years for participants in the multiple risk factor intervention trial: findings related to a prior hypothesis of the trial. *Journal of the American Medical Association*, **263**, 1795.

Paterson N. (1994). *Cyberfeminism.* http://echonyc.com.70/0/cul/cyber/paterson.

Quitkin, F. M., Stewart, J. W., and McGrath, P. J. (2001) Gender differences in treatment response (letter). *American Journal of Psychiatry*, **158**, 1531–1532.

Ridker P. M., Cook N., Lee I.-M., *et al.* (2005). A randomized trial of low-dose aspirin in the primary prevention of cardiovascular disease in women. *New England Journal of Medicine*, **352**, 1293–1304.

Rose H. (1994). *Love, Power, and Knowledge: Towards a feminist transformation of the sciences.* Bloomington, Indiana University Press.

Rosser, S. V. (1986). *Teaching Science and Health from a Feminist Perspective: A practical guide.* Elmsford, NY: Pergamon Press.

Rosser S. V. (1988). 'Women in science and health care: a gender at risk' in S. V. Rosser (ed.) *Feminism within the Science and Health Care Professions: Overcoming resistance* (New York: Pergamon Press), 3–15.

Rosser S. V. (1990). *Female-Friendly Science* (New York: Pergamon Press).

Rosser S. V. (1994). *Women's Health: Missing from U.S. medicine* (Bloomington: Indiana University Press).

Rosser, S. V. (1997) *Re-engineering Female Friendly Science.* New York: Teachers College Press.

Rothfield P. (1990). 'Feminism, subjectivity, and sexual difference' in S. Gunew (ed.) *Feminist Knowledge: Critique and construct* (New York: Routledge), 121–144.

Silver, D. (2000). 'Margins in the wires: looking for race, gender, and sexuality in the Blacksburg Electronic Village' in M. McCaughey and M. Ayers (eds.) *Cyberactivism* (New York: Routledge), 133–150.

Sorenson K. (1992). Towards a feminized technology? Gendered values in the construction of technology. *Social Studies of Science*, **22**, 5–31.

Spanier, B. (1995). *Im/Partial Science: Gender ideology in molecular biology.* Bloomington, IN: Indiana University Press.

Steering Committee of the Physicians' Health Study Group (1989). Final report on the aspirin component of the ongoing physician's health study. *New England Journal of Medicine*, **321**, 129–135.

Suchman L. (1994). 'Supporting articulation work: aspects of a feminist practice of technology production' in A. Adam, J. Emms, E. Green and J. Owen (eds.) *Women, Work and Computerization: Breaking old boundaries—building new forms* (Amsterdam: North-Holland).

Suchman L. and Jordan B. (1989). 'Computerization and women's knowledge' in K. Tijdens, M. Jennings, I. Wagner and M. Weggelaar (eds.) *Women, Work and Computerization: Forming new alliances* (Amsterdam: North Holland).

Thoresen K. (1989). 'Systems development: alternative design strategies' in K. Tijdens, M. Jennings, I. Wagner and M. Weggelaar (eds.) *Women, Work and Computerization: Forming new alliances.* Amsterdam: North Holland.

Tong R. (1989). *Feminist Thought: A comprehensive introduction* (Boulder, CO: Westview Press).

Trivers R. L. (1972). 'Parental investment and sexual selection' in B. Campbell (ed.) *Sexual Selection and the Descent of Man* (Chicago, IL: Aldine).

U.S. Department of Health and Human Services (2000). National Institutions of Health. Implementation of the NIH Guidelines on the Inclusion of Women and Minorities as Subjects in Clincal Research. Comprehensive Report. (Fiscal Year 1997 Tracking Data) 2nd Revision. May 2000.

Vergano D. (2006). Study: medical manual's authors often tied to drug makers. *USA Today*, 20 April, 6A.

Wajcman J. (1991). *Feminism Confronts Technology* (University Park, PA: Pennsylvania State University Press).

Weber R. (1997). Manufacturing gender in commercial and military cockpit design. *Science, Technology and Human Values*, **22**, 235–253.

Webster J. (1995). *Shaping Women's Work: Gender, employment and information technology* (New York, Longman).

Williams P. and Crissman L. (1994). 'Colonial discourse and post-colonial theory: an introduction' in P. Williams and L. Crissman (eds.) *Colonial Discourse and Post-colonial Theory* (New York: Columbia University Press), 1–20.

Wilson E. O. (1975) *Sociobiology: The new synthesis* (Cambridge, MA: Harvard University Press).

Winner L. (1980). Do artifacts have politics? *Daedalus*, **109**, 121–136.

Young, A. H. (2001) Gender differences in treatment response to antidepressants. *British Journal of Psychiatry*, **179**, 561.

Young, A. H., Dow, R. C., Goodwin, G. M., *et al.* (1993). The effects of adrenalectomy and ovariectomy on the behavioural and hypothermic responses of rats to 8-hydroxy-2(di-n-propylamino)tetralin (8-OH-DPAT). *Neuropharmacology*, **32**, 653–657.

Chapter 6

The critical theory of psychopharmacology: the work of David Healy and beyond

Douglas Porter

6.1 Introduction

David Healy has written extensively on the subject of psychopharmacology. His work makes an important contribution to the critical theory of this technology. The strength of Healy's criticism is that he never loses sight of the social benefit of psychopharmacology. Too often, the critique of technology amounts to nothing more than a lamentation over the inevitably alienating aspects of technological progress. A meaningful critique of technology must go beyond these parameters and critically examine the resolution of social contingencies in the development of technology. The question shifts from whether technology is good or bad to whether our technology is being designed for the better or for the worse. David Healy is in a position to engage in such critique because first and foremost he is a historian of psychopharmacology. Healy's historical approach in narrating the advent of psychopharmacology undermines any illusion of material inevitability in the development of this technology. A careful history of psychopharmacology debunks the notion of inevitability by revealing contingencies in the development of this science-based technology that are resolved according to social values. Healy carefully documents how social values have impacted supposedly narrow technical issues like research design, interpretation of data, even the meaning of cause and effect as applied to this technology. The presence of social contingencies in technological development brings up normative questions regarding which social values should be incorporated into our technologies.

Healy's work is highly critical of the influence that the pharmaceutical industry is having on the development of psychopharmacology. At times Healy seems to suggest that the marketing imperatives of industry are corrupting science that would otherwise develop in a value-neutral manner.

Ultimately, I believe the notion of 'value-neutral' science undermines the type of technological reform that Healy advocates. Modern technology has become virtually synonymous with applied science, and epistemological suppositions about science have had an impact upon the way we understand technology. A scientistic epistemology that views good science as objective, value-neutral, and determined solely by the facts precludes a critical analysis of the social values that play a necessary role in the production of science. In fact, the notion that objective science is value-neutral invites moral skepticism by suggesting that values are merely subjective and arbitrary. Healy's work stands in stark opposition to a stance of moral skepticism. His work is important, not because of its neutrality, but because it is imbued throughout with a concern that psychopharmacology fulfill its therapeutic potential instead of deteriorating into a technological tool of social engineering.

A concern for the moral legitimacy of psychopharmacology works implicitly in Healy's critique. Healy's concept of a 'science of therapeutics' adds a specifically moral concern to the traditional scientific concern for objective truth. The notion of therapeutic science injects an additional requirement that our science be developed according to the interests of patients. Developing a formal theoretical conception of moral legitimacy will help clarify what is at stake and imperative in Healy's critique of psychopharmacology.

Encompassing a critical concern for the social values and the more narrowly conceived technical issues that intersect in the formation of technology requires moving toward a more 'social' epistemology, an epistemology that can appreciate the rational nature of argumentation about objective truth and moral legitimacy. It then becomes apparent why concerns for objectivity, efficiency and moral legitimacy are not only compatible but form necessary counterparts in good technological design. Healy's recommendations for technological reform work in this direction.

6.2 Social contingencies in technological development

In an attempt to unpack the social dimensions of psychopharmacology and challenge the notion that the development of this technology in its specific form was somehow inevitable it is helpful to focus on the 1962 amendments to Food and Drug Administration (FDA) regulations related to the licensing of medication. This is a pivotal historical moment referred to repeatedly in Healy's work (Healy 1997, 2002, 2004) that set off a cascade of institutional relations. Together this institutional nexus of relations goes a long way to explaining why psychopharmacology has taken the specific shape that it has. It also reveals the presence of alternative pathways of development, suggesting that the very nature of psychopharmacology would be changed if different social values were emphasized in its development. Healy characterizes the 1962 amendments to FDA regulations as a response to the tragic events associated with thalidomide. The teratogenic effects of thalidomide brought home the grave risk associated with the use of pharmaceuticals. The regulatory amendments attempted to offset the risk associated with the use of pharmacology in part by requiring that medication be of proven benefit in the treatment of a specific disease. If a medication cured a disease its potential benefit would be clear and significant. Where substantial benefit is foreseen, substantial risk is more justifiably taken (Healy 1997).

Fatefully, the FDA chose the randomized controlled trial (RCT) as the method for proving that a medication was an effective treatment for a specific disease. Healy openly questions this interpretation of the meaning of the RCT. The strength of the RCT is related to the null hypothesis and providing evidence that a medication is, in fact, doing nothing. As such, the RCT can reign in unjustified therapeutic enthusiasm. For example the RCT was instrumental in demonstrating that cortisone was ineffective in the treatment of schizophrenia. The RCT can make clear when a medication has no effect. However, it is quite a leap from showing that a medication has an effect to demonstrating that a medication cures a disease (Healy 2001*a*). For example, the Hamilton scale for depression appealed to the makers of imipramine and was implemented by them in clinical trials because the scale emphasized characteristic effects of treatment with imipramine, changes in sleep and appetite.[1] The Hamilton scale will help demonstrate how imipramine does 'something' and separates from placebo in a controlled trial. However, to infer from this difference from placebo that imipramine is a specific cure for the specific disease of depression does not follow. Imipramine will also affect the sleep and appetite of people who do not have depression. The specificity of imipramine treatment for the disease of depression simply does not exist in the manner implied (Healy 1997).

Simplified theories that characterized depression as a shortage of serotonin, or schizophrenia as an excess of dopamine, belied the clinical heterogeneity of patients carrying the same diagnosis. People carrying the same diagnosis would have markedly different responses to treatment with the same medication, some getting better, some actually growing worse. Just as there is good reason to question the homogeneity of patients, there is good reason to question the homogeneity of classes of medications such as the 'antidepressants.' As opposed to the magic bullet model of antibiotics, 'The antipsychotics and the antidepressants are neither specific in the sense of specific to one disease nor specific in the sense of working regardless of the nonspecific milieu in which they are delivered' (p. 257). Nonetheless, psychopharmacology evolved according to the regulatory demands of a specific treatment for a specific disease. The pragmatic significance of the RCT for the pharmaceutical industry was established and with it a new call for specificity, 'Randomized control trials of the kind that are used to register pharmaceuticals demand standardized rating scales, operational criteria, and the standardization of psychiatric diagnoses. After 1962 a standardization of diagnostic practice was all but inevitable' (p.100).

Healy wonders that things could be radically different with 'a stroke of the regulatory pen.' Rather than the specificity of categorical and medical models, dimensional models of psychopathology could emphasize the tonic quality of medications. Rather than correcting a lesion, psychopharmacology could be conceived of as modulating a constitution (Healy 1997, 2002). Healy notes that the therapeutic significance of medications that straddle the categories of antidepressant and antipsychotic are largely lost because of the need for specificity. And, chemicals such as substance p, ritanserin and ketanserin that may have therapeutic significance are never developed into psychopharmacology because they fail to show the necessary specificity (Healy 2002).

Certain drugs would suddenly fall under the rubric of psychopharmacology; perhaps others never would have come under the rubric of psychopharmacology. It seems clear that the nature of psychopharmacology would be different. Of course, just because things would be different does not mean that things would be better.

6.3 **Normative considerations**

Debunking the notion that the development of psychopharmacology as it stands was inevitable raises the normative question, 'Is this the best of all possible technological worlds?'. Healy clearly feels that it is not. He introduces convincing evidence that the pharmaceutical industry has benefited more than the community at large from the scientific and regulatory status of the RCT. The production of an RCT is extraordinarily expensive. With the loss of public funding for research, the pharmaceutical industry came to the fore as the only entity with sufficient resources for their undertaking. The status of the RCT as the only valid form of scientific evidence would indirectly evolve into extraordinary pharmaceutical industry control of evidence and the flow of information. The industrial influence on the production of science was reflected in the increasing amount of pharmacological studies designed to support industry interests in marketing. The atmosphere became one in which scientific ideas were acceptable only if they had commercial value.

Healy criticizes the growing divergence between data produced in accordance with industry interests and data that could meaningfully inform clinical practice as 'hardly being value-free' and goes on to state that, 'Good science will result only from studies that are designed to answer scientific questions rather than from ones designed to support regulatory applications and market penetration' (Healy 2001*a*). One could certainly infer from this comment that Healy believes that ideological considerations are interfering with what should be the unbiased, value-neutral production of science. The implication is that our technology would improve if only our science was value-neutral. This is where Healy leaves himself open to legitimate criticism. Healy focuses on the pernicious influence of the pharmaceutical industry on scientific research, but conflicts of interests also arise in publicly funded research (Spece *et al.* 1996). Criticism of Healy has noted that Healy himself has conflicts of interests created by his consultant work in litigation against pharmaceutical companies (Coyne 2005). The insinuation here is that Healy's work also fails to live up to the ideal of being value-free and therefore can be discounted. I believe the strength of Healy's work lies not in its neutrality, but in its tireless effort to reinvest the science-based technology of psychopharmacology with the interests and values of patients. Appreciation of this strength requires discarding the epistemic ideal of value-neutrality. Healy's jab that the fashionable call for 'evidence-based' medicine actually amounts to a call for 'evidence biased' medicine (Healy 2001*b*) remains paradoxical if objective science is regarded as value neutral. The idea of 'evidence biased' medicine points out that scientific evidence may be objectively true yet biased toward particular values and interests.

Progress in making the best of all possible technologies requires shifting from a vain search for the chimera of value-neutral science to the more fruitful struggle for morally legitimate science. The direction and manner in which the scientific lens should be focused is far from transparent. The ideal of value-neutral science is illusory. In fact, the illusion that social values have no impact upon the development of science and technology is often employed as an excuse to avoid democratic accountability and conceal the values that eventually become 'concretized' in our science-based technologies (Feenberg 1999). Healy concludes that the, 'evisceration of the science of psychiatric therapeutics by pharmaceutical corporations leads to therapeutic decline' (Healy 2002: 312). The notion of a 'therapeutic science' infuses science, and the technology on which it is based, with a specific and peculiar concern for moral legitimacy. To clarify the notion of morally legitimate science and demonstrate its presence in Healy's work we will have to overcome the thoroughly entrenched notion that good objective science is equivalent to value-neutral science and embark on a more careful consideration of epistemological issues.

6.4 An epistemological detour

A concern for objective truth is at the heart of the scientific enterprise. An unfortunate consequence of the rigid dichotomies associated with a scientistic epistemology is that objective truth is defined in opposition to subjective values. The result is the 'Either/Or' thinking characteristic of the 'science wars' where science is either reduced to a relativistic exercise of political power or characterized as a value-neutral exercise progressing in an inevitable fashion determined solely by the facts.[2] The illogical impact of this rigid dualism has become most readily evident in healthcare in our knowledge of pathology. The is and the ought, the descriptive and the prescriptive, the factual and the evaluative, the objective and the subjective all appear to become entwined in the categories of pathology. Pathological phenomena are of course objective phenomena, but then so are the physiological or 'normal' phenomena that fall outside the realm of the pathological. If objectivity is our sole criterion for validity the means to discriminate between normal and pathological phenomena disappears. If we remain purely descriptive there would be no line between the normal and the pathological. The pathological, as such, would not exist as a potential realm of knowledge (Canguilhem 1991).

Common sense dictates that what sets pathological phenomena apart from the normal is the negative value we attach to these phenomena. If we adhere to a dualistic epistemology in which values are subjective and in that sense arbitrary, then the ramifications for the science of pathology are dire. If pathology is a reflection of underlying value judgments then it resembles arbitrary opinion more than scientific fact. K.W.M. Fulford combats this view in *Moral Theory and Medical Practice* by tracing the necessary and productive role that negative social values must play before any factual demarcation of a diseased biological state can take place. He notes that what allows us to ignore or forget the implied value judgments in mental and physical illness and talk about disease as strictly a factual state of affairs is, '…the extent to which the criteria for the value judgment expressed by it are settled or agreed – the more settled the criteria, the less marked (by and large) are its evaluative connotations' (Fulford 1989: 61). The evaluative dimension may be forgotten, but in the case of pathology social values provide a necessary element in the disclosure of objective knowledge.

Recent developments in social epistemology have emphasized the necessary and productive role that social values play in the production of knowledge. Phillip Kitcher (2001) offers the analogy of the cartographer. In creating a map of a mountain we may be concerned with or guided by the value of getting across the mountain as quickly as possible. Taking this value seriously will, of course, require that our map be objectively accurate. However, it is also possible to be guided by a concern for exploring indigenous flora on the mountain. Our map would look quite different, but would still be objectively accurate. These maps are not merely social constructs in the sense that they have nothing to do with the objective reality of the mountain. However, an important shift has developed. Objectively accurate knowledge is not a passive, value-neutral representation. In this context our values promote a pragmatic interest in accuracy and the disclosure of relevant facts. Values are not merely a source of bias but rather engage us in the world. Values help us to disclose and make manifest aspects of the world that would otherwise go unnoticed, and they do this with an eye toward potential paths of action and intervention (Longino 1990).

Social epistemologists note that background assumptions replete with value judgments play a necessary role in the production of scientific knowledge and by no means do they preclude a cooperative search for objective truth. The ramifications for the meaning of 'good science' are complex. The concern for objectivity remains. However, any naiveté about the neutrality of our knowledge must be relinquished. Recovering the social process of knowledge production reveals that 'objectivity' is no guarantee that our knowledge is value-free and unbiased. Reflective scientific practice now has the additional burden of critically examining the values in which it is grounded. To return to the map analogy, if someone dogmatically decreed that only maps disclosing routes of alacrity should be produced, the maps would be objectively accurate but they would be biased toward the interests of travelers in a hurry. We must move from the either/or thinking that science is *either* objective, value-neutral and apolitical *or* that science is subjective, evaluative, political and irrational to the idea that science can aspire to be both objectively accurate and grounded in morally legitimate values. The notion of science grounded in morally legitimate values is foreign to a scientistic epistemology that defined objective science in opposition to subjective values. The rigid dichotomies associated with a scientistic epistemology have the unfortunate consequence of inviting moral skepticism with the portrayal of 'values' adhering to a subject in an arbitrary, irrational manner. It is no wonder then that the discourses of the sciences have not typically contained the language of moral legitimacy. The language of rational argumentation offers more promise in this regard.

6.5 **Rational argumentation**

The discourses of science and technology are always mixed. The ramifications of science and technology extend beyond a concern for empirical accuracy. The maps we create are not only descriptive; they delineate a prescriptive path for future travel. It is well recognized that our science-based technologies ultimately impact the structure of our world and the social roles we come to play. Elements of description and prescription, the 'is' and the 'ought' become entwined in our science and technology. Treating technology as merely technical requires abstracting from the larger social context in which the production and appropriation of technology is always already embedded. The development of psychopharmacology involves a complex mixture of clinical and bench science that intersects with multiple social institutions. The interests of the pharmaceutical industry, medical and other scientific professions, government regulation, and insurance reimbursement all intersect with complex interpretations of patient needs to affect the shape that psychopharmacology eventually takes. Luckily, as the philosopher Calvin Schrag (1992) has noted, the complex mixed nature of our discourses never outstrips the 'resources of rationality.' Rationality here is not identified with adherence to a particular scientific method. Rationality is instead recognized in those forms of argumentation that are based upon criticizable validity claims. 'From physics to morality, from mathematics to art criticism, our cognitive accomplishments form a continuum within the common, though shifting, terrain of argumentation in which validity claims are thematized' (Habermas 1993: 30). The logic of argumentation may change when we shift from making empirical assertions to making assertions about the authenticity of our values or the moral legitimacy of our institutional norms. However, all these forms of argumentation remain rational to the extent that they rely strictly upon the persuasive force of good reasons.

Processes of rational argumentation play a crucial role in the development of the objectively accurate science that technical feasibility requires. Processes of rational argumentation also prove indispensable in the clarification of social needs and interests, and establishing the moral legitimacy of our institutional norms. In terms of empirical assertions, epistemologists have shifted from the view of the sole researcher achieving true belief by strict adherence to the proper method. The nature of the proper method is in fact open to rational debate depending upon the object of inquiry (Pera 1994; Peukert 1986). Instead of the object being accurately represented in the subject, social rules for argumentation are emphasized as pivotal in arriving at true beliefs about the world (Rehg 1998; Goldman 1999). Helen Longino notes that the objectivity of our scientific knowledge hinges upon social processes of argumentation and public scrutiny. There should be access and appropriate response to '...recognized avenues for the criticism of evidence, of methods, and of assumptions and reasoning;' (Longino 1990: 76). I believe Healy's view of science is compatible with these assertions, '...the empirical nature of the enterprise does not stem from the qualities of one individual but from the fact that the enterprise is a collaborative one. Left to their own devices without a peer group to winnow the wheat from the chaff even the most eminent of scientists lose touch with reality' (Healy 1990: 216).

Rational argumentation regarding authentic values should be familiar to healthcare practitioners from the elaboration of informed consent. According to the doctrine of informed consent healthcare should be deployed in a manner consistent with the values of the patient. In practice this does not amount to blind submission to a preset nexus of values that happen to be contained in the subjectivity of the patient. In making sure that medical practice is proceeding according to the needs and interests of the patient, the patient's values may be made explicit or elucidated for the first time in a novel situation. At times the patient's values are subject to revision on the basis of deliberation and rational argumentation. Although values were considered subjective, arbitrary and irrational in terms of a scientistic epistemology, rational argumentation about values plays a pivotal role in the practice of informed consent (Applebaum and Grisso 1998). The human capacity to reason about values does not equate to an expectation of sharing the same values. In the absence of coercion universal consensus over the 'right values' is not to be expected. As Ezekiel Emanuel puts it, 'To affirm reasoned discussion on fundamental ideals is not to suggest that there is only one true set of ideals or only one true interpretation, only that it is possible to discuss ethical values rationally' (Emanuel 1991: 163).

The Kantian tradition differentiates issues of morality from other values. Moral legitimacy entails proceeding in a manner that is equally good for all in view of our differences. Kant's categorical imperative, to treat humanity, universally, as ends and never simply as means, links morality to respect for free and equal moral persons in all their diversity. Transcribing this conception of morality to the institutional level entails social institutions inscribed with respect for the plurality of people they affect (Ricoeur 1992). Habermas's version of critical theory (Habermas 1990, 1998) does a great deal to clarify the pivotal role that rational argumentation plays in establishing the moral legitimacy of our institutional norms. The logical emphasis in argumentation here shifts from questions of authenticity to establishing universalizability. If the people impacted by a particular institution can agree in a process of rational argumentation that the norms guiding the institution reflect everyone's interests, the moral legitimacy of the institution can be inferred (Rehg 1994). Habermas's emphasis on inclusion in dialogue in order to obtain impartiality has been referred to as an intersubjective reformulation of the Kantian categorical imperative (Baynes 1992). Habermas's work establishes the regulative moral ideal of the un-coerced participation of affected parties in establishing institutional norms. The moral legitimacy of our institutions, even our scientific institutions, hinges upon their ability to accommodate the diverse needs and interests of the people they impact.

The fact that science and technology evolve in a contingent manner according to social values raises questions of moral legitimacy for our science and technology. Philip Kitcher in *Science, Truth and Democracy* specifically invokes a notion of a 'well-ordered science' in which scientific inquiry continues to attend to the traditional scientific concern for objective accuracy but also 'should satisfy the preferences of the citizens in the society in which it is practiced' (Kitcher 2001: 117). The moral legitimacy of science is attained when the pursuit of science reflects the interests of the citizenry whose lives are directly impacted by the course of scientific development. The interests of the citizenry are not transparent in this complex context. Forums for deliberation and citizen participation are needed if our sciences and technology are to be inscribed with the values of the citizenry. The extensive discourse on the democratization of science and technology hinges upon this conception (Feenberg 1999; Kitcher 2001; Kleinman 2000; Remedios 2003; Sadler 2002; Sclove 1995). For people that find their interests marginalized by scientific and technological norms in healthcare and elsewhere, whether for reasons of class, gender, orientation, or race; participation in research is seen as a pivotal tool in remedying injustice (Harding 1991; Haynes and Smedley 1999; Hogg 1999; de Koning and Martin 1996*b*; Minton 2002; Navarro 1976; Salmon 1990).

In view of our revised epistemological considerations the desire for a value-neutral science seems counterproductive. It can only serve to conceal and preclude reflection upon the social values that inevitably play a necessary role in the production of science and science-based technology. Reflection upon social values does not prohibit concern for the objective accuracy of our knowledge. In terms of a theory of argumentation a rigorous science now has the tools to expand its purview and strive for moral legitimacy in addition to the traditional concerns for objective accuracy. Morally legitimate science and science-based technology must be developed according to the interests of the citizenry affected. This exercise, far from value-neutral, obtains its impartiality by accommodating the values of those affected. As David Kaplan puts it, this calls for discourse that '...involves taking the perspective of others since valid norms must be acceptable to everyone, as a shared expectation that would resolve conflicts of interests. Argumentation is therefore inseparable from the interpretation of needs and interests' (Kaplan 2003: 72).

6.6 **Whose science? Whose technology?**

Now that we have developed a notion of epistemology that can accommodate rational truth claims about empirical and moral matters we are in a better position to appreciate Healy's critique of psychopharmacology. Pivotal to Healy's critique is his demand that psychopharmacology be developed according to a rigorous science of therapeutics. The notion of therapeutic science contains the traditional scientific concern for objectivity but points toward additional requirements related to issues of moral legitimacy. A therapeutic science by definition should be developed according to the needs and interests of the patients that it most intimately affects. Understanding these needs and interests requires the active participation of the patients themselves. The concern for empirical accuracy is not free standing in this context. It is grounded by the pragmatic demand to relieve the suffering occasioned by illness. Even at his most critical, Healy self-consciously avoids a romanticist dismissal of the potential benefits of psychopharmacology. The pragmatic therapeutic interest seems to allow Healy to encompass a concern for the potential misuse of power in the resolution of design contingencies without becoming skeptical about the merit of scientific and technical argument.

Healy laments that the historical developments that granted so much control of the production of science to industry undermined the production and recognition of good scientific arguments. Scientific ideas 'would rise and fall not so much because of the careers of forceful personalities and good arguments within the field of psychiatry, but because of the laws governing patent duration' (Healy 2002: 217). Advocates of participatory research have noted that pivotal value judgments intersect with the production of science in terms of which questions are asked, how they are asked, in determining what counts as evidence and how the data is eventually interpreted (de Koning and Martin 1996*a*). An effort to uncover conflict between marketing and therapeutic interests on all these levels is apparent in Healy's work. In terms of scientific evidence of therapeutic effect Healy questions how effects on a 'Brief Psychotic Rating Scale' or a 'Hamilton Depression Scale' can be seen as translating into evidence of clinical effectiveness in view of rising rates of depression and rising mortality rates for schizophrenia (Healy 2002). There has been a de-emphasis on patient based quality of life scales. Manufacturers of SSRIs have published less than ten per cent of quality of life data developed, suggesting a gross failure in this regard (Healy 2001*a*). Clinical trials could be designed to demonstrate the proportion of patients who are likely to find a particular therapy both beneficial and acceptable but no such trials have been undertaken (Healy 2002).

In terms of the interests determining which scientific questions are simply never asked there is the example of the question of Prozac induced suicidality. It is hard to argue that this is a question without therapeutic significance. Representatives of Lilly, the makers of Prozac, met with representatives from the FDA and there was general agreement that to investigate this question scientifically, a prospective rechallenge study, in which patients who developed suicidality would be randomized to Prozac or an alternative noradrenergic medication, was needed as was an appropriate scale sensitive to suicidality. Protocols for this study were developed and an appropriate scale for suicidality designed but neither were ever implemented (Healy 2004). Healy stresses the overall importance of the patent in the development of the science of psychopharmacology. For example, knowledge about withdrawal from benzodiazepines was popularized when Mead Johnson had an incentive to publicize evidence of these problems to give their anxiolytic product buspirone a competitive edge. Similarly, the makers of Prozac popularized knowledge of withdrawal phenomenon associated with SSRIs because their product was not susceptible to the phenomenon (Healy 2002). Although here there was a confluence of therapeutic interest and competitive market interest, Healy frets that when all the treatments on patent for a particular condition share a particular side effect, knowledge of that side effect will never see the light of day. Healy believes this may be true in the case of certain SSRI side effects. When a company does not have a financial interest in producing scientific knowledge, the knowledge will not be developed. Although scientific information on older, off patent, or non-prescription medications would clearly be therapeutically relevant Healy laments that finding this information at a scientific meeting is like finding 'snow in the Sahara' (Healy 2004).

Pharmaceutical companies clearly recognize the importance of being in control of the science. A medical information company that wrote fifty-five articles on behalf of sertraline [Zoloft] describes its mission to…'Deliver scientifically accurate information strategically developed for specific target audiences' (p. 116). The practice of 'ghostwriting' in which company personnel draft an article and later get a clinical author to 'sign off' on the final version is growing in importance. Control of the science extends beyond what is asked to how the data is prepared and tabulated. Often the clinical author that signs off on an article never sees the raw scientific data associated with the article. Healy cites the example of coding agitation associated with SSRI treatment as 'failure to respond' rather than as a side effect and emphasizes that, 'By the time the data have been tabulated by the company, the issue of what the data show may have been settled' (p. 115). 'Ghostwritten' articles designed by industry personnel may be of questionable scientific merit. However, the practice of attaching a prominent clinicians name as author, publication in prominent journals, and an efficient system of distribution means these articles are actually the most widely referenced (Healy 2003). Over-publication of positive results and suppression of negative results leads to a predictable pattern of overestimating the therapeutic qualities of these biotechnologies and underestimation of side effects.

Scientific studies can be done until desired results are achieved. In terms of FDA regulations, separation from placebo on the basis of a rating scale in two separate studies is considered evidence of psychopharmacological efficacy. However, there is no limit on the total number of studies undertaken to achieve two studies of statistical significance. Healy notes that Zoloft was approved as an antidepressant on the basis of two positive studies. Six studies were undertaken. Four failed to demonstrate difference from placebo. One of the 'positive' studies claimed superiority on the basis of relapse of depression when patients were taken off of Zoloft, but what was termed relapse of depression may have been more accurately characterized as withdrawal from the Zoloft (Healy 2004). The proprietary nature of the scientific data has meant that unfavorable results can be suppressed. Financial sponsorship of a published study is the greatest predictor of outcome (Healy 2002, 2003). This 'science' more closely resembles an exercise in wish fulfillment for the pharmaceutical industry than any serious grappling with objective reality.

6.7 **Market ideology**

Healy's work underscores a conflict between marketing interests and therapeutic interests in the development of psychopharmacology. This assertion contradicts some of the more democratic pretensions of what I will call market ideology. Market ideology asserts that the marketplace can work behind our backs to efficiently respond to the needs and interests of the citizenry through a supply and demand scenario. It is interesting to note that market ideology can grant that, far from being value-neutral, science and technology evolve in a contingent manner depending upon particular needs and interests. However, because science and technology are developed according to a profit motive, they should evolve in a manner that is specifically responsive to consumer needs and interests. The impact of this ideology can be measured to some extent by a change in healthcare nomenclature. Patients are now referred to as consumers with the belief that patients were merely passive recipients of healthcare while consumers are empowered to shape their healthcare systems.

There can be little doubt that market imperatives affect the shape that science and technology ultimately take. In his book *America by Design: Science, technology, and the rise of corporate capitalism* (Noble 1977), David Noble carefully chronicles how manipulations of patent law have historically affected which technologies are developed and which technologies are never developed.

Marcia Angell points out that pharmaceutical corporations are no strangers to such patent manipulation (Angell 2004). A question remains as to whether or not a profit imperative necessarily leads to morally legitimate science-based technology. Does technology based upon consumer demand reflect the interests of those being affected? Developing healthcare according to a consumer model marginalizes certain needs and interests. The needs of patients must be formulated in terms fit for consumption. The interest in profit means that healthcare needs must be devised in a manner that facilitates readily commodifiable solutions often to the exclusion of the underlying social and ecological origins of illness (Salmon 1990). However, even readily commodifiable technological products developed according to a profit motive will not evolve in a way that corresponds to the scope or severity of health care needs because, unlike people, not all consumers are created equally. A proliferation of copycat treatments for gastroesophageal reflux and erectile dysfunction while nonprofitable but devastating pandemic illness goes largely unaddressed can hardly be said to meet criteria for moral legitimacy (Angell 2004; Farmer 2005). In terms of the regulative moral ideals generated by Habermas's critical theory, all the parties affected by these decisions would not and could not agree that these norms meet the needs of all those being affected by our decisions.

Because of the inherent inequality of consumers, technology developed according to consumer needs and interests would not necessarily be morally legitimate. However, it is far from a given that technology does develop according to consumer interests. Stuart Ewen in his book *Captains of Consciousness: Advertising and the social roots of the consumer culture* (Ewen 1976) examines the long history of industrial attempts to manipulate the perception of need through advertising. Rather than following a passive 'supply fulfilling a demand' scenario as dictated by market ideology, industry works hard at creating demand for its product by creating the perception of a need. Healy finds this scenario applicable in the case of psychopharmacology. Regulations were meant to curb the misuse of pharmacology by restricting their use to cases of disease. The industrial response to this restriction has been to market the disease itself in order to increase the sales of their product. For example Healy notes (Healy 1997), in attempting to increase the sale of its antidepressant, amitriptyline, Merck publicized the idea of depression by buying and distributing 50,000 copies of *Recognizing the Depressed Patient*. Sometimes marketing and therapeutic interests do coincide. An 'education' campaign regarding obsessive–compulsive disorder consisting of sponsored patient support groups, conferences, journal supplements, and distribution of *The Boy Who Couldn't Stop Washing* ensued when five companies received licenses to treat the disorder. Healy notes that, 'a good argument can be made that these efforts have...redressed an imbalance' (Healy 1997: 207). However, a thousandfold increase in the incidence of depression in the wake of SSRI marketing from 0.5 per cent in the 1950s to 10 per cent in the 1990s (Healy 2002) leads Healy to conclude that these companies are fashioning a social lock to fit their psychopharmacological key (Healy 2004). Healy leaves us with a disturbing rhetorical image, 'biomedical developments take place in a world where the corporate capacity to colonize the consciousness of citizens, physicians, regulators, outstrip the capacity to bring real benefit'(p. 287). When the interests of industry take precedence over the interests of patients our science and technology fail to be therapeutic. Instead, they deteriorate into a form of social engineering.

6.8 **Citizen participation for better technology**

Healy's work never dismisses problems with psychopharmacology as a consequence of an inevitably alienating intrusion of 'technology'. Criticisms that label technology as inherently alienating may ironically be perpetuating the alienation they lament if they disguise the very possibility of more democratically organized technologies that can play a pivotal role in self-actualization (Sclove 1995). David Noble is worth quoting at length here:

> The development of technology, and thus the social development it implies, is as much determined by the breadth of vision that informs it, and the particular notions of social order to which it is bound, as by the mechanical relations between things and the physical laws of nature. Like all others, this historical enterprise always contains a range of possibilities as well as necessities, possibilities seized upon by particular people, for particular purposes, according to particular conceptions of social destiny.
>
> (Noble 1977, xxii)

Our technology can be developed for the better or for the worse. Andrew Feenberg (Feenberg 1999) suggests in his work that rather than a post hoc, take it or leave it, approach to technology it is far more productive to 'question technology' as to what and whose interests become encoded and objectified in its design. It should be clear by now that Healy thoroughly interrogates psychopharmacology and he concludes that the corporations producing these new biotechnologies answer ultimately to shareholders, not the community. 'Medical research would follow the money potentially benefiting the favored few rather than the community at large' (Healy 2004: 255).

Modern medicine has become something of a poster child for the potential therapeutic impact of applied science and technology. To fulfill this therapeutic potential our science and technology has to be critically examined not only for objective accuracy but also for moral legitimacy. Science does not obtain moral legitimacy by remaining value neutral. Morally legitimate science and technology reflects the interests of the citizens affected. We cannot rely on the free hand of the marketplace to confer this type of moral legitimacy to our technology. Empowering patients does not entail pigeonholing them as consumers so much as recognizing their right as citizens to shape healthcare according to their values (Hogg 1999). Recognition of the moral dimensions of science and technology has led to calls for its democratization. Citizen participation is an institutional means of inscribing our science and technology with the values of those being affected. Healy never gives up on the idea that psychopharmacology can be shaped to fulfill its claim as a therapeutic technology. Healy's sums up his view of science as follows, 'the vaunted objectivity of science lays not in any method so much as in scrutiny by a community—ordinarily a community of scientists, in the first instance, but in the final analysis by the community at large' (Healy 1997: 105). No one is affected by the science of therapeutics more intimately than patients. Yet, Healy notes, 'In this case the data that are typically neglected are the data of what depressed, manic, and schizophrenic subjects actually say' (Healy 1990: 131). As an alternative, Healy envisions neuropsychological research that, '...would enable psychiatric patients to...become empirical investigators and managers of their own disorders' (p. 117). In Healy's view an appropriate evolution of science, '...would be for some individuals affected with schizophrenia to be awarded scientific recognition for their work on schizophrenia from the inside' (p. 218).

An important historical example of an alternative approach to therapeutic science evolved in AIDS research. As Healy characterizes it, 'researchers, medical ethicists and AIDS activists sat around the table and hammered out agreements about what needed to be done and what could be done' (Healy 1997: 105). Epstein's work *Impure Science* invokes this situation as pivotal in demonstrating the potential benefit of citizen participation in what were heretofore considered the unimpeachable confines of scientific and technical expertise. Activists challenged and 'transformed the procedures by which drugs are tested, the ways in which test results are interpreted, and the processes by which those interpretations are then used in the licensing of drugs for sale' (Epstein 1996: 33). The result of communication between scientists and the people most intimately affected by therapeutic science was not a political sullying of 'pure' science. Rather, '...by working toward methodological solutions that satisfy, simultaneously, the procedural concerns of researchers and the ethical demands of the patient community, AIDS activists have, at least in specific instances, improved a tool for knowledge in ways even researchers acknowledge' (p. 341).

In the wake of the positive impact of citizen participation in AIDS research, the National Institutes of Health has acknowledged the benefit of public participation in health research and proposed the formal institutionalization of this participation. While endorsing such actions as giving patients equal ownership rights to the data produced in research and recommending that patient cooperatives take over the design and management of clinical trials (Healy 2004), Healy is not naïve about potential shortcomings to patient participation when this participation is co-opted from the start. Industry has taken an interest in patients not only with 'direct to consumer' advertising, but with sponsorship of patient groups that correspond to industry interests. Industry has targeted groups such as the National Alliance for the Mentally Ill specifically because of their power as lobbyists (Healy 2002). Healy notes we live in an era when industry spends £1000 per day to send delegates to find out how to form and influence patient groups (Healy 2004). Rebecca Dresser in her book *When Science Offers Salvation* grapples with the difficulties of institutionalizing public participation at the NIH in a meaningful and fair manner. She notes that guaranteeing a formal right to participation actually gives an undue advantage to the wealthy and powerful who have the resources to employ lobbyists at will. Aspects of deliberative democracy must be combined with features of procedural justice in order to legitimately address the complex intersection of ethical and technical issues that occur in health research (Dresser 2001).

6.9 **Concluding remarks**

David Healy's historical account of psychopharmacology is a critical one. Healy's concern for therapeutics prompts his careful and critical examination of historical contingencies in the development of this peculiar form of technology. To appreciate the depth of this critique and how it makes an important contribution to the overall critical theory of technology it becomes necessary to overcome an epistemology that would have us believe that good science is a value neutral affair. Social values form a necessary element in the production of science and science-based technology but do not preclude the cooperative search for empirical truth or technical feasibility. It is possible to argue rationally for morally legitimate values in which to ground our science based technology. It is clear that therapeutic advocacy must extend beyond narrow technical concerns and incorporate a concern for the moral legitimacy of our science and technology. This moral concern is evident in Healy's work.

Healy points out how and where psychopharmacology has diverged from patient interests in order to fulfill marketing imperatives. If psychopharmacology is to fulfill its potential as a therapeutic technology it must be developed according to the needs and interests of the patients it affects. The alternative is for psychopharmacology to deteriorate into the technological tool of a pernicious form of social engineering. In keeping with the tradition of critical theory, the point of our work is not only to understand our world, but also to change it. Healy's work is punctuated with recommendations for reform that would help the technology of psychopharmacology become inscribed with the values of the people it is meant to help. We have the opportunity, with the help of the affected community, to reinvest in our technology so that it can fulfill its therapeutic potential. Healy's work does a great deal to point the way toward a psychopharmacology of, by, and for the community.

Endnotes

1 A move to replace the Hamilton scale has developed because the Hamilton scale does not emphasize the actions of the newer antidepressants. See Bender, K. (2005). Throwing out the gold? Reconsidering the HAM-D. *Psychiatric Times*, April, 1–6.

2 For more on the nature of the 'science wars', see the website http://www.zmag.org/ScienceWars/index.htm.

References

Angell M. (2004). *The Truth about the Drug Companies: How they deceive us and what to do about it* (New York: Random House).

Applebaum P. and Grisso T. (1998). *Assessing Competence to Consent to Treatment: A guide for physicians and other health professionals* (New York: Oxford University Press).

Baynes K. (1992). *The Normative Grounds of Social Criticism: Kant, Rawls and Habermas* (Albany: State University of New York Press).

Canguilhem G. (1991). *The Normal and the Pathological* (New York: Zone Books).

Coyne J. (2005). Lessons in conflict of interest: the construction of the martyrdom of David Healy and the dilemma of bioethics. *American Journal of Bioethics*, 5, W3.

Dresser R. (2001). *When Science Offers Salvation: Patient advocacy and research ethics*. (New York: Oxford University Press).

Emanuel E. (1991). *The Ends of Human Life: Medical ethics in a liberal polity* (Cambridge, MA: Harvard University Press).

Epstein S. (1996). *Impure Science: AIDS, activism, and the politics of knowledge* (Berkeley and Los Angeles: University of California Press).

Ewen S. (1976). *Captains of Consciousness: Advertising and the social roots of the consumer culture* (New York: McGraw Hill Book Company).

Farmer P. (2005). *Pathologies of Power: Health, human rights, and the new war on the poor* (Berkeley: University of California Press).

Feenberg A. (1999). *Questioning Technology* (London and New York: Routledge).

Fulford K. (1989). *Moral Theory and Medical Practice* (Cambridge: Cambridge University Press).

Goldman A. (1999). *Knowledge in a Social World* (Oxford: Clarendon Press).

Habermas J. (1990). *Moral Consciousness and Communicative Action* (Cambridge, MA: MIT Press).

Habermas J. (1993). *Justification and Application: Remarks on discourse ethics* (Cambridge: MA, MIT Press).

Habermas J. (1998). *The inclusion of the other* (Cambridge, MA: MIT Press).

Harding S. (1991). *Whose science? Whose knowledge?: Thinking from women's lives.* (Ithaca, New York: Cornell University Press).

Haynes M. and Smedley B. (eds.) (1999). *The Unequal Burden of Cancer: An assessment of NIH research and programs for ethnic minorities and the medically underserved* (Washington, DC: National Academy Press).

Healy D. (1990). *The Suspended Revolution: Psychiatry and psychotherapy re-examined* (London, Faber and Faber).

Healy D. (1997). *The Antidepressant Era* (Cambridge, MA: Harvard University Press).

Healy D. (2001*a*). The dilemmas posed by new and fashionable treatments. *Advances in Psychiatric Treatment*, 7, 322–327.

Healy D. (2001*b*). Evidence biased psychiatry? *Psychiatric Bulletin*, 25, 290–291.

Healy D. (2002). *The Creation of Psychopharmacology* (Cambridge, MA: Harvard University Press.

Healy D. (2003). Interface between authorship, industry and science in the domain of therapeutics. *British Journal of Psychiatry*, 183, 22–7.

Healy D. (2004). *Let them Eat Prozac: The unhealthy relationship between the pharmaceutical industry and depression* (New York and London, New York University Press).

Hogg C. (1999). *Patients, Power and Politics: From patients to citizens* (London, Sage Publications).

Kaplan D. (2003). *Ricoeur's Critical Theory* (Albany: State University Of New York Press).

Kitcher P. (2001). *Science, Truth, and Democracy* (New York: Oxford University Press).

Kleinman D. (ed.) (2000). *Science, technology, and democracy*. Albany, State University of New York Press.

de Koning K. and Martin M. (1996*a*). 'Participatory research in health: setting the context' in K. de Koning and M. Martin (eds.) *Participatory Research in Health: Issues and experiences* (London: Zed Books), 1–18.

de Koning K. and Martin M. (eds.) (1996*b*). *Participatory Research in Health: Issues and experiences* (London: Zed Books).

Longino H. (1990). *Science as Social Knowledge: Values and objectivity in social inquiry* (Princeton: Princeton University Press).

Minton H. (2002). *Departing from Deviance: A history of homosexual rights and emancipatory science in America* (Chicago: The University of Chicago Press).

Navarro V. (1976). *Medicine under Capitalism* (New York: Prodist).

Noble D. (1977). *America by Design: Science, technology, and the rise of corporate capitalism.* (Oxford: Oxford University Press).

Pera M. (1994). *The Discourses of Science* (Chicago: The University of Chicago Press).

Peukert H. (1986). *Science, Action, and Fundamental Theology: Toward a theology of communicative action* (Cambridge, MA: The MIT Press).

Rehg W. (1994). *Insight and Solidarity: The discourse ethics of Jurgen Habermas* (Berkeley and Los Angeles: University of California Press).

Rehg W. (1998). 'Argumentation theory and the philosophy of science since Kuhn: the rationality of theoretical advance,' paper presented to Seminaret i Vitenskapsteori, Universitetet i Oslo, Oslo, Norway, August 1998, available at the University of Oslo website: www.tf.uio.no/etikk/artikler/rehgonscience.htm.

Remedios F. (2003). *Legitimizing Scientific Knowledge: An introduction to Steve Fuller's social epistemology*. (Lanham, Maryland: Lexington Books).

Ricoeur P. (1992). *Oneself as Another* (Chicago and London: The University of Chicago Press).

Sadler J. (2002). 'Values in developing psychiatric classifications: a proposal for the DSM-V' in J. Sadler (ed.) *Descriptions and Prescriptions: Values, mental disorders, and the DSMs* (Baltimore, MD: The Johns Hopkins University Press), 301–322.

Salmon J. (1990). 'Profit and health care: trends in corporatization and proprietarization' in J. Salmon (ed.) *The Corporate Transformation of Healthcare: Issues and directions*, vol. 1 (Amityville, NY: Baywood Publishing Company), 55–77.

Schrag C. (1992). *The Resources of Rationality: A response to the postmodern challenge* (Bloomington, Indiana: Indiana University Press).

Sclove R. (1995). *Democracy and Technology* (New York: The Guilford Press).

Spece, Jr R., Shimm D., and Buchanan A. (eds.) (1996). *Conflicts of interest in clinical practice and research* (Oxford: Oxford University Press).

Chapter 7

Toward a post-technological information theory

Donald Mender

7.1 Introduction

The technological assumptions upon which 21st century psychiatry rests are instrumentally informational. In Foucault's terms, the general historical sequence of production modes has developed into a post-industrially instrumental 'mode of information,' which finds special expression in today's psychiatric reduction of mind to a data-processing instrument equated with a computer-like brain.

Yet instrumental information theory as it now stands is peculiarly ill-suited to the task of dealing with the ontologically situated meaning of psychological subjectivity: information theory's foundational formalism, explicitly inaugurated by Claude Shannon and continued in current practice, excludes intentionality from its own rubric, while the contingently instrumental reasoning of computer programming fails to engage the plenary challenges of existential necessity.

This paper will argue that a meaningful, non-instrumental reconstruction of information theory incorporating ontic intentionality is possible. The key to such an advance involves a shift from Shannon's formalism and computational instrumentalism to a semantically holistic and ontologically rooted adaptation of meta-theoretical constructs borrowed from post-Newtonian physics.

These constructs, which include gauge fields, spontaneously broken symmetries, path integrals, and quantum state collapse, can address both the semantic conundra and the existential gaps arising from current instrumentally informational paradigms. Moreover, such approaches imply radical new diagnostic and therapeutic possibilities for the future of psychiatry.

7.2 The current hegemony of techno-psychiatry

In recent years the emergence of myriad technologies has reshaped psychiatry. Twenty-first century researchers have developed macroscopic brain scanning machines, microelectrode recording arrays, biochemical assays, genetic markers, quantitative behavioral inventories, and double-blind protocols in order to illuminate putatively objective features of both normal and abnormal human psychology; the cyber-engines of all these investigative modalities are increasingly powerful digital computing machines. At the same time, psychopharmacologists have been enlisting potent new drugs in order to suppress many psychiatric symptoms; driving the use of these new 'magic bullets' is the perceived promise of cost-efficiency.

As a result of such developments, proponents and users of technology now enjoy almost hegemonic avenues of influence within academic psychiatry. 'Evidence-based' guidelines derived from technologically grounded research have become the gold standard of scholarly psychiatric thinking, mechanistic neuroscience has come to dominate academic psychiatry, and psychopharmacology increasingly monopolizes the career paths of psychiatric residents seeking university posts. Meanwhile, older 'vague' psychoanalytic approaches to the understanding and management of psychopathology, using existential hermeneutics and the somatic intentionality of signal anxiety rather than programmed technology, have been almost entirely relegated to the extreme margins of psychiatric discourse and practice, beyond the pale of scholarly respectability (Mender 1994).

It is important to view all of the above developments in a larger social context. Our present world economy is not merely an *ad hoc* technological one; its very foundation rests upon an agenda of informational instrumentalism (Poster 1984). The aim of informational instrumentalism is relentless, minimally entropic cost-efficiency. This normative target is promoted by productivity-driven cultural superstructures arising from a globally competitive base of semiconductors and fiber-optic cable. It should thus be no surprise that psychiatry marches in lockstep with the general demands of an enveloping informationally instrumentalist world. The contours of ontological meaning within that world are flattening ineluctably under the constraints of soullessly cost-efficient gigabyte transduction and thereby squeezing existential polysemy into oblivion, both within and outside the psychiatric community.

There is a large price to pay for this totalizing trend. Informationally instrumentalist paradigms have come to define our very sense of self, and organized psychiatry increasingly endorses and contributes to such constraining self-definition. The process entails contemporary psychiatry's acquiescence in allowing the investigative biases of informational instrumentalism to deform the conclusions of its research according to a strictly 'functionalist' view of the mind. This functionalist perspective likens the psychologically germane operations of living, sentient humans beings to one among many possible material instantiations of a generic computing mechanism. People are viewed as neurobiological data processers, equipped with carbon-based 'wetware' whose efficiency has been honed by natural selection to serve instrumental ends analogous to those served by silicon chips in artificial computers. Functionalists therefore feel justified in assigning to brains a 'digital' design, whose ability to calculate behavioral 'outputs' relies on discrete and countable micro-units in the form of neurons that can be purposefully manipulated and transformed according to the rules of arithmetic and Boolean logic. Most recently, the architectures of computing 'systems' thought to model the brain's operation have morphed from serial to parallel processing networks coordinating variegated computational modules, but functionalism remains the underlying dogma.

As a result, almost all contemporary theories about the causes of mental illness can be translated into a species of reduction to faulty computing mechanisms. To the extent that researchers view neurons as computational nodes and their transmitter substances as media connecting those nodes, many neuroscientific ideas about psychiatric disease have come to assert a functional correspondence between psychiatric disease and the notion of a damaged logic board, chip, or network architecture.

For example, the hypothesis that defective neural network modulators such as acetylcholine, serotonin, norepinephrine, and dopamine cause mental abnormalities is now widely accepted among psychiatrists. Concepts of modulatory failure in depression, mania, anxiety disorders, attention deficit syndromes, and schizophrenia have come to dominate psychiatric discourse.

This domination has arisen despite the fact that even empirical support for the relevant models is flawed. Abnormal findings in the brains of psychiatric patients cannot suffice to show that underlying 'glitches' cause mental illnesses. One must also consider the reverse possibility that the behavioral effects of mental illnesses like schizophrenia, perhaps through poor nutritional habits and hygiene, generate brain abnormalities as non-etiological byproducts.

Nevertheless, computational neuropsychiatry shows no sign of giving ground in the face of these objections or other more conceptual criticisms like Searle's Chinese Room analogy (Searle 1990), Merleau-Ponty's arguments for the embodied intentionality of mind (Kearney 1986), and the ontological rejoinders of Hubert Dreyfus (Dreyfus 1991). Today's neuropsychiatrists cannot even begin to consider the possibility of accommodating existential meaning because the foundational inflexibility of contemporary psychiatric neuroscience supports neither ontological nor semantic understanding (Mender 1994).

7.3 Instrumental information theory and bad faith in psychiatry

The underlying rigidity of informationally instrumental technology has two limiting properties that keep current psychiatric thinking in an intentionally and ontically impotent straightjacket. One limit is the contentless formalism of standard information theory; the other limit is the instrumentally reified character of contingently imperative reason, namely the 'if…, then…' instructional language of computer programming. These two problematic features are inextricably interrelated at their core by a common lack of ontological referentiality.

Standard information theory, which undergirds both computing and communications technologies in wide use today, was first codified by Claude Shannon in the early 1950s. Shannon defined information as a number expressing the unlikeliness of one among all possible arrangements of the elements comprising any system. For example, according to Shannon's formulation, the information contained in a 'heads' result as one of two possible outcomes in a coin toss is greater than the result of rolling a 2 on a die which has six possible outcomes. The most striking feature of information as Shannon conceived it is its lack of attention to corporeal content; only the form of the arrangements in a system is addressed, while the specific nature (embodied kinds such as nickels versus quarters in coin tosses) of components is ignored. In other words, Shannon's notion of information quantifies the amount of syntactical order (negative entropy) of a system but does not account for the semantic referents of that system's physical building blocks as concrete signifiers (Seife 2006).

Contingently imperative reason, the computational complement of formalistic information theory, is an instrumental feature of all technology but reveals itself in purest form through the abstractly formulated, disembodied programming of generic computing mechanisms ('universal' Turing machines). Contingently configured algorithms involving arbitrarily chosen conditions ('if…') married to consequently triggered instructions ('then…') determine the flow of logic in Turing programs. Such instructions, because they are imperative rather than declarative sentences, can therefore refer to no ontologically independent truth values. Moreover, because the imperatives of those instructions are contingent, they cannot engage the molar plenum of existential necessity. Hence, ontic referentiality eludes them.

Standard information theory and contingently imperative instrumental reason are methodologically embraced by today's psychiatric leadership because of a misperception that they lend a scientific patina to psychiatric inquiry and practice. Nothing could be farther from the truth. In their opaqueness to existential semanticity, standard information theory and contingently imperative instrumental reason stand in stark opposition to authentic science. Committed scientific inquiry is an ontological endeavor entailing the courageous exploration of nature's meaning and, through that avenue, of human subjectivity's place within the manifold of existence. Heidegger's derogations of science notwithstanding, the history of scientific progress has demonstrated time and again characteristics of Heideggerian good faith.

The existential authenticity of the scientist reveals itself in interrogatively open praxis, rather than restrictively predicative declaration, to both express and work through empirically falsifiable scientific hypotheses framed as uncompromisingly self-challenging 'postulates of the impossible' (e.g., the quantum-mechanical assertion that one cannot in principle measure both the position and momentum of a particle at the same time). Scientific good faith is especially evident during seminal paradigmatic 'revolutions,' when actively perturbative physical probings through critical experimentation dethrone dominant working mythologies about the centered scientific subject. Examples include Copernican displacement of the geocentric observer, Einstein's extension of relativistic epistemology from Galilean dynamics into optics, and matrix-mechanical entwinings of the quantum experimentalist with observed objects. Such shifts in understanding the self's place in nature can occur without warning when unanticipated empirical observations, like those of the convention-shattering Michelson-Morley and double-slit experiments, force an anxiety-laden crisis upon established scientific convention and thus strip consensual orthodoxy of its instrumentally 'ready-to-hand' veneer. The complacent subject of the previous scientific paradigm is thereby jolted off center, and the impact brings home the potential fallibility of everyone involved (Bronowski 1977; Hall 1993; Losee 2001).

If the informationally instrumental psychiatry of our times is to transcend its present limits and become a truly scientific discipline, then psychiatric thinkers must begin to grapple with the formalistic pitfalls and existential bad faith of misapplying standard information theory and contingent computational imperatives to the existence and intentionality of the psychiatric subject. A new approach, retaining the precision of current psychiatric research methodologies while also reaching out to incorporate notions of meaning and onticity, will be needed. The expanded perspective will require a logic flexible enough to link the potentially paradoxical referentiality of semantics and the non-reifiably protean concreteness (Barrett 1958) of existence. Successful expansion will have to bridge a still yawning chasm between two fundamental extremities delimiting human life: on one hand, those pre-existing objects, including vulnerable human neural tissue, comprising the world into which birth throws us, and, on the other hand, the horrifically self-nullifying meaning of that world's capriciousness for the ultimately mortal psychiatric subject. In other words, the future growth of psychiatry into an existentially meaningful science must be able to enfold a semantic understanding of personal ontological limitation into our intrinsic sense of self.

The importance of the term 'intrinsic' cannot be emphasized enough here. Shannon's formalism and the contingently imperative reasoning of computer programming, by attempting to banish both semantics and ontology from their discourses, render ontic meaning extrinsic to instrumental information. The informational instrumentality of the computational algorithm allows no intrinsic room for existential intentionality. To see why, the logics behind both semanticity and existence must be understood in detail.

The synonymous terms 'semanticity', 'intentionality', and 'meaning' all tautologically denote by their common definition a signifier's reference to something other than itself. Such denotation, when applied to a formal proposition whose intentional referents are bounded by the universal quantifier 'for all...,' must point to something outside the universalized proposition itself (Bronowski 1978). This sort of extra-propositional reference, when applied to the universally vetted symbols and rules comprising a logical algebra, must refer in turn to a meta-algebraic entity extrinsic to the logical algebra's own formal self.

Gregory Chaitin illuminated the relevance of this reasoning to computer programming through the use of a *reductio ad absurdum*. He demonstrated the semantic paradoxicality of a generically self-contained algorithm hypothetically constituted by a completely meaningful, that is, totally non-redundant, digital instruction (Barrow 1999). Attempts at such an impossibly 'pure,' universally irreducible formulation in the algebraic language of a digital computer must lead the logician into an infinite regression of ever-receding chimerical self-reflections always outside the boundaries and beyond the internal reach of the sought-after construct.

The absurdity put forward by Chaitin highlights the self-defeating role played by the universal quantifier in trying to contain intentionality as a property putatively intrinsic to an algorithmic process. In fact, the universal quantifier's closure of contextual possibilities for interpretation is by the very nature of its own definition the culprit separating formal propositional logic from meaning introduced by generic outside references.

An important ontological implication issues from these considerations. Propositions utilizing the universal quantifier can be always reformulated without logical distortion in terms of the existential quantifier 'there exists...' (Guttenplan 1997), which, like meaning shorn of external context, eludes essentialistic or hypostasized predication. Existence and predicatively non-contextual semanticity can be seen logically as no more than mirrors of each other, mutually complementary aspects of Kant's non-predicative sentential 'copulae.'

Would-be conservators of computational psychology have endeavored in vain to find a 'nonlinear' way around the self-referently paradoxical bottleneck of predicatively non-contextual semantics and by implication onticity. Such attempts have been challenged epistemologically by Searle's Chinese Gym critique (Searle 1990). A more algebraically oriented challenge, arising from the open-ended addition of 'fuzzy-logical' terms to binary 'on/off' Boolean states, provides a benchmark of the extrinsic way that current non-linear formalisms necessarily defer ad infinitum rather than make tractable the intrinsically problematic aspects of meaning and their ontic reflections.

Strategies attempting to anchor nonlinear logic in the physical domain have generated their own externalizing regressions. Extrinsically engrafting the concept of energy as a would-be carrier of ontological intentionality on to instrumental information has given rise to the seductive nonlinear idea of algorithmic 'depth,' which incorporates notions of programmed complexity by quantifying the number of 'valleys' delineating stable minimal states separated by 'mountainous' energy barriers throughout the thermodynamic 'landscapes' of systems under scrutiny. However, the extrinsic nature of energy in this paradigm does not quietly disappear, tamed and tethered beneath non-linear thermodynamic landscapes. Instead, non-linear thermodynamics must resort to regressively reduplicative extrinsic 'baths' as free energy sources and heat sinks to make the open, 'far-from-equilibrium' systems work (Prigogine 1996).

7.4 Symmetry and information theory

Hence, it appears that neither the mechanistic approaches of Boolean algebra, Shannon's formalism, computational contingency, 'fuzzy logic,' nor nonlinear thermodynamics can make existential meaning seamlessly intrinsic to instrumental information. A new perspective is needed. One candidate may be the mathematics of abstract symmetry.

Symmetry in this general sense is defined as a property that remains unchanged while the system being considered is in some way transformed. For instance, the appearance of a square is symmetrical under ninety-degree rotations. A circle has greater rotational symmetry than a square possesses in that the circle's shape is invariant under rotational transformations through any arbitrary number of degrees. According to this criterion, the square demonstrates a larger amount of constrained order than the circle. That is, a square's lower degree of symmetry imbues it with a larger rotational information content than that of a circle. This principle can be generalized beyond simple geometrical parameters to any kind of conserved property subject to some chosen transformation. Examples include the unchanging configuration of an electrical field under an interchange of negative and positive charges, the conservation of a system's total energy despite alterations in potential and kinetic components, and the constancy of physical laws in the face of shifting dynamical reference frames. In all such cases, the degree of symmetry relates inversely to the amount of information.

Physicists find it particularly useful to distinguish two types of symmetry: global and local. We shall see that the relationship between global and local symmetry is also crucial to the project of embedding ontic intentionality intrinsically within the rubric of a new, non-instrumental, non-formalistic kind of information theory.

The term 'global' symmetry refers to invariances under transformative changes that are the same everywhere, i.e. globally, throughout the system under consideration. One illustrative example might involve the rigid surface of a hollow steel sphere, which is globally symmetric to the extent that its shape is preserved after all the points on its surface rotate the same number of degrees in the same direction.

'Local' symmetry, on the other hand, requires a stricter invariance under transformations that may differ in degree or direction from place to place throughout the system studied. For instance, local symmetry applies insofar as the shape of a thin rubber spherical surface, perhaps the skin of an inflated balloon, might in principle remain unaltered after selected points are each carefully rotated a different distance or in a different direction across its surface.

Global and local symmetry thus differ, as illustrated in the above examples, by virtue of transformations proceeding identically at each location throughout the relevant system in the 'global' case and non-identically from point to point in the 'local' case. This difference in transformational uniformity constitutes scaffolding for the intrinsic properties of a system. Such scaffolding in general is expressed through the abstract notion of a 'gauge field.'

The illustrative cases of rigid and rubber spheres provide a specific example of a concrete gauge field: the configuration of elastic tensions across the rubber sphere undergoing locally varying rather than globally uniform point-to-point surface transformations. Other instances of gauge fields are generated by different types of global-to-local symmetry contrasts in a variety of systems and domains, most notably those governing subatomic particle interactions; these particular sorts of gauge fields can be understood as the fundamental forces of physics.

In general gauge fields may be seen as abstract 'curvatures,' created by the localization of global symmetries and intrinsic to their structural architecture.

The abstract quasi-differentiability of these localized symmetries enable the equations describing them to serve as overarching 'differential laws' from which a broad range of instantiated 'solutions' can be deduced by generalized integrative methods. The intrinsic character of a gauge curvature flows from its origin in topologically internal connections (Bernstein and Phillips 1981) among components of the germane system which, without such topology, would serve merely as an embedding external 'context' for the relevant invariances.

A concrete geometric example can serve to provide an intuitive illustration of what is generally meant by the intrinsic nature of an abstract curvature. One can ask how an imaginary 'flat' surveyor would go about detecting any curvature that might happen to bend the two-dimensional surface in which he or she lives. The surveyor could proceed by picking three different points, drawing the straightest possible lines between them to form a triangle, and then measuring the angles at the triangle's three vertices. If the surface were flat or were wrapped around a cylinder, the number of degrees in those angles would total 180. If the surface were wrapped around a sphere, the total number of degrees would be expected to exceed 180. The 'flat' surveyor would not have to leave the familiar surface of the sphere and travel in an alien third-dimensional direction to detect a departure of the spherical surface's curvature from the null value of the flat surface, although he or she would be forced to resort to three-dimensional (i.e., extrinsic) geometry to distinguish cylindrical curvature from total flatness. Only in the case of the spherical surface's finite but unbounded topology could the flat surveyor make measurements capable of detecting nonzero curvature while remaining within the intrinsic structure of the relevant two-dimensional 'universe.'

In that sense, the curvature of the cylinder's surface can be considered geometrically extrinsic, while the curvature of the sphere's surface may be regarded as intrinsic (Icke 1995; Mender 1994). In a similar sense, the generic curvature of a gauge field is an intrinsic property of any system displaying symmetries under not merely global but also local versions of pertinent transformations.

7.5 Intentionally intrinsic information and subjective existence

The project of enlisting symmetries and gauge curvature to help develop a new, existentially relevant kind of information theory in which meaning is intrinsically embedded must begin with the global invariances implicit in the phenomenology of Edmund Husserl. Husserl's inquiry into the structure of subjective experience involved thought experiments that bracketed as methodologically irrelevant distinctions between real and illusory objects of perception. His approach endeavored to obstruct the epistemic access of an investigating subject to the ontological status of any object as 'real' versus 'non-existent.' For Husserl, the objective truth and falsity of a subjective experience hence became equivalent, much as affirmative and negative truth values are equivalent in relation to a paradoxical statement. One might say that Husserl's research program rendered any phenomenologically permissible statement made by a perceiving subject invariant under the quasi-paradoxical exchange of objectively affirmative and negative truth values.

Husserl formulated his epistemological proscriptions expressly to facilitate methodical introspection, which to him implied both purposeful application and, with respect to any 'real' subject under consideration, standardized reproducibility. One can consider the resulting symmetry of the Husserlian object to be global because the ontologically uniform subjective state implicitly allowed by Husserl is restricted to that of an 'existing' rather than 'unreal' perceiver. In such a globally symmetrical context, meanings, though constituting a link between subject and object, must remain an extrinsic connection, topologically 'flat' in the absence of any gauge curvature.

Husserl's globally symmetrical, methodically standardized mode of inquiry remains phenomenologically 'uncurved' because it lacks one key ontic element: the involuntary spontaneity of existential meaning, which infuses anxiety into lived, experienced information actually valued as crucial to a subject's survival. Herein lies a critical potential nexus between the existentially charged informational demands of 'fight-or-flight' arousal systems in the living human brain and ontological meaning for Dasein, the subject of Heidegger's life and death phenomenology.

Heidegger, like Husserl, comprehended the value of bracketing the gap between existence and non-existence in a quasi-paradoxical manner. However, the existence and non-existence bracketed by Heidegger applied most germanely not to the intended object but instead to the intending subject. Heidegger framed the latter bracketing as a diffusely grounded understanding of mortality by every subject, each in his or her own idiosyncratic way. According to Heidegger, this mortal intuition flies in the face of the self-contradictory proposition that 'I do not exist' (Hoffman 1993). Such an existential absurdity contains within its very paradoxical nature a symmetrical relationship to its own truth and falsity.

The symmetry of Heidegger's existential paradox is not merely global in the manner of Husserlian invariance. Heidegger's symmetry is maintained across the 'locally' idiosyncratic variations distinguishing disparate perspectives on subjective existence. Despite these variations, according to which different subjects at different times of their lives appear to exhibit different kinds of receptivity to intimations of their own mortality, the 'care' underlying Dasein's investment in his or her own existence always rests on a fundamental, personal understanding of life's finitude. What maintains Heideggerian symmetry in the face of apparently varying subjective perspectives about death is fluctuation in the compensatory existential meaning attached to each different life situation. Some semantic fluctuations entail authentic anxiety, others inauthentic retreat into the narcosis of comforting mass delusions and fashions. All such varied meanings inhere intrinsically within the subject's existence and extend Heideggerian symmetry from globality into the manifold localities of individual subjective interpretation; for these reasons such meanings may be said to constitute an existentially intentional gauge field.

What form would a revised understanding of information theory have to assume in order to grow naturally from a Heideggerian gauge field of ontological meaning? To answer this question and hence build a bridge fully interrelating the information-intensive workings of brain arousal systems and Heideggerian existentialism, our understanding of symmetry and gauge curvature must be supplemented by yet another abstract idea from mathematical physics: spontaneous symmetry breaking.

In general terms, spontaneous symmetry breaking arises when the differential equations delineating any kind of symmetry generate at least some integrative solutions which fail to display that symmetry. To grasp the abstract concept of spontaneous symmetry breaking in a more concrete way, consider as one example a marble dropping into a fully symmetrical bowl whose lowest interior point, and hence the locus of least potential gravitational energy, is at the center. The marble will rapidly roll to that minimum spot and then stay there. However, if the bowl is instead shaped like a sombrero, the marble will settle not at the center, which is no longer the lowest point, but instead somewhere on a continuous circle of energetically minimal locations between the bowl's center and rim. The hump in the middle of the sombrero shape breaks the bowl's energetic symmetry.

Another example of a broken symmetry can be gleaned from a collection of fine oblong iron filings lying on a level tabletop. In the absence of a magnetic field, the orientation of each filing's long axis will be independent of the others. An average of randomly surveyed filings will point in no particular preferred direction. However, if a magnet is introduced underneath the tabletop close to the filings, they will orient themselves along the magnetic field's lines of force. One can say that the orientation of the filings when non-magnetized has a high degree of rotational symmetry, but the magnet 'breaks' that symmetry. In the process of magnetic symmetry breaking, a greater amount of rotational order is imposed on the filings, and the system thereby acquires more information.

Symmetry-breaking influences of any sort, including the magnetic behavior of iron, are all very close conceptually to the notion of a hump in a sombrero. Generalizations of symmetry-breaking 'humps' are the 'hills' that intervene between minimal 'valleys' within the abstract 'landscapes' of a given system. Each such 'hump', in that it breaks an entropy-laden symmetry, imbues its system with information.

Select 'humps,' namely those that break local symmetries under so-called 'non-Abelian' transformations and thereby intrinsically load gauge-theoretical systems with nonlinearly self-transcendent information, should by virtue of those select, nonlinearly self-transcendent properties be candidates able to support the general structure of a new kind of information theory with built in ontological meaning. However, such Heideggerian information, though broadly capable of capturing and conveying the life and death meanings suffusing existential phenomenology, must find specific instantiation through the language of biophysics, delineating the physical principles by which living systems, including the human brain, break non-living entropy-laden symmetries.

The most basic physical science relevant to this instantiating task is quantum-theoretical, insofar as energetic information increments associated with biological symmetry breaking correspond to quanta situated within a single narrow preferred frequency band of energy magnitudes among all the random possibilities across the radiative spectrum. That single narrow band bears the quantum-mechanical characteristics of visible light and thus resonates with the life-sustaining processes of energy capture by photosynthesis, energy transfer by electron transport, energy storage by ADP and related phosphates, and energy reorganization by the myriad configurational changes implicit in the quantum chemistry of carbon chains (Loewenstein 1999).

The Heideggerian symmetry which transcends the existential paradox 'I (as a living subject) do not exist' can achieve biophysical instantiation by dovetailing with Darwinian aspects of systems that are chemically sustained by quanta of visible light but also anticipate their own potential extinction by photons from other frequency bands, such as thermally disruptive microwaves and mutagenic gamma rays. This symmetry constraint requires the rare occurrence (events which are virtually but not literally impossible in accordance with the concept of zero set-theoretic measure) of evolutionarily adaptive innovations that grapple with quantum physical phenomena in regions of the electromagnetic spectrum not limited to visible light. Those rare innovations serve to re-schematize the lethal components of radiation into life-affirming incarnations within the visible frequency band, much as X-rays are converted into computed tomography scans and DNA diffraction images, or as the radiative products of nuclear fusion have been reinterpreted by the human intellect into heuristic models of the strong and weak forces.

Propagation of such biophysically instantiated Heideggerian symmetry in conformity with the demands of each subjective evolutionary perspective must proceed through the translation of information from one reference frame into another, effectively amplifying and reducing frequencies and commensurate mass-energies of quanta across the entire radiative spectrum as needed for adjustments to differing requirements conditioned by varying naturally selective contexts. Transformations based on the spacio-temporal dilatations and contractions of special relativity and its quantum-statistical expression in the continuous frame shifts of quantum field theory offer possible vehicles for this kind of adaptive compensation.

7.6 **Ontologically meaningful information and the future of psychopathology**

Inclusion of quantum field theory in the above model introduces both a complication and an opportunity into our nascent formulation of Heideggerian information theory. The complication consists of a statistical blurring that rules out the feasibility of a deterministically comprehensible structure for ontologically meaningful information. The opportunity flows from the existentially therapeutic possibilities inherent in probabilistic risk.

On the complicating side, quantum field theory expands the number of possible gauge fields from a single deterministic option to a cacophonous multiplicity of variations in accordance with the notion of 'path integrals' (Icke 1995). The concept of path integration, formulated by Richard Feynman and now enshrined in the standard methodology of physics, specifies that every quantum-field-theoretic process must proceed through disparate but simultaneous intermediate stages along an infinite number of possible parallel 'paths,' all beginning and ending with a common initial and final state. Each individual component path can be considered a distinct gauge field, and each can be assigned its own 'probability amplitude' of occurrence. The sum of all such probability amplitudes for a given process must equal a certainty value of 100% and represents the 'superposed' path of the total system.

However, because quantum field theory is subject to Heisenberg's famous quantum-mechanical uncertainty principle, any experimental attempt to assay the progress of such a process collapses the system's total 'superposed' state into one of its component pathways. Exactly which component path is selected by any specific collapsing act of experimental observation is always governed by random chance. This randomness is a manifestation of Heisenbergian uncertainty, adapted for quantum field theory through so-called 'second quantization.'

There is one path associated with each superposed multitude that can be uniquely understood as an 'extreme' gauge field. This single pathway constitutes an analogy to the idea of a 'shortest route' between the initial and final state of the system. In that sense, all alternative paths are longer 'detours.'

Such a distinction between an extreme path and detours hints at a possible opportunity to identify an existentially normative standard for intentionally gauged information. The French philosopher Paul Ricoeur (Kearney 1986) has distinguished between, on one hand, the ontological semantics of Heidegger as the 'shortest' route to meaning and, on the other hand, alternative paths of interpretation, which he designates as hermeneutic detours. An isomorphism thus emerges between physical path integration and the hermeneutic alternatives inherent in informational intentionality. This isomorphism suggests that quantum field theory's bio-instantiation of ontologically significant information among all possible informational intentionalities normatively represents the 'shortest' possible gauge-theoretic path of life's hermeneutic enterprise.

Herein lies an enticing potential for the enhancement of both diagnostic and therapeutic clarity in the normative understanding of the human mind. If future psychiatrists avail themselves of the opportunities now latent within the idea of an improved information theory, able to incorporate biophysically ontological semanticity into its own intrinsic structure, then the normativity implied by Feynman path integration in tandem with Ricouer's contrast between the shortest hermeneutic route and detours will offer a new way of distinguishing an ontologically optimal process from hermeneutic engagements undertaken in various degrees of existential 'bad faith.' This kind of distinction, married to elements of the quantum field-oriented psychophysics already under development by Globus (2003), Jibu and Yasue (1995), and Vitiello (2001), might lead to novel, phenomenologically informed insights concerning the quantum-pathophysiology of mental illness.

Moreover, a 'gravitonic' neurocognitve hypothesis advanced by Penrose and Hameroff (Penrose 1989) suggests that extension of existentially intentional information theory beyond the biophysical implications of quantum field theory into the frontier of quantum gravity might provide future psychiatrists with currently unanticipated therapeutic advances. Penrose and Hameroff have postulated that quantum-gravitational influences reaching a critical threshold in the brain mediate the collapse of superposed states, including path-integrated sums of component gauge field probability amplitudes, into single components in a manner heretofore attributed solely to Heisenberg uncertainty. According to the principles of general relativity, such gravitonic mediators of collapse should be capable of 'lensing' radiative quanta into and out of any given frequency band, including but not limited to the biologically preferred frequencies and associated mass-energies of visible light photons. Hence, it seems reasonable to hope that quantum gravity might eventually provide a means of enabling Heisenberg-like 'leaps' from detoured bio-hermeneutic pathways to the normatively extreme route of existentially authentic understanding.

Although Penrose and Hameroff have portrayed gravitonic collapse as a non-random phenomenon determined by 'objective' factors buried beneath the fabric of space-time, any future mobilization of their ideas in the pursuit of bio-existential healing will likely evade the deterministic bad faith of technological control. If 'objective' Penrosean factors were proved to exist, their therapeutic exploitation would require access to extraordinarily miniscule, 'sub-Planck' scales of length, which most probably will remain beyond the reach of instrumental physics. Hence, any practical instantiation of quantum-gravitational psychotherapeutics will have to operate in an effectively randomized fashion. It is also possible that the 'factors' postulated by Penrose and Hameroff will be found to arise from the decentered subjectivity of the quantum measuring agent and not from any occult objective influences (Mender 2007). In that case, the random aspects of existential risk will inhere ineradicably in any trials of psychiatric therapies inspired by gravitational collapse.

In any event, future psychotherapeutic transformations of existentially meaningful information, shaped by either practical or principled limits on the determinacy of quantum gravity, will effectively resist any retrogressive slide back into the present psychiatric pseudo-world of technological objects and agendas. Consequently, exploratory approaches to the optimization of Dasein's brain (Globus 2003) may become free to develop and mature. Over time, ontologically intentional informational constructs of mental health and pathology, of psychiatric diagnosis and therapeutics, and perhaps of professional identity among psychiatrists themselves may blossom along radically statistical lines.

Such future developments could well render the field of psychiatry unrecognizable to the sensibilities of our own technological era.

Acknowledgments

Acknowledgment and appreciation are extended to Gordon Globus, Emeritus Vice Chair of Psychiatry and Professor of Psychiatry and Philosophy, University of California at Irvine, and James Phillips, Associate Clinical Professor of Psychiatry, Yale University School of Medicine. Both contributed critical suggestions during the development of this manuscript.

References

Barrett W. (1958). *Irrational Man* (New York: Anchor), 161–163.

Barrow J. (1999). *Between Inner and Outer Space* (Oxford: Oxford University Press), 85–98.

Bernstein J. and Phillips A. (1981). Fiber bundles and quantum mechanics. *Scientific American*, **245**, 123–137.

Bronowski J. (1977). *A Sense of the Future* (Cambridge, MA: MIT Press), 74–103 and 221–234.

Bronowski J. (1978). *The Origins of Knowledge and Imagination* (New Haven: Yale University Press), 67–89.

Dreyfus H. (1991). *Being-in-the-World* (Cambridge, MA: MIT Press), 117–119.

Globus G. (2003). *Quantum Closures and Disclosures—Thinking Together Postphenomenology and Quantum Brain Dynamics* (Amsterdam and Philadelphia: John Benjamins), 4–165.

Guttenplan S. (1997). *The Languages of Logic* (Oxford: Blackwell), 175–177.

Hall H. (1993). 'Intentionality and world: division I of *Being and Time*' in C. Guignon (ed.) *The Cambridge Companion to Heidegger* (Cambridge: Cambridge University Press), 122–140.

Hoffman P. (1993). 'Death, time, history: division II of *Being and Time*' in C. Guignon (ed.) *The Cambridge Companion to Heidegger* (Cambridge: Cambridge University Press), 195–214.

Icke V. (1995). *The Force of Symmetry* (New York: Cambridge University Press), 80–99 and 200–204.

Jibu M. and Yasue K. (1995). *Quantum Brain Dynamics And Consciousness* (Philadelphia: John Benjamins), 73–191.

Kearney R. (1986). *Modern Movements in European Philosophy* (Manchester: Manchester University Press), 73–112.

Loewenstein W. (1999). *The Touchstone of Life* (Oxford: Oxford University Press), 54–60.

Losee J. (2001). *A Historical Introduction to the Philosophy of Science* (Oxford: Oxford University Press), 153–156 and 198–202.

Mender D. (1994). *The Myth of Neuropsychiatry* (New York: Plenum), 1–30 and 101–113.

Mender D. (2007). Decentering the subject of physics. *Neuroquantology*, **5**, 175–181.

Penrose R. (1989). *The Emperor's New Mind* (Oxford: Oxford University Press), 248–449.

Poster M. (1984). *Foucault, Marxism and History: Mode of production versus mode of information* (Cambridge: Polity Press), 44–94.

Prigogine I. (1996). *The End Of Certainty* (New York: The Free Press), 55–72.

Searle J. (1990). Is the mind's brain a computer program? *Scientific American*, **262**, 26–31.

Seife C. (2006). *Decoding the Universe* (New York: Viking), 56–87.

Vitiello G. (2001). *My Double Unveiled: The dissipative quantum model of the brain* (Amsterdam and Philadelphia: John Benjamins), 67–145.

Part 3

Technology and psychiatric disorders

Chapter 8

Technology and mental disorders: a clinical probe into the differential impact on individuals

Douglas W. Heinrichs

And out of what one sees and hears and out
Of what one feels, who could have thought to make
So many selves, so many sensuous worlds,
As if the air, the mid-day air, was swarming
With the metaphysical changes that occur,
Merely in living as and where we live.
(Wallace Stevens, from *Esthetique du Mal*)

8.1 Introduction

Philosophic perspectives on technology's impact on human life have most often relied on monolithic and abstract characterizations both of technology itself and of human nature. This is true both of those following from the critique of Heidegger (1977) as well as those within a Marxist frame of reference. In such discussions technology is typically talked about as if it were a definable and unified process unfolding with progressive intensity and intrusion into human life. In this way of thinking, it ought to be possible to identify specific attributes of technology that have consistent and mounting consequences on human beings. The human beings in turn are viewed as having certain effects imposed upon them by technology that can be understood in terms of their nature qua human beings as opposed to their specific, unique attributes as individuals. At most there may be some discussion of differential impact on large segments of the human community, usually based upon economic class.

An exception to this general pattern has been those discussions flowing from the perspective of social constructionism. Here there is frequently an analysis of the role of different groups of individuals within the society, with their particular perspective and interests, influencing the emergence and characterization of specific pieces of technology. This goes some way toward providing a more specific and concrete sort of analysis. However, it tends to look at influences only in one direction, focusing on how specific interests within the larger culture contribute to the successful development of a particular bit of technology (Winner 2003). These analysis tend not to be informative about the unique impact of particular instances of technology on particular sorts of individuals.

There is no reason to assume that technology is a monolithic unfolding process that is uniform, even at the qualitative level, in its influence on persons. Although it is to be expected that there are some uniformities in the impact of a particular technological development on large groups of individuals in a given society, there are nonetheless sufficient differences in individual attributes to create considerable differential impact for any particular technological event. The purpose of this discussion is to begin an initial exploration of a complimentary approach to the more traditional ones. The goal is to identify and characterize the differential impact of particular facets of technological development on the adaptation and functioning of individuals, based on subtle or not so subtle differences in their mode of engaging the world. One way to locate some such differences is by considering variations that have been defined as forms of psychopathology. This has the advantage that articulated characterizations of the cognitive, affective, and interpersonal patterns found in these conditions already exist in the clinical literature. Furthermore, many of these individuals are engaged in treatment relationships where environmental factors influencing their functioning are already a focus of ongoing attention.

It should be stressed at the outset that there is nothing limiting or even privileging the application of this approach to psychopathological variations. The same considerations can be applied to any variation in the strengths, weaknesses, and stylistic preferences that individuals bring to the task of engaging and adapting to the world. Which of these forms of life are given diagnostic labels and hence pathologized is based on many factors, including changes in society. For instance, would attention-deficit disorder without hyperactivity ever have become a psychiatric diagnosis except in a world where most better employment opportunities require extensive periods of formal education that place high attentional demands on individuals?

Considerations of this general sort are not without precedent. Cross-cultural studies of outcome in schizophrenia by the World Health Organization and other groups since the 1970s, for instance, showed that although the incidence of the illness was fairly constant across cultures, the outcome varied dramatically. The outcome was far worse in more technologically and industrially developed societies and better in pre-industrial traditional societies (Kulhara 1994). It was speculated that traditional cultures reduce the need to adapt rapidly to change and increase the portion of important relationships that are with persons well known to the patient who can help him adapt and will be more tolerant of his deviance. Finally it was felt that traditional societies could accommodate more periods of dysfunction without totally removing the patient from productive work.

Even this sort of approach, however, starts with quite coarse differences in functional outcomes between groups and then speculates as to possible explanatory mechanisms. By contrast, the intent here is to illustrate a hypothesis generating approach that moves in the opposite direction. Individual clinical examples are used to identify the impact of discrete technological developments on persons with particular sorts of psychopathology. I have intentionally chosen rather microscopic instances, and some of the consequences may seem quite trivial, but their purpose is to illustrate specific hypothesized mechanisms of impact. The magnitude and generalizability of such effects would need to be the object of further systematic study on a larger scale.

The sort of questions asked here can be seen as broadly Darwinian in nature. When focused on the big picture, Darwinian approaches typically highlight the flourishing of one species at the expense of another or the evolution in the overall form of the prototypical member of a given species. Of course it is important to remember that in the short time frame, and more microcosmic perspective, Darwinian thinking is based upon variation between individual members of a species and the relative advantages or disadvantages of their individual traits in the specific environmental context in which those individuals live. Hence, in considering technology we start with populations of individuals that contain variability in cognitive, affective, and relational features. We then can consider a specific technology-induced change in the environment, and ask which individuals have their functioning and adaptation improved by this technology-induced change and which individuals are disadvantaged. This parlays into clinical questions and strategies, as improving the functional capacity of our patients is one of the key goals of treatment. How can we exploit beneficial technologies and compensate for disadvantaging ones with this particular sort of patient?

To be truly Darwinian, of course, the individual advantages and disadvantages exposed by this sort of approach would have to translate into differential reproductive success for the individuals involved. Whether this is in fact the case will be discussed later in this paper. The value of this approach in understanding technological impact does not depend upon that feature.

It would still be quite useful and informative as an approach to technology if it only applies in a pseudo-Darwinian sense where the selective advantage and disadvantage is in terms of human flourishing rather than reproductive success. In the discussion below the sorts of hypotheses that can be generated by this approach will be illustrated by considering examples from my clinical practice representing three diagnostic conditions: attention-deficit disorder, Asperger syndrome and affective disorder.

8.2 Attention-deficit disorder

Attention-deficit disorder (ADD) is characterized most essentially by an impaired ability for sustaining volitional attention. It is expected that some evidence of this problem begins in childhood and in most cases continues to be apparent throughout life, although in some individuals it seems to spontaneously lessen in adulthood. Individuals with this condition are able to pay attention for long times to things that interest them intrinsically. Difficulty comes in choosing to pay attention to something that is not compelling to them, but is important. The attractiveness of the stimulus appears to dictate where the individual's attention goes rather than the individual's decision to attend based on understanding the importance of a particular feature of the environment to the person's larger goals. Because school is filled with the latter sort of instances, it is not surprising that academic settings are most often where attention-deficit problems are noticed. Because complicated goals often involve multistep planning of this sort, individuals with ADD frequently demonstrate what has been characterized as executive dysfunction, namely the difficulty in putting together and following through on the execution of multiple steps towards a desired outcome. The attraction to immediately appealing stimuli often results in a rather impulsive cognitive and interactive style in individuals with ADD, as they frequently say and do things before thinking through the consequences. Some individuals with this condition also show considerable motor hyperactivity, including restlessness and fidgeting. At least as this condition has come to be characterized in the USA, hyperactivity is not considered an essential feature of this condition and is not always present. From a neurobiological perspective, individuals with ADD appear to show differences in the activity of dopamine systems in the prefrontal cortex, and the range of pharmacologic interventions that have been shown useful with this condition have in common the ability to modulate dopamine activity in the frontal cortex (Faraone and Biederman 2004). Apart from the argument about whether one would want to pathologize individuals with this condition, it clearly characterizes a particular variant in cognitive, affective, and relational style. How might particular technological features differentially affect such individuals?

> William is currently a 22-year-old man diagnosed since middle school with ADD inattentive type. He is quite intelligent but did marginally in high school and dropped out of college his first year. He has shown some periods of dysthymia as well as intermittent alcohol and cannabis abuse. When he was 19 he showed some sustained hypertension despite no change in his stimulant medication. He has a strong family history of hypertension and I strongly urged him to contact his family physician for further assessment and treatment of his elevated blood pressure. In keeping with his parents' recent strategy to encourage his assumption of adult responsibility, they refrained from making the appointment for him and simply reminded him to make it. On two subsequent visits I asked him if he had seen his doctor and he reported that he had not yet done so. At the first visit I simply stressed the importance of dealing with his blood pressure. At the second visit I pushed him as to what the problem was. He then told me that he had in fact twice called the doctor's office. His physician was part of large group practice and he was immediately confronted with a complex phone system with layers of options and no easy way to access a live person. Both times he proceeded through two or three choices and hung up. He described increasing feelings of frustration and irritability but also a vague sense of confusion as if he did not know where he was going with all this. It was this growing unpleasant feeling that appeared to precipitate his hanging up.

Such phone systems are bits of technology that irritate many of us, but I suggest that they expose a particular form of vulnerability in persons with ADD. The nature of this can be seen by using the distinction offered by Daniel Dennett between the 'design stance' and 'intentional stance' (Dennett 1971). The design stance begins by looking at how some object or process is put together and then inferring from the relationship of the parts to what that item can do. Thus a clever person could take apart an alarm clock and infer that this device could be used to awaken one at a specific time. The intentional stance makes sense of a situation by beginning with the intentions and goals of a putative agent, either as expressed by the agent or inferred by the observer. Individuals with ADD typically have a form of executive dysfunction in which they are locked to immediate goals and intentions. They have trouble putting together a series of steps that ultimately lead to a more remote goal, namely generating a behavioral design that leads to an end. Using Dennett's distinction one can say that they have difficulty assuming the design stance as a way of ultimately implementing an intention.

Consider again William's dilemma in calling his doctor. In former times a real person would answer the phone. William would state the purpose of his call. The person at the other end would grasp his intention and use his or her knowledge of the design of the office procedure to implement that intention, namely, making an appointment. With the automated system he calls with an intention but is confronted with an elaboration of the design, multiple layers of options nested in a particular way that can be used to achieve multiple goals. He must exploit the design through sequential steps directing it towards his ultimate intention. This is where he bails out. In our discussions of this, William related to me how he had lost two of his four choices for classes at the community college because he got frustrated trying to register online and waited until a friend returned from vacation to do it for him. By that time, two of the classes were filled.

This contrasts sharply with William's success with video games. They in fact are one of his passions and in an attempt to find some basis of relating to him his father had once bought him a new game and suggested they learn to play it together. This ended in mutual frustration, however, as the father attempted to work through the instructions while William immediately began to play, trying move after move until the game became clear by induction. In short, he was continuously focused on an immediate goal until by the process of protracted induction the larger design became clear. His father's approach of studying the design first by reading the directions was intolerable for William.

The vast multiplication of technological strategies that confront individuals with the need to work through designs might be expected to pose significant challenges for individuals who have that variant in how they engage the world that we label ADD. For those of us involved in trying to treat individuals with this condition, attention to the development of compensatory strategies in dealing with this sort of challenge become an important part of treatment. At the larger societal level this mechanism may serve to identify a group of individuals who will be progressively disadvantaged in their attempts to flourish in a society filled with technologies of this sort.

As an aside, this kind of mechanism offers an alternative way of characterizing the whole notion of psychiatric nosology. Social constructionists have persistently challenged the view that categories of mental illness constitute true categories of nature. They suggest that these categories emerge from the imposition of particular frames of reference by groups with some degree of power and dominance in the society as a way of furthering their own interests and preservation, in this case the medical and psychiatric establishment (Gergen 1985, 1990). An alternative formulation is to concede that, although conditions like ADD do not represent intrinsic or universal disease states, it is enough that there are, among those variations in cognitive and affective style based on whatever mechanisms, some that include, for instance, reductions in volitional sustained attention. If individuals live in a social environment where this variant does not impose an excessive comparative disadvantage on the individual, it is not likely to be pathologized. If, however, the individual lives in a world where this variant is sufficiently disadvantageous, and at least some psychological or biological strategies for its ameliorization have been developed that can be broadly characterized as medical, the condition is likely to receive a designation as a mental disorder. That designation itself carries a range of consequences for individuals so labeled; some are desirable whereas others are not. Among the desirable ones include some acknowledgment of the comparative disadvantage that makes the person eligible for certain accommodations by the larger society. Indeed this goes a long way toward defining what constitutes justice for these individuals.

8.3 **Asperger syndrome**

Asperger syndrome (AS) is a condition that has received increasing attention in recent years. It is generally characterized as being on the relatively mild end of the spectrum of autistic disorders. Impairments in social interaction are hallmarks. Individuals with this variant typically show great difficulty reading social expectations and intentions accurately. They have trouble receiving accurate information from body language, voice intonation, facial expressions, and other forms of nuanced communication. They tend to have difficulty appreciating humor and/or irony in verbal communications, being prone to literal and concrete interpretations of language. They tend to make very little eye contact when interacting with others. They have a hard time inferring the mental states and intentions of others. Hence, they are prone to misread situations and respond in ways that others feel are inappropriate. This frequently leads to interpersonal conflict, ridicule, and a judgment that they are insensitive and uncaring about the needs of others. They are prone to repetitive, obsessive-like behavior and interests, often having accompanying tics and other stereotypic movements that further make them stand out. As a result they frequently, early in life, develop patterns of social isolation and are often picked on and scapegoated in group settings. They often do best with impersonal information and subject matter and frequently do very well with abstract systems such as mathematics. In fact, they and their relatives are overrepresented in certain professions such as mathematics and engineering (Baron-Cohen *et al.* 1998).

Andy is a 23-year-old young man who presented to me for treatment of a depression secondary to the impending divorce of his parents. He had been diagnosed in elementary school with AS and received extensive therapy and social rehabilitation treatment in the intervening years. A bright young man, he has acquired remarkable knowledge of his condition and has worked to develop compensatory strategies. In reviewing his history for prior episodes of depression he described an extended period of angry dysphoria in middle and high school related to troubled peer relations. He described

> his difficulty reading non-verbal cues in others and how this led to responding in ways that induced ridicule. It also led him to distorted inferences about the intentions of others resulting in what he described as a 'paranoid view'. He described getting increasingly anxious in the face of confusing interpersonal stimuli, and as he got more anxious he got more paranoid. When I asked him how he overcame all of this to the extent that he has, he cited his relationships on the Internet. After developing a series of long-distance friendships at the encouragement of his parents, he came to rely extensively on Internet communications even with local peers. He appreciated the absence of facial expression, body language, and prosody. This freed him to focus on the text with minimal anxiety. If he did get anxious, he could pause before responding to regroup and consider. When confused by a communication, which happened especially with irony, humor, and extensive use of unspoken assumptions, he learned to ask explicitly for clarification rather than jumping to questionable and often paranoid conclusions. Over time he actually learned to apply some of these strategies to face to face dealings with others. He described a gradual shift away from paranoid assumptions to the expectation that, with clarification, the intentions of others were usually benign.

It has become commonplace to hear complaints, particularly by parents, bemoaning the dehumanizing influence on our children of so extensively using online communication with text alone. However, for Andy and numerous other individuals with AS whom I have seen, the simplification and communicative poverty of this medium is precisely what allows space for developing compensatory strategies that facilitate successful participation in their interpersonal world. Hence we may have the interesting situation where a feature of technology that may in fact have some potential disadvantages for interpersonal relationships in society overall nonetheless can constitute a distinctive comparative advantage for a group of individuals with a particular variant in their mode of living such as the one we characterize as AS. These types of technology can provide other advantages for these individuals as well. The vast increase in a technological establishment necessary to sustain computer-based technology and similar developments creates a host of well-paid employment opportunities that play to the strong suit of individuals with AS. There has been an explosion in our society's needs for computer scientists, engineers, and others with similar technical expertise. Hence it is likely that the chances of an individual with AS, who is otherwise bright and motivated, to achieve financial success in our current culture is greatly increased.

This is obviously very good news for individuals with AS. A more interesting question is whether this could actually represent an instance of a truly Darwinian mechanism. There has been much recent attention to what appears to be a dramatic increase in AS and other manifestations of the autistic spectrum (Dales *et al.* 2001; Kaye *et al.* 2001; Yeargin-Allsopp *et al.* 2003). There are many possible explanations for this, including increased sensitivity to making the diagnosis but if, as many experts believe, there is a true increase in the frequency of this variant, one possible explanation is that in recent generations the heightened chances of an individual with AS achieving sufficient financial success to be seen as a desirable mate would lead to increased reproduction by these individuals, resulting in an increased frequency of the condition in the population. This is obviously speculative but it illustrates the more general point that the pseudo-Darwinian approach based upon comparative advantages in flourishing can easily translate into comparative advantages in reproductive success.

8.4 **Affective disorders**

In the discussions of ADD and AS the focus was on the consequences of direct interactions with certain technological features by persons with certain cognitive and affective attributes. In considering affective disorders, I want to highlight another mechanism: the ability of technological advances and the resultant social changes to alter key values and expectations in terms of which people judge each other. As Aristotle noted, how we assess how good a person or object is depends heavily on our view of the function or that person or thing. I hypothesize that although technology was intended to help us function better, it frequently has the effect of changing our view of how we are to function. In some ways functioning well has come to mean functioning like a good machine. What exactly are machine virtues? I posit that at least the following two are included. (1) A good machine consistently functions at optimal or near optimal efficiency all of the time it is in operation. (2) It should be able to function as much of the time as possible, ideally continuously, with minimal 'down time' and minimal maintenance. A good machine meets our desire that it be constantly available to produce optimally. However, for optimal efficiency, the individuals working with these machines must also be constantly available to optimally produce. They are conceptualized as part of the 'standing reserve' that is at the center of Heidegger's concept of 'enframing' (Heidegger 1977). One can think about this issue in the larger terms of its impact upon all of us. However, is there a differential impact on certain individuals with particular moods of life?

Mary is a 52-year-old marketing and advertising executive. She has a bipolar disorder that has been well controlled for decades. Nonetheless she is prone to subtle but noticeable shifts in energy, creativity, and efficiency. For two decades she worked for a midsized family-owned business and was a highly valued employee. Her creativity and enthusiasm, heightened during periods of mild hypomania, were appreciated. Her intermittent periods of low energy and mildly decreased productivity were tolerated as she more than made up for them when she was doing well. Ten years ago the

> business was sold to a large corporation. Her new supervisor tracked indices of productivity and became distressed by her variability of performance. During a period of mild anergy her boss observed her sitting at her desk for 10 to 15 minutes staring off into space and doing nothing. He accused her of 'slacking off' and confronted her with what he regarded as her inadequate recent productivity. She pointed out that at other times her productivity was quite high and that overall she was at least comparable to her peers. He retorted that her periods of high performance simply pointed out what she could do and that she should be functioning at that level all of the time. Her failure to do so represented a bad attitude. Shortly thereafter she was laid off in a downsizing. She has held multiple jobs since then but never reaching her former level of success. She describes how difficult it has become to find a setting that will tolerate her variability in performance, even though at its worst it meets at least the minimum standards.

Even persons without mood disorders show more fluctuations in performance over time than the good machine. This kind of fluctuation represents the cyclical quality characteristic of many aspects of biological systems. Despite this fact, which is well recognized even in folk psychology, we are being increasingly subjected to the machine value for unvarying peak performance. This represents an unnatural demand on all of us. Nonetheless there are certain individuals who will be especially disadvantaged by this demand. Individuals with mood disorders, even when optimally stabilized on medications, as Mary is, tend to show greater fluctuations in energy, intellectual speed, and efficiency than most persons. When given sufficient room by the environment, most individuals with mood disorders can learn to compensate for these fluctuations and be quite productive. It is noteworthy that Mary's boss was troubled by the cyclical nature of Mary's productivity rather than the overall level of it. Clearly this reveals his expectation that humans should be able to function like machines, maintaining optimal productivity in a consistent and continuous manner. Her periods of high productivity, rather than being seen as compensatory, simply served to condemn her as working below her potential the rest of the time. Individuals with affective disorders are particularly unable to approximate this machine virtue, and excessive attempts to do so are fraught with peril.

> Darryl is a 45-year-old project manager for a biotech firm. His bipolar disorder takes a different form than Mary's. He is rarely depressed and then only after bouts of full blown mania. Most of the time he is slightly hypomanic. His thoughts move fast; he is quite expansive and driven. Other than mild impatience and irritability it causes him little trouble. In fact he is extraordinarily productive, working tremendously long hours. He is a charismatic team leader, bright and creative. However, every few years there is a crescendo in his behavior and he evolves into a full-blown manic episode. Then he is unable to work and at times requires hospitalization with hallucinations and grandiose delusions. I have for years pushed Darryl to look at what is a clear pattern of progressively escalating his hours at work and overextending himself at the urging of his

supervisors from whom he receives mounting praise until he spins out of control into full mania. I, along with his very supportive wife, stress the need for balance and moderation, adequate sleep, and time for rest and relaxation as part of managing his illness. He complies for a while but is gradually seduced by the praise and rising expectations of his bosses. Even supervisors who have witnessed his manic episodes seem unable to see his increasing intensity and efficiency as problematic. Like the good machine, if he can do it now he can keep doing it and with less and less 'down time.'

Over and above appropriate pharmacological management, it is well established that behavioral strategies that stress the balanced structuring of a person's life, and most especially the avoidance of sleep deprivation, are critical to the successful management of bipolar disorder. Unfortunately even individuals who understand this well when they are in a state of normal mood tend to lose an appreciation for this need for balance as they become hypomanic. The hypomanic state is frequently so exhilarating for patients that they are unable to consider the possibility that this could in any way be bad for them. Indeed, persons such as Darryl find the machine values of constant optimal productivity quite reasonable and sensible when they are hypomanic. Hence a work environment that espouses these values is particularly difficult for such individuals.

At one level the application of machine values in the workplace appears to be simply a pragmatic exploitation of workers without regard for their welfare. It is all too easy to begin to see employers as simply coldly and insensitively willing to extract all they can from workers, allowing them to self-destruct and simply be replaced. Although this attitude does undoubtedly at times occur at the conscious level, it is most likely that the overall problem is much more insidious, and is buried in the unconscious assumptions that are becoming increasingly typical of our technological society. If that is true, one would expect to see these values being applied even in settings where there is in fact little practical economical advantage.

Monica is a 63-year-old housewife with grown children. She has a long history of recurrent major depression that has been well controlled in recent years, and, she considers herself in sustained remission. That is, she did until her husband's recent retirement. A mechanical engineer, he has been supportive and devoted to his wife and family although she has long complained that he is not the world's best communicator. He looked forward to retirement to spend more time with Monica and to visit his children and grandchildren. Shortly after retiring, however, he began to complain about what he characterized as her frequent bouts of depression and insisted she talk to me about a change in medication. She denied any sadness or dysphoria. She had a consistently good hedonic capacity. What she cited as the source of his concern was a lifelong pattern of mild fluctuations in energy and drive. She has periods lasting a few days, occurring a couple of times per month, when she is less inclined to do housework or take on projects and less inclined to go out socially. When her children were young she generally pushed herself through these times meeting her obligations.

Now she sees little reason to do so, but enjoys reading and relaxing during these periods. After a few days her energy increases and she returns to her usual activity level. She easily gets done all that she needs to and her husband has no complaints about how she cares for the house or for him. When pressed, it is the fluctuations themselves that he sees as problematic. Within couples therapy he was able to recognize how he had come to value consistency of output as an unquestioned ideal in his work life and how he unwittingly imposed it on his wife.

The above examples suggest mechanisms by which individuals with affective disorders are particularly disadvantaged in a social environment imbued with machine values. As the salience of these values increase in our society, it is likely that we are all subject to these deleterious effects, but that they impact on individuals with affective disorders sooner and more severely. This suggests another potential advantage to a strategy examining the differential impact of technology on individuals with particular variants in their cognitive, affective, and relational mode of life. In a sense they serve as canaries in the coal mine. Just as the increased sensitivity of the birds to atmospheric toxins served as a warning to the miners, the adverse impact on these individuals with affective disorders should send a warning to us all. Indeed it is not surprising that, looking through the pattern of onset and frequency of depression throughout the twentieth century, individuals born in successive decades show both an earlier age of onset and higher lifetime prevalence for depression than individuals in the decades preceding them (Klerman and Weissman 1989). It is hard to imagine that this represents any kind of true evolutionary change in the population. That would require identifying an extremely powerful environmental factor leading to progressive increases in reproductive success in individuals with affective disorders. This seems extraordinarily improbable. A much more likely explanation for the data is that society is changing in ways that progressively stress individuals carrying some genetic predisposition to affective disorders such that it is more likely to be manifested and at an earlier age.

8.5 **Discussion**

It is the goal of this discussion to illustrate the use of clinical material from the treatment of those individual variants in cognition, affect, and relating that have been identified as mental disorders in exploring the complex impact of various technologies on individual members of a society, as opposed to the global impact of technology on a society at large. The choice to look at forms of psychopathology is one of convenience given the ready availability of detailed characterization of these variants and clinical material that allows the exploration of the impact of technology on individual lives. This approach could be applied, however, equally successfully to any variation in the cognitive, affective, and interpersonal styles of individuals. The important point to note is that this sort of exploration can complement in useful ways the analysis of a more global view of technology on society. Sometimes such differential effects can constitute warning signs for possible ill effects on a more global level; namely, the canary in the coal mine phenomenon, as illustrated with affective disorders. At other times this approach can remind us that even technological change viewed as having an overall and typically adverse effect can at the same time represent distinct benefits for certain subgroups in the population. This is illustrated in the consideration of the impact of online communication in the case of AS.

In addition to its contribution at the descriptive level to characterizing the impact of technology on individuals in our society, this approach can inform certain evaluative activities as well. At the most immediately pragmatic level identifying particularly disadvantageous technological developments for particular individuals can lead to the elaboration of individually designed compensatory strategies for those persons. In the case of variants characterized as psychopathology this work often occurs in the context of clinical treatment. For other variants it could occur in other settings, such as educational ones. At a more general level of public policy, the identification of adverse impacts on subgroups of individuals can raise concern about possible negative impacts on larger groups if the technological trend is allowed to continue unopposed. In these cases, such as the intrusion of machine values into our society, more general attempts to use public policy and public forms of persuasion to reduce the negative impact would be possible. Finally the appreciation of the differential impact of technological developments on various subgroups of people can be an informative perspective on the complex problems of justice as applied to individuals with disabilities. It makes the concept of disability more fluid and context sensitive and hence may add a useful dimension to this aspect of justice (Nussbaum 2006).

The evaluative prospective is in fact quite intrinsic to this model in the sense that is best characterized as pseudo-Darwinian. Although it focuses on the variability within the population and the differential advantage and disadvantage of technological developments on those variations, it is in the realm of human flourishing that those advantages and disadvantages are defined. That eudaimonistic concept is, of course, intrinsically evaluative. This approach is fully justifiable on these terms. Over and above that, however, there may be times when the model has something to say that is truly Darwinian. This occurs in those circumstances where the differential effects on individual flourishing also have an impact on the differential reproductive success of persons.

References

Baron-Cohen S., Bolton P., Wheelwright S., *et al.* (1998). Does autism occur more often in families of physicists, engineers, and mathematicians? *Autism*, **2**, 296–301.

Dales L., Hammer S. J., and Smith N. J. (2001). Time trends in autism and MMR immunization coverage in California. *Journal of the American Medical Association*, **285** 1183–1185.

Dennett D. C. (1971). Intentional systems. *Journal of Philosophy*, **8**, 87–106.

Faraone S. V. and Biederman J. (2004). 'Neurobiology of attention deficit hyperactivity disorder' in D. S. Charney and E. J. Nestler (eds.) *Neurobiology of Mental Illness*, 2nd edn (New York: Oxford University Press), 979–999.

Gergen K. J. (1985). The social constructionist movement in modern psychology. *American Psychologist* **40**, 266–275.

Gergen K. J. (1990). Therapeutic professions and the diffusion of deficit. *Journal of Mind and Behavior*, **11**, 353–367.

Heidegger M. (1977). 'The question concerning technology' in J. G. Gray (ed.) *Martin Heidegger: Basic writings* (New York: Harper and Row), 283–318.

Kaye J. A., Melero-Montes M. M., and Jick H. (2001). Mumps, measles, and rubella vaccine and the incidence of autism recorded by general practitioners: a time-trend analysis. *British Medical Journal*, **322**, 460–463.

Klerman G. L. and Weissman M. M. (1989). Increasing rates of depression. *Journal of the American Medical Association*, **262**, 899–900.

Kulhara P. (1994) Outcome of schizophrenia: some transcultural observations with particular reference to developing countries. *European Archives of Psychiatry and Clinical Neuroscience*, **244**, 227–235.

Nussbaum MC. (2006). *Frontiers of Justice: Disability, nationality, species membership* (Boston: Belkamp).

Winner A. (2003). 'Social constructivism: opening the black box and finding it empty' in R. C. Scharff and V. Dusek (eds.) *Philosophy of Technology: The technological condition.* (Oxford: Blackwell), 233–244.

Yeargin-Allsopp M., Rice C., Karapurkar T., Doernberg N., Boyle C., and Murphy C. (2003). Prevalence of autism in a US metropolitan area. *Journal of the American Medical Association*, **289**, 49–55.

Chapter 9

Frontal fatigue: how technology may contribute to mental illness

Mark D. Rego

9.1 Introduction

I shall start with a quotation.

> ...when the environment contains distractors; when ambiguity and conflict are high; when appearance and significance are at odds; when events must be interpreted in light of contextual peculiarities; when prepotent response tendencies must be restrained for some long term purpose; when decision trees have multiple branches; and when the egocentric point of view must be transcended
>
> (Mesulam 2002)

This could easily be a description of the challenges of life in the modern world. Or perhaps it is a critique of an overly technological society, which has lost its roots of tradition and culture. To clarify let me add the beginning of the quotation,

> The manifestations of prefrontal damage become particularly prominent when...

This summarizing statement is from *Principles of Frontal Lobe Function* (Stuss and Knight 2002), an edited volume on the neurophysiology and function of the prefrontal cortex (PFC). The relationship between PFC function and the stresses of modern life is clearly suggested in this quotation. The question for this chapter is whether this relationship can be extended to elucidate an association between stress and mental disorders.

This increased prevalence of mental disorders is most often attributed to 'stress', which in turn is attributed to 'modern life.' Although these may be accurate descriptive attributions, they leave many questions open. Some that will be considered in this essay are: what is it about modern life (where time-saving, work-reducing, shortage-eliminating, and safety-providing technology are plentiful) that is stressful? What is it that is being stressed? Finally, what is it about stress that may contribute to the development of mental illness?

In this chapter I will approach these questions by substituting proxies for modernity on the one hand, and stress vulnerability and consequent mental disorder on the other. These are, respectively, technology and the functions and dysfunctions of the human prefrontal cortex.

Much of what we call modernity can be traced to advances in technology. The result of these advances, however, has placed increasing and, I will argue, different types of stress on individuals than during previous eras. Briefly, technology has detached us from the immediate demands and constraints of our environment and culture. These needs can be mundane such as what to wear and eat each day, or they can be complex, such as how we define ourselves in various roles (e.g., gender, age, ethnicity, social and work roles).

This detachment, though liberating in many ways, puts new demands on the individual. By cutting off the demands and constraints of the environment and culture technology also cuts us off from a wellspring of information about the world and ourselves. The modern individual is then left to constantly redefine, reformat, and reconstruct who they are and how they live their life.

The work of this constant restructuring falls predominantly on the very advanced human capacities of prefrontal cortical function (as does the building a technological society in the first place. This reciprocity will have important implications in this discussion). The PFC and its attendant functions is the area of higher human function, other than language, which is vastly advanced over primates. A brief review of PFC function will be given with an emphasis on its ability to create and integrate multiple layers of symbolic representation (Mesulam 2002). In addition, the near-ubiquitous role of the PFC in psychopathology will be reviewed.

Finally a relationship will be proposed between the detachment from environmental and cultural information afforded by technology and the pressures upon the individual to use the PFC to reconstitute this needed information. The resulting 'frontal fatigue' will be proposed as a mechanism of stress that may produce or exacerbate mental disorders. Potential mediating mechanisms will also be discussed.

9.2 **Mental illness**

I shall begin with some observations about the problems of mental illness and our current era. It is a common and empirically supported assumption that the incidence of common mental disorders is increasing (Klerman and Weissman 1989; Fombonne 1994, 1998). Various studies have the documented the increased incidence and prevalence over the course of the twentieth century. Some associated factors such as urbanization (Bocker Pedersen *et al.* 2001; Peen 1997; Sundquist *et al.* 2004) and migration (Cantor-Graae and Selten 2005) to industrialized societies and earlier age of onset of illness through the course of the twentieth century have been consistently associated with these increases. In addition, previously small areas of concern have blossomed into epidemics of clinical and scholarly activity over the past generation. These include eating disorders, attention-deficit disorder and pervasive developmental disorder.

Although there may be many contributing factors such as increased awareness among treators and the public, as well as increased availability and promotion of biological therapies, most epidemiologists believe the increases noted to be, at least in part, independent of these factors. The 'true' increase is then commonly attributed to various forms of 'stress', which in turn are attributed to different dimensions of 'modern life.'

The solutions to debates about and delineations of stress and modernity are no doubt complex and cannot be shouldered by one perspective. Various psychological, social, and philosophical explanations have been have been recently put forth in attempts to conceptually accommodate these changes in society and perhaps offer solutions (Arendt 1958; Borgman 1984; Easterbrook 2003; Honorés 2004; Lane 2000; Schwartz 2004; Sennett 1998). My approach will be narrower but will, I hope, be more generally applicable to other perspectives.

To forge some explanatory connection between modernism and mental disorder I shall narrow the field of consideration by using proxies for both areas. For modernism I will substitute technology; and for mental disorder I will substitute the function and dysfunction of the human PFC.

9.3 **The human prefrontal cortex**

The human PFC is the most recently evolved part of the human brain and, with language, stands greatly superior in its capacities to all other animals. It is only the past three decades that much of the function of the PFC has become known. In general the PFC receives information from all sensory and motor structures of the body, as well as limbic input of affective and recalled information. The PFC does not contain the sites of sensory perception, motor perception or control, affect, or memory. Rather, it integrates these sources of experience and information to form representations and conscious states that guide action, intent, and interpretation. Rather than focus on the anatomical structure of the PFC, I shall concentrate on functional characteristics. This large part of the neocortex is organized in various schemes.

Schemes that emphasize the integrative functions of the PFC, such as that described immediately below, generally mirror anatomy (Mesulam 2002). More complex schemes, which describe higher, more abstract functions, do not reflect anatomy but give a more explanatory psychological perspective on

PFC function (an example of this follows further below). A standard integrative scheme is as follows:

- Primary sensorimotor: provides the integration of perceptual and proprioceptive information to create an interface with the physical environment.
- Unimodal: receives input from individual perceptual organs and performs the necessary integration to create percepts.
- Hetermodal: receives input from all perceptual organs to provide fuller representations of the environment as generally experienced in consciousness.
- Paralimbic: has no external input at all, connects PFC to limbic areas of affect and memory.
- Limbic: regulation of the internal milieu of the CNS.

The unimodal, heteromodal, and paralimbic are the three modules of function that form the interface between the external world, previous experience and consciousness. When we speak of the more psychological aspects of the PFC, we are speaking almost entirely of the paralimbic and heteromodal areas.

However, the PFC is not merely like a sophisticated digital device, which puts together large amounts of divergent data to create impressive images. Rather, it takes the data and in an iterative manner constantly recontextualizes it to reach more and more subtle and complex pictures, plans, and understanding to follow the shifting needs and perspectives of the individual. To better explicate this it is necessary to describe the more abstract psychological functions of the PFC. To do this I shall describe the basic capacities afforded by the PFC and then elaborate the higher functions built upon them.

The three basic functions of the PFC are: selective focus on a one or several stimuli with the intentional exclusion of others (i.e., concentration); the formation of symbolic representations from integrated data; and the flexible manipulation of these symbols in working memory into novel patters of thought and effectively executed action. These functions are the basis for what is commonly referred to as executive function. They are experienced by most people as the ability to concentrate, formulate a problem, conceptualize alternatives, and execute them in an efficient fashion. Attention-deficit disorder is the paradigmatic disorder of the PFC, but PFC dysfunction is ubiquitous in psychiatric disorders as well as in common experience. We have all experienced the breakdown of these capacities in times of fatigue, stress, or emotional upheaval (e.g., indeciciveness, difficulty following a conversation, poor concentration, deficient immediate memory, and losing a train of thought are common examples).

With these capacities in mind, we can construct a hierarchy of abilities that more clearly illustrate the full range of the PFC. In essence, these constitute the human capacities to refrain from a default mode of function (i.e., that which would link a stimulus to some automatic, instinctual or impulsive response) (Mesulam 2002).

- The constraint of distractibility, perseveration and disinhibition. The limitation of these types of response allows time to consider and execute action (or not).
- The ability to approach and tolerate novelty, uncertainty and choice. Novelty seeking and playfulness increase up the phylogenic tree and decrease in a given individual as a task becomes more familiar. This function demands the ability to withhold a response, tolerate the unfamiliar and even enter into it to explore possibilities.
- The affective emotional coloring of action. By integrating past and present experience we are not left with actions that are preordained by immediate limbic imperatives.
- Significance, context and ambiguity. A situation may demand subtle differences in interpretation and thus demands a high degree of integration with context to ascertain its significance. People with PFC damage often lose the 'gist.'
- The ability to switch perspectives and to maintain mental relativism. The ability to assess a situation from other vantages including other minds. Without this capacity it is difficult to maintain or develop mature judgment, interpersonal skills and empathy.

There are two final points to be made about the PFC. First, it is not a stress-response organ. The PFC disengages in times of stress. Cogitating and planning are shifted to other cortical areas or dimensions of experience during times of stress. Researchers have been able to observe the behavioral manifestations of the breakdown of PFC function under stress in animals and to describe some of the physiological mechanisms of this disengagement (Arnsten 2002). Again there is a common experience of this phenomenon in which we find ourselves unable to concentrate, find the right words, or execute multi-step or complex tasks while under stress, unduly fatigued or overwhelmed.

Lastly, the PFC has been almost universally implicated in every imaging and structural study of the common psychopathologies. It is now assumed that dysfunction of frontal–subcortical circuits are integral to the development of common axis I pathologies (Akiyoshi *et al.* 2003; Blumberg *et al.* 2003; Cavallaro *et al.* 2003; Cummings 1993; Baving *et al.* 2002; Mayberg 2002; Powell 1995; Soares 2003; Moritz *et al.* 2002; Ursu *et al.* 2003; Voeller 2001;

Zubieta *et al.* 2003) (It is notable in this regard that the PFC is the only brain area that when lesioned produces change of function—changes that are reminiscent of psychopathology—rather than wholesale loss of function.) This does not suggest that the PFC is the sole locale of psychopathology; nor that there is some central root to all disorders (making for a unitary disorder unsupported by current knowledge). It merely locates within the PFC some core aspects and/or connections necessary for the development of axis I disorders. (Speculations about the nature of these and their relationship to normative function are at the end of this essay.)

9.4 **Technology**

Generally speaking, technology frees us from the boundaries of environmental and cultural conditions. In most developed countries, a person can survive with very little attention paid to the physical environment. Environmental relationships (and therefore constraints) such as that between time and space are largely loosened. Fast travel, cellular phones, and email have, for example, recently severed many of these time–space connections (e.g., distance does not dictate time needed to communicate). These loosening of constraints have greatly impacted the influence of accidents of birth such as gender, physical size, and disability, as well as accidents of nature such as abundance and shortage.

In addition, cultural prescriptions and proscriptions on matters such as what to eat and what role to play in society no longer require consultation before venturing out in the world.

There are certainly other factors responsible for what we may now call modernism. Along with technology, developments in the politics of civil society figure chiefly in these changes. It can be said though that technology has contributed not only in the ease and efficiency it has brought to modern life, but has facilitated these other social and political developments. (This is largely indirect by removing barriers erected by accidents of birth such as physical capacities and locale, and by making cultural assumptions about the significance of race, gender, and so on untenable.) As there have been many philosophical perspectives elaborated to explore aspects of technology, I will not review them here. Rather, I shall borrow from several, most notably Albert Borgman's, device paradigms.

As Borgman (1984; see also Tijmes 1999) describes it, the hurdles described above have been surmounted by the use of devices. Devices have the character of separating means from ends. They are developed with only ends in mind and therefore do not embody the problem they solve nor do they generally follow the linguistic and symbolic traditions of a culture. The classic example given by Borgman is acquiring water from a well as opposed to a spigot. In the case of the well, the person getting the water is familiar and has direct contact with the mechanics of the pail and the pulley as well as knowledge of the condition of the well itself. When turning on a spigot most of us have little idea how the whole thing works and little knowledge about the condition of the water supply. The end of getting water and the means of going about it have been officially severed.

In this sense, modern technology does not reveal itself in the way things like wells do. Devices are not imbedded in the physicality of the environment, but rather exist self-referentially in the world of other similar devices. Will archeologists in distant millennia know what we did with the carburetors, motherboards, and under-arm deodorant they dig up from our long forgotten cities? (Most people alive today depend these three items daily but do not know what the first two do or how the third does its job.) Information technology has only expanded this abyss.

Although devices have created a world in which physical needs and the limitations of our constitutions can be partly surmounted, it has done so by disengaging us not only from the physical environment but also from previous sources of information about ourselves and our worlds. By extending into the realm of limitations dictated by roles, gender, size, physical ability, age, language, and so on, devices have also disconnected us from cultural sources of information that would previously guide self-understanding and the many plans that make up a life.

Where you lived, your age and gender, your station in society, your culture and language, down to the materials and recipes of daily living, have for most of human history provided the mental, interpersonal, and societal structures that organize our lives. Technology, through its direct effects and its indirect contribution to social reform, has made these structures increasingly obsolete. Although most, including me, applaud these changes; they have come with new demands.

Freedom from all the above predefined roles and limitations has brought about the need to choose what was previously given. These choices include things like how and what we should eat; how to insure the health and safety of our bodies; how to parent, love, befriend, and partner; how to relax and be entertained; how to choose forms of energy for heat and light; how to get from one place to another; how to appear; how and whether to worship; and finally, just how to be. We even must choose how to get information and thus how to choose. (Schwartz 2004) This list is obviously abbreviated. It is important to note that these choices may be quotidian, life encompassing and everywhere between.

A technological society also maintains a pressure to continually choose by offering multiple alternatives, marketing to attract consumer favor and influence values about choices, and by emphasizing the maximization of choices by producing technology that is ever more efficient.

As an example I offer a day in the life of a middle-aged psychiatrist, who has benefited greatly from and exploits the advantages of technology. I awaken early to exercise, as my sedentary life style afforded by an advanced technological society leaves no protection from rapid physical decline. This is made more complicated by some physical injuries—due to weaknesses generated by dependence on effort-saving technology—that have moved me through various forms of exercise and special exercise machines to one that seems to fit the bill. For now, I then eat a carefully chosen breakfast as the surplus of food provided by technology has made my past eating habits unwise. I check my email (this speaks for itself), read two newspapers—one a national paper published in another state, drive one mile to my office in my very safe car which I felt compelled to purchase even though I did not need to, but because the new safety features were quite advanced. There, as I see patients and return calls, I must re-prioritize my day countless times to accommodate the incoming flux of information and problems. I will glance at the medical journals in the day's mail to see what I need to learn to maintain good care and then answer more emails. I will troubleshoot insurance (born of a system that is immensely complex and bears no resemblance to the act of being paid for my services) and office problems, many of which are essentially computer problems. I pick up my daughter and shuttle her around to dance class and help her with homework (now done on the computer). I take stock of how tired I am to plan the night, part of which will likely include thinking about the day. I will think about the way I manage my many roles and whether or not it is in need of rethinking. I catch up with my wife about her day and may work on training the new voice-recognition program I have for my computer so that I can avoid the task of typing this paper, which I did not do because I was too busy. To avoid more work I will call someone far away on my cell phone as it is free after 8:00p.m. Finally I may browse my 144 channels of digital cable and on-demand movies, and unable to decide on what to watch I will read a book and fall asleep (and if not, take a pill). This is also an abbreviated list.

In the face of this cacophony of choices I shall attempt to distill out some basic demands placed upon us by a technological society. The first is complexity. Within our vast array of choices, there is much to keep track of, organize, scrutinize, and organize again. I call this the number-of moving-parts problem. There are just too many of everything.

The second demand is that of the conceptual or abstract nature of the environment in which we interact. As Borgman points out, the means are now somewhat independent of the ends and the technology is not self-revealing. We must abstract out the nature of these systems and choices before they are useful to us. (A bucket declares itself without hesitation; while visiting a friend recently, I had to confess after thirty minutes' effort that I could not get the shower to work.)

Lastly is the demand of reformatting. Amid the number of choices and their increasingly abstract nature is the constant updating of information, systems, tasks, goals, roles, identities, and so on. Again, these mental gymnastics are both quotidian and ongoing projects of lifelong significance.

These very demands push society to create solutions, solutions that organize and streamline choice, further conceptualize abstract ideas and help in reformatting all that this implies. The solutions, as can be seen by this description, are likely to be more technology. They demand more of the same.

The triad of complexity, abstractness, and reformatting describes not only the demands of a technological society but also the function of the PFC. A quick review of the functions of the PFC shows that maintaining working memory of various objects of consciousness, abstracting, and integrating different sources of information to create new representations (e.g., goals, plans, roles) and manipulating multiple symbols in memory into new combinations to circumvent prescribed paths or invent ones is exactly what the PFC does *and* exactly what technology demands.

9.5 **Prefrontal cortex and the world**

This similarity is, I think, not coincidental. As we have exploited our powerful PFCs to solve problems, we have also imposed the PFC upon our world. The devices we create more and more mirror PFC function, place demands on the PFC, create PFC-like solutions to previous demands, and on and on. We are not only increasingly cut off from environmental and cultural sources of experience, but we are creating a world that mimics the way in which we conquer its limitations.

Here we can begin to sense the stress building as our minds are cut off from non-technological and less PFC-intensive sources of experience. It is intuitive to say we simply are not built that way and will begin to feel the strain. However, are there more specific things that can be said about the ways in which this stress may manifest? Why would our brains not like a world fashioned after its highest function? I will propose two answers here that, although theoretical, are grounded in established understanding of PFC function.

The first is the observation mentioned earlier that the PFC is not a stress organ. When stressed, the PFC is largely diminished in its capacities to mediate responses. Yet the solutions to stress are more and more PFC based; more choices, more complexity, more abstractness, and more reformatting. This would seem to defeat some of the ways we are inherently equipped to cope with stress (e.g., interpersonal support, the structure of tradition and the fatalistic luxury of having *no* choice). By altering the world along PFC lines we are also altering and limiting our abilities to respond to stress.

Second, if the PFC is being taxed, it is reasonable to conclude that vulnerabilities within the PFC may begin to manifest as significant deficits. As stated above, the PFC has been found to be ubiquitously associated (most clearly with functional magnetic resonance imaging in recent years) with all major psychiatric disorders. The stress of inherent vulnerabilities is easily observable in schizophrenia and attention-deficit disorder. A stress–diathesis model, like that used by most clinicians and researchers, would also be predicted by this conceptualization of PFC attempts at adaptation. In such a model the classical and ever more complicated nature–nurture is not replaced by a stress-PFC model, but made more specific and explanatory. The 'nature' in this more specific model is the psychophysiology of the PFC (and its probable undergirding of the normative functions that go awry in most psychopathology); whereas the 'nurture' is the PFC-like, abstract technological world we are building. Pathology results when excesses and consequent limitations of the latter impact the range of responses from the ever more isolated former.

9.6 **Further thoughts**

I close with two theoretical descriptive mechanisms by which the taxation of the PFC may lead to mental disorders. I have already mentioned the central role of the PFC in the development and maintenance of psychiatric disorders. Taking this empirical finding as a foundational point of departure for both a biological and a philosophical perspective, I shall theoretically explore the breakdown of the structure of consciousness, which is key to the development of mental disorders.

Biologically speaking, the PFC is highly integrated with all other aspects of the neocortex and subcortical areas. Most of these connections are bidirectional. Our normal experiences in consciousness contain within them a sense of fit between the object of consciousness and our experience of it. I see what I assume I am looking at, I feel what I touch, I am saddened by what, in my world, seems sad. I call this the intentional fit of experience. It is not the result of reason or inference. Rather, it is intuitive: the *feel* of experience.

A perceptual experience that seems anomalous immediately strikes us as out of place. 'Did I really see that mouse out of the corner of my eye?' we might ask ourselves. Similarly, psychiatric patients, upon deeper discussion will usually describe a sense that what they think or feel is not quite right. A person may state the he is aware that his sadness does not seem to fit his life. Even people with auditory hallucinations will often be aware that these are 'voices' and not actual people. We may refer to this as insight, but I think it is insight of a different kind. It is awareness of the loss of fit in the intentionality of the experience. Realizations of these discordances may be viewed as an underpinning for the efficacy of cognitive therapy (i.e., noticing 'irrational' or automatic thoughts may be taking note of this intuitive lack of intentional fit, rather than pure reason itself). This will obviously vary from one modality to another, among individuals and among disorders, but nonetheless there remains a sense of a natural connection between the object of consciousness and consciousness itself.

What I propose here is that normal dependence of the PFC upon other areas of experience (i.e., cortical and subcortical input) creates intentional constraints upon the ways in which it can represent the world. The result of such constraints is an intuitive sense of fit between what is in consciousness and what is real. These areas of input are mostly affective experience (past and present) and episodic memory, but of a highly organized and refined kind. They are experiences and interpretations of being in the world. The physicality of the environment (and its consequent meaningfulness and ability to reveal itself) and cultural experience that brings with it large degrees of interpretive power stand out most here. When these inputs are cut off by our growing dependence on a technological-PFC world, the normal intentional constraints are lost or weakened. The mind, unable to make sense of its own experience of the world, now turns inward towards the powerful PFC to solve the problem (Arendt 1958). It feels sad, finds no intentional fit for the feeling (owing to the loss of input or interpretive power from physicality and culture), and looks for objects of its sadness; it is anxious and follows suit. Such new objects will also not be a product of inference, and although containing personal qualities, will reflect structures available to the PFC. Similar cases can be made for the normative neuropsychology of the sense of completeness and the development of compulsions (Fear and Healy 1997; Ursu *et al.* 2003) as well as an overly sensitive process of conclusion formation and a propensity to delusions (Colbert and Peters 2002; Dudley and Over 2003).

The second theoretical mechanism here is philosophical and suggests that the folding in of the PFC onto itself creates a certain kind of anxiety that is new to our era. The existentialists have long warned us of the despair or nihilism resulting from a world in which we are alone and without meaning. A world built by, for, and similar to the PFC creates a world that is a step beyond this. It is a world without a world. The mind is alone and in need of creating a world for itself. This type of anxiety transcends loneliness and may be the propel us beyond the grasp of more technology and more PFC function toward a replacement of meaning not with meaninglessness, but with confusion; despair with a desperation to act or reach a conclusion that has no place to begin.

References

Akiyoshi J. *et al.* (2003). Frontal brain hypoactivity as a biological subsrtate of anxiety in patients with panic disorder. *Neuropsychobiology*, **47**, 165–170.

Arendt H. (1958). 'The vita activa and the modern age' in H. Arendt (ed.) *The Human Condition* (Chicago: The University of Chicago Press), 329.

Arnsten A. F. T. (2002). 'Neurochemical modulation of prefrontal cortex and functional observations' in D. T. Stuss and R. T. Knight (eds.) *Principles of Frontal Lobe Function* (Oxford: Oxford University Press), 51–84.

Baving L. *et al.* (2002). Frontal brain activation in anxious school children. *Journal of Child Psychology and Psychiatry and Allied Disciplines*, **43**, 265–274.

Blumberg H. P., *et al.* (2003). Frontostriatal abnormalities in adolescents with bipolar disorder: preliminary observations from functional MRI. *American Journal of Psychiatry*, **160**, 1345–1347.

Bocker Pedersen C. and Mortensen P. B. (2001). Evidence of a dose–response relationship between urbanicity during upbringing and schizophrenia risk. *Archives of General Psychiatry*, **58**, 1039–1046.

Borgman A. (1984). *Technology and the Character of Contemporary Life*. (University of Chicago Press, Chicago).

Cantor-Graae E. and Selten J.-P. (2005). Schizophrenia and migration: a meta-analysis and review. *American Journal of Psychiatry*, **162**, 12–24.

Cavallaro R. *et al.* (2003). Basal corticofrontal circuits in schizophrenia and obsessive–compulsive disorder: a controlled, double dissociation study. *Biological Psychiatry*, **54**, 437–443.

Colbert S. M. and Peters E. R. (2002). Need for closure and jumping-to-conclusions in delusion-prone individuals. *Journal of Nervous and Mental Disease*, **190**, 27–31.

Cummings J. L. (1993). Frontal–subcortical circuits and human behavior. *Archives of Neurology*, **50**, 873–880.

Dudley R. E. J. and Over D. E. (2003). People with delusions jump to conclusions: a theoretical account of research findings on the reasoning of people with delusions. *Clinical Psychology and Psychotherapy*, **10**, 263–274.

Easterbrook G. (2003). *The Progress Paradox* (New York: Random House).

Fear C. F. and Healy D. (1997). Probabilistic reasoning in obsessive–compulsive disorder and delusional disorders. *Psychological Medicine*, **27**, 199–208.

Fombonne E. (1994). Increased rates of depression: update of epidemiological findings and analytical probelms. *Acta Psychiatrica Scandinavica*, **90**, 145–156.

Fombonne E. (1998). Increased rates of psychosocial disorders in youth. *European Archives of Psychiatry and Neuroscience*, **248**, 14–21.

Honoré C. (2004). *In praise of slowness. How a worldwide movement is challanging the cult of speed.* Harper, San Francisco and New York.

Klerman G. L. and Weissman M. M. (1989). Increasing rates of depression. *Journal of the American Medical Association*, **261**, 2229–2235.

Lane R. L. (2000). *The Loss of Happiness in Market Economies* (New Haven: Yale University Press).

Mayberg H. S. (2002). 'Mapping mood: an evolving emphasis on frontal–limbic interactions' in D. T. Stuss and R. T. Knight (eds.) *Principles of Frontal Lobe Function* (Oxford: Oxford University Press), 376–391.

Mesulam M. M. (2002). 'The human frontal lobes: transcending the default mode through contingent encoding' in D. T. Stuss and R. T. Knight (eds.) *Principles of Frontal Lobe Function* (Oxford: Oxford University Press), 8–31.

Moritz S. *et al.* (2002). Executive functioning in obsessive–compulsive disorder, unipolar depression and schizophrenia. *Archives of Clinical Neuropsychology*, **17**, 477–483.

Peen J. D. (1997). Admission rates for schizophrenia in the Netherlands: an urban/rural comparison. *Acta Psychiatrica Scandinavica*, **96**, 301–305.

Powell K. B. (1995). Frontal lobe dysfunction in affective disorders. *Clinical Psychology Review*, **14**, 525–546.

Schwartz B. (2004). *The Paradox of Choice. Why more is less* (New York: Harper Collins).

Sennett R. (1998). *The Corrosion of Character. Personal consequences of work in the new capitalism* (New York: W. W. Norton & Company).

Soares J. C. (2003). Contributions from brain imaging to the elucidation pathophysiology of bipolar disorder. *International Journal of Neuropsychopharmacology*, **6**, 171–180.

Stuss D. T. and Knight R. T. (eds.) (2002). *Principles of Frontal Lobe Function* (Oxford: Oxford University Press).

Sundquist K. *et al.* (2004). Urbanisation and incidence of psychosis and depression. Follow-up study of 4.4 million women and men in Sweden. *British Journal of Psychiatry*, **184**, 293–299.

Tijmes P. (1999). 'Albert Borgman: technology and the character of everyday life' in H. Achterhuis (ed.) *American Philosophy of Technology. The empirical turn* (Bloomington: Indiana University Press), 11–36.

Ursu S. *et al.* (2003). Overactive action monitoring in obsessive–compulsive disorder: evidence from functional magnetic resonance imaging. *Psychological Science*, **14**, 347–353.

Voeller K. S. (2001). 'Attention-deficit/hyperactivity disorder as a frontal–subcortical disorder' in D. G. Lichter (ed.) *Frontal–Subcortical Circuits in Psychiatric and Neurological Disorders* (New York: Guilford Press), 334–371.

Zubieta J.-K. *et al.* (2003). Regulation of human affective responses by anterior cingulate and limbic μ-opiod neurotransmission. *Archives of General Psychiatry*, **60**, 1145–1157.

Chapter 10

Bored to tears? Depression and Heidegger's concept of profound boredom: a postpsychiatry contribution

Phillip Sinaikin

10.1 Introduction

In their recently published book, *Postpsychiatry*, clinical psychiatrists Patrick Bracken and Philip Thomas (Bracken and Thomas 2005) characterize academic psychiatry at the end of the twentieth century as firmly rooted in a reductionistic model of the human mind and its aberrations in 'madness and distress'. This has resulted in a technological framing of emotional and cognitive problems as decontextualized clusters of symptoms arising from causal biological processes that can be scientifically studied and manipulated. This biopsychiatric approach has allowed for a consolidation of power and authority in the medical psychiatric profession and, to its legions of zealous supporters, has allegedly brought scientific 'objectivity' and technologically grounded progress to this formerly floundering medical specialty. As practicing clinicians, however, Bracken and Thomas find that 'reductionistic approaches cannot account for the sort of problems we encounter in our day-to-day practice'. In particular, they say, the focus on decontextualized clusters of symptoms minimizes or ignores the central role played by meanings, values, and context in human emotional life and distress. They therefore propose an alternative, a 'postpsychiatry', grounded in a postmodern hermeneutic that assigns central importance to a recognition of the validity of multiple perspectives, to meaning as a primary human reality not reducible to causal explanation and to the bodily, temporal and cultural context of presentations of madness and emotional distress. To establish a foundation for their proposed 'hermeneutics of distress' they turn to the philosophy of Martin Heidegger.

Heidegger has famously expressed deep concern about the role of technology in modern life (Heidegger 1971). He defines the current epoch of man's existence as '*Gestell*', which is usually translated as a particular kind of 'enframing' of reality in which the dictates of utility, order, control and efficiency (what he calls the technological attitude) surmount all other concerns. As Lovitt puts it, 'Technology treats everything with 'objectivity'. The modern technologist is regularly expected, and expects himself, to be able to impose order on all data, to 'process' every sort of entity, nonhuman and human alike, and to devise solutions for every kind of problem. He is forever getting things under control' (Heidegger 1971: xxvii). Although Heidegger expresses grave concern about the dehumanizing impact of *Gestell*, modern biopsychiatry, with its singular focus on order, efficiency and control in its diagnostic and treatment practices, could be said to embody it. In this paper I will examine how the hegemony of biopsychiatry is not only dehumanizing but is also increasingly creating practical, logical and moral dilemmas and roadblocks for both providers and users in everyday clinical practice. To illustrate this I will examine the recently published results of the STAR*D study of the pharmacological treatment of major depression. I will then offer a radically contrasting conceptualization of major depression interpreted as a manifestation of an encounter with the Heideggerian primordial mood of profound boredom.

10.2 **State-of-the-art biopsychiatry 2006**

Academic psychiatry is currently running a multicenter trial funded by the National Institute of Mental Health (NIMH) of antidepressant treatment of depression called the STAR*D, an acronym for Sequenced Treatment Alternatives to Relieve Depression (NIMH press releases 2006). There are 2,876 participants in 23 psychiatric and 18 primary care treatment sites. The cost of the study is estimated to be around $35 million. STAR*D promotes itself as devoted to the goal of developing a definitive algorithm for the medical treatment of all cases of depression, including so-called 'treatment resistant' depression, through a logical sequencing of medication and augmentation strategies. This algorithm is desperately needed by many psychiatrists and other physicians whose sole method of treatment for depression is to prescribe antidepressants and find themselves faced by case after case of partial responders, non-responders, and previous responders whose medication has 'stopped working'. The study further touts its clinical relevance because of its real-world setting in medical clinics and doctor's offices, and the inclusion of a broader array of complicating variables such as substance abuse and concurrent psychiatric disorders.

Results for all four phases of the study have been published. Because efficacy studies of antidepressants and treatment strategies for resistant cases have been the topic of innumerable publications during the past twenty years, the

STAR*D study allows an opportunity to assess how far biopsychiatry has truly progressed in that time in developing more reliable and effective diagnostic and treatment strategies for the providers and users of mental healthcare.

In STAR*D, subjects were selected on the basis of scoring 'high enough on a standard depression rating scale to be diagnosed with major depression'. In phase one all subjects were treated for 12 to 14 weeks with the selective serotonin reuptake inhibitor (SSRI) Citalopram, with dosage adjustments made if indicated. Clinical data were obtained by interview, rating scales, and (symbolic of just how deeply the technological attitude has taken hold in biopsychiatry) by automated phone questionnaires. As if further evidence were needed that this type of study is dehumanizing, A. John Rush, the principal investigator in STAR*D, has been quoted as saying that patient self-reports about whether they feel better on antidepressants cannot be trusted because they 'are not going to be accurate' and that patients 'cannot be precise' (MacNeil 2006: 7). There is no placebo group in this study design. The desired endpoint is identified as remission, defined as 'virtually free of all symptoms of depression'. For those who do not achieve remission, various options are available in phases two and three and beyond for augmenting or changing treatment.

In phase one it has been reported that about 30 per cent of the subjects achieved remission. In phase two, of the 70 per cent of patients who did not achieve remission in phase one, 575 subjects elected to drop out of the study. Of the 1,438 subjects left, about 25 per cent of those who chose to switch antidepressants were symptom free at the end of another 14 weeks whereas 30 per cent who opted for augmentation recovered in the same time frame. Much to the chagrin of clinicians (and eagerly waiting pharmaceutical companies), no particular pharmacologic agent or augmentation strategy separated out as superior to others in the phase two data. In phase three a new set of somatic treatment options are tried on those subjects who did not get well in phases one or two. A much larger percentage of remaining subjects dropped out of the study between phases two and three. Of the 1,006 non-responders from phase two, only 376 elected to enter phase three. So 630 subjects had dropped out, which was probably a good decision because only about 15 per cent of phase three subjects achieved remission. Finally, of the 319 hearty souls who still did not get better in phase three, only 108 elected to go on to phase four where they were treated to a drug cocktail of Effexor and Remeron or treated with the MAO inhibitor tranylcypramine. Although receiving little focal attention from the researchers, it has also been reported that in analyzing phase one data it was observed that 'being well educated, employed, married, white, and female, with fewer complicating problems, were factors associated with a better antidepressant response' (NIMH press release, 1 January 2006).

So what do the users and providers of mental healthcare (and the taxpayers who funded the study) get out of this $35 million, often labeled 'landmark', study? They found out that in a non-placebo controlled study over the course of nearly a year around 50 per cent of compliant and cooperative patients get better. I am not sure what the lesson is, but we have also learned that, at least in this case, the longer the study the higher the percentage of drop-outs at each choice point. However, from my perspective as a veteran practicing clinician, I can answer what I learned in one word: nothing! There is absolutely nothing in this study about diagnosis or treatment that teaches me something that I did not already know or have not seen written about for years. Put into simple terms, STAR*D is, in essence, recommending that clinicians should diagnose major depression by using standardized criteria (or better yet, rating scales), initiate treatment with an antidepressant, and if that does not work raise the dose, try a different medication, or try an augmentation strategy; it does not matter which option is chosen, they all have an equal chance of working, or not.

The next obvious question from the medication-oriented clinician looking for guidance from academic psychiatry is what to do after all reasonable medication trials and augmentation strategies fail? Should the case be re-formulated into a psychodynamic, interpersonal, cultural, or spiritual problem with a radical shift in treatment recommendations? Those who understand how dominant the biopsychiatric discourse has become know that this is not going to be the answer. More likely will be a recommendation to either re-diagnose the patient (it is currently very common to see non-responsive depressed patients re-diagnosed as bipolar) or to turn to 'state-of-the-art' technology and the growing number of machines and devices being used to stimulate brain activity. Although not a new technology, electroconvulsive therapy (ECT) has been enjoying a revival in popularity. Repetitive transcranial magnetic stimulation (rTMS) involves passing strong magnetic pulses through the brain. This procedure has not yet been approved in the USA but is available in Canada. Finally, there has been Food and Drug Administration (FDA) approval granted to an invasive surgical procedure for treatment resistant depression. It is called vagal nerve stimulation (VNS) and involves the surgical implant of a pacemaker under the skin on the chest wall that is then connected by a wire to the vagus nerve in the neck to send electrical signals directly into the brain. The 'psychiatrist' (if it is still appropriate to use that label) must then make frequent adjustments to the pacemaker, (a 'billable procedure' my sales representative tells me), titrating side effects (such as hoarseness, change in voice, coughing, and neck pain) against clinical benefits, often felt only after many months of treatment (Splete 2005).

10.3 The hegemony of biopsychiatry

The dilemma that I, my fellow clinicians, and all users of mental healthcare face is clearly rooted in the singular dominance of the medical model in psychiatry. A medical model by definition requires starting with a definitive diagnosis that then predicts the course of the illness and guides its treatment. Critics of biopsychiatry rightly argue that human emotional distress is simply too complex and multilayered a phenomenon to yield to a simplistic symptom checklist method of diagnosis. Most locate the genesis of the hegemony of biopsychiatry in American (and world) psychiatry as the development and unrelenting promotion of the symptom based, allegedly 'value-neutral' and 'atheoretical' diagnostic system in the Diagnostic and Statistical Manual of the American Psychiatry Association, Third Edition (DSM III). Expanding on Kutchins and Kirk's scathing critique of DSM (Kutchins and Kirk 1997), Lewis characterizes the DSM diagnostic model as bad science whose influence is spread by bad rhetoric motivated by bad politics (Lewis 2006). I will use this same format to evaluate why STAR*D similarly fails to offer any definitive direction or help to those suffering from emotional distress or to the clinicians trying to help them.

10.4 Bad science

Despite the long list of distinguished academic psychiatrists who designed the study, STAR*D is clearly bad science. Leaving aside the yet unresolved, overarching question of the validity of psychiatric diagnoses, STAR*D is bad science on many other levels. For example, having no placebo group in the study falsely skews any positive results in favor of drug treatment. Most antidepressant studies show placebo response rates in the 20–40 per cent range (Fink 2006). In many antidepressant studies, medication response is no better or barely better than placebo. There is a growing literature questioning the overall legitimacy of antidepressants based on their characteristically narrow margins of separation from placebo (Greenberg and Fisher 1997). That there was no placebo group in the STAR*D study allowed this extremely problematic issue to essentially be ignored.

A second element of bad science in the STAR*D study is the lack of acknowledgement of even the possibility of a spontaneous recovery or personal growth accounting for the improved rating scores in at least some of the study subjects who achieved remission. It has always been a source of amazement to me how the rating scales and diagnostic criteria for depression are so disconnected from everyday lived experience. I have yet to see a rating scale inquiring whether someone who is displaying signs and symptoms of depression has or has not broken up with a girlfriend/wife/boyfriend/husband/lover in the recent past. Nor does any scale inquire whether a remission of depression coincided with a reconciliation of the relationship. This is just one of an infinite number of environmental, psychosocial, and cultural variables that affect moods in living humans. The idea in STAR*D that the only variable that could possibly account for remission of depression is medication is not only another example of bad science but highlights how the authors openly ignore their own data that antidepressant response is positively correlated with education, marital status, employment, race, and 'fewer complicating problems'!

10.5 **Bad rhetoric**

It has been said we live in the era of spin. What kind of spin or rhetoric can be attached to a $35 million study that essentially resulted in outcomes not much better than placebo and completely failed in its goal to formulate a rational sequential treatment strategy for medication non-responders? The following are some quotes from the NIMH newsletters released to report the results of STAR*D. (I have italicized the rhetorical terms.)

> These trials match the NIMH *vision* of developing *personalized care.*
> (Dr Thomas Insel, head of NIMH, quoted in 1 January 2006 NIMH newsletter.)
>
> These findings provide important treatment options to mental health clinicians and *millions of Americans who struggle* with treatment resistant depression.
> (NIH director Elias A. Zerhoun quoted in 23 March 2006 NIMH newsletter.)
>
> STAR*D continues to provide valuable real-world information about treating depression. Not only are the results *enlightening,* but they are telling us that more research is needed to help people with this *debilitating illness,* especially those who have tried several treatments and the treatments have failed.
> (Dr Thomas Insel, quoted in 6 July 2006 NIMH Newsletter).

And finally:

> Patients who do not respond to two antidepressant treatment trials *should not give up.*
> (Dr Thomas Insel, quoted in 6 July 2006 NIMH Newsletter).

The purpose of the persuasive rhetoric in these statements is clear and very familiar to anyone who follows biopsychiatric literature. With enough time, enough money, and enough research the pharmacologic (or electrical or magnetic) manipulation of neuronal activity will eventually 'cure' everything from crack cocaine dependence, to depression, to painful shyness, to road rage, and nighttime bingeing. Of course, persuasive rhetoric can go both ways. Suppose an anti-medication advocate was asked to report on the results of the STAR*D study. Without distorting the facts the STAR*D results could be summarized as follows: 2,876 subjects suffering from major depression participated in the study. For the first 12–14 weeks all subjects were treated with the SSRI Citalopram. This medication failed to relieve the depression in 7 out of 10 (70 per cent) of the subjects. The more than 2,000 subjects who remained depressed were then given the choice of several options, including changing to other medications or adding medicines to the Citalopram to augment its effect. After another 12–14 weeks, around 70–75 per cent of this group still did not recover from their depression. For those who chose to not give up and try yet another medication for 12–14 weeks (a total now of over 9 months since starting the study) 80–90 per cent failed to get better.

That is the power of rhetoric. Restate the facts with a negative spin and it looks like the study is an abysmal failure. However, why is it that this negative spin on the data is rarely, if ever, heard? Why do doctors and patients alike only seem to be exposed to positive spins on psychiatric medication studies? That brings us to politics.

10.6 **Bad politics**

Nearly every study or paper that I read in psychiatric journals says somewhere in the summary that 'more research is needed'. The fact that more research being needed is an assessment made by people who make their living doing research speaks to what Lewis (2006) identifies as the political elements involved in the hegemony of medical model psychiatry. Living, breathing people with personal and political agendas created the medical model, and people with personal and political agendas continue to support and propagate it. That the self-interests of academic psychiatrists, managed-care health systems, and ultimately the incredibly powerful and profitable insurance and pharmaceutical industries are best served by an exclusionary medical model in psychiatry is beyond question. The packaging and marketing of emotional wellbeing as a purchasable commodity fits perfectly into the profit driven hyper-reality of twenty-first century life.

The as-yet unassailable dominance of biopsychiatry can best be understood as an instance of the relationship between power and knowledge so clearly explicated by Foucault. As Bracken and Thomas summarize it: 'According to Foucault, in modern societies, power is exercised most often through "regimes of truth": expert discourses through which we understand ourselves and our motives, our desires and our behaviors. Furthermore, such discourses have their expert commentators, advisors and judges. We come to live our lives through these discourses and think about our priorities and values in terms that are given to us. Because they are "regimes of truth" they provide the backdrop to our ethical debates and through them it becomes possible to utter the "truth". In fact, what is regarded as true or false is set by these discourses.' (Bracken and Thomas 2005, 93). Foucault was an historian, so he not only explained how regimes of power and 'truth' operated throughout history, he (and other philosophers such as Thomas Kuhn) shed light on how regimes are toppled and new ones take their place. Biopsychiatry is not immune.

Despite the best efforts of those who profit from the exclusivity of biopsychiatry, the continual emergence of negative data and increasingly implausible narratives (e.g., bipolar disorder in two-year-olds: *Time* magazine, 19 August 2002) is beginning to erode its persuasiveness as being a legitimate member of the larger medico/scientific 'regime of truth'. First, there is the obvious lack of progress in concretely and convincingly demonstrating that psychiatry is a true medical science. No definitive pathological lesion or biochemical process underlying psychiatric illness has been demonstrated. No biological or laboratory test has been developed to test for the presence or absence of disease. Response rates below 50 per cent have not been improved upon in decades. The lack of concrete proof of a disease process combined with the ongoing hubris of psychiatrists and pharmaceutical companies has opened biopsychiatry to increasingly visible critical attacks both from within and outside the profession. Even a source of critique as impeachable as Tom Cruise and scientology can lend a measure of legitimacy to their anti-psychiatry rhetoric by arguing against the chemical imbalance rhetoric so enthusiastically endorsed by mainstream psychiatry. The only thing that seems to be 'progressing' in psychiatry, in fact, is the number of morbidities and mortalities being caused by treatment. We are now being warned that treatment with antidepressants can increase the risk of suicide. A new warning was just issued in 2005 regarding birth defects and Paxil, an SSRI that has been in use since 1992 (FDA News 2005). The number of people being asked to simply accept and cope with sexual dysfunction grows each time another SSRI is prescribed. Some of the second-generation antipsychotics are proving to have risks of metabolic side effects equal to or more serious than the risks of extrapyramidal side effects in first-generation drugs (Robert Freedman, quoted in Pre-2006 Archives of AHRP, 20 September 2005). We are also warned not to use second-generation antipsychotics to control behavior and psychosis in demented elderly patients because, simply (and without any causative connection), it can kill them (FDA Public Health Advisory 2005). A recent NIMH funded $60 million multi-center study, the Clinical Antipsychotic Trials of Intervention Effectiveness (CATIE) reported a 64–82 per cent non-compliance rate in schizophrenics treated with the allegedly more tolerable and effective (and incredibly more expensive) second-generation antipsychotics. The growing trend of diagnosing ill-defined bipolar 'spectrum' conditions in adults and now increasingly in children is resulting in the widespread prescribing of 'mood stabilizing' medications that have serious side effects and, for some, black-box warnings of potentially fatal complications. Biopsychiatry is spinning out of control but still, few seem to be noticing. That is because the Foucauldian power of the biopsychiatry discourse has so far effectively muffled the voices espousing alternative perspectives on human emotional health and distress. Muffled, yes...but not silenced.

10.7 **Enter postpsychiatry**

There are a growing number of legitimate and thoughtful voices being raised in criticism of the hegemony of biopsychiatry. Organizations of professionals such as the Association for the Advancement of Philosophy and Psychiatry, the International Center for the Study of Psychiatry and Psychology, the Constructivist Psychology Network, the Critical Psychiatry Network and Division 32 of the American Psychology Association hold meetings, give papers, and publish articles and books critical of the medical model. User groups such as Mind Freedom, Mad Pride, and Hearing Voices Network as well as individuals from many non-psychiatric disciplines are openly and publicly voicing their concerns about the dehumanizing impact of biopsychiatry. Although sometimes expressing widely divergent views, one thing that these critical voices have in common is the call for the establishment of a multi-perspectival foundation for mental healthcare. It is in the spirit of this postmodern turn and in support and agreement with Bracken and Thomas' grounding of postpsychiatry in a Heideggerian inspired hermeneutic that I offer an interpretation of major depression as a manifestation of an encounter with what Heidegger conceptualizes as the primordial mood of profound boredom. I begin with a personal anecdote.

10.8 **My panic attack**

It happened about thirty years ago when I was a graduate student in psychology. I was taking a break from schoolwork, sitting in the den watching television when suddenly, for no apparent reason, I was gripped by an overwhelming feeling of terror and dread. My heart started pounding and I could barely breathe or think straight. What stands out most vividly in my memory of that day, however, was the visual phenomenon I witnessed. The television set appeared to physically move away from me and shrink in size as it receded to a more distant location across the room. Simultaneous to this movement I experienced the television undergo a strange perceptual transformation from the familiar, entertaining and comforting entity it had been for me into a cold and impersonal mere physical object. I now literally 'saw' the television as just a box of wood around a panel of glass with two dimensional images emitting sounds, neutrally sitting there among other familiar yet now eerily foreign objects in the room. What was happening to me? For that matter, what was happening to the world?

Medical model mental-health professionals will, of course, readily recognize what happened to me that day. I had a panic attack. The sense of unreality and loss of familiar meaning of everyday objects I experienced was a symptom of that panic attack called derealization.

The panic attack eventually subsided, but the memory of the derealization experience continued to haunt me and I sought to understand more deeply and fully its meaning and significance. The circular definitions offered in DSM and similar texts were of little explanatory value. Nor could I just blindly accept the medical model's ungrounded theorizing that derealization is merely an epiphenomenon of the abnormal chemical processes underlying a panic attack. These facile explanations did not come close to accounting for the profundity and impact of my lived experience of derealization. To search for a more comprehensive understanding I turned to philosophy.

Perhaps what I had experienced was akin to what happened to Roquentin in philosopher Jean Paul Sartre's novel *Nausea* (Sartre 1949). When Roquentin had his panic attack on a bus, the world was stripped of all meaning and sensibility; everyday objects were no longer familiar or recognizable. However, that was not quite right. I did not see the so-called 'in-itself' being of the television; it was not transformed into some viscous mass of meaningless matter. I still saw the television as a television; it was simply no longer my television, no longer a familiar 'friendly' thing entertaining and relaxing me.

A more accurate and intuitively valid description of what I experienced that day comes from the philosophy of Martin Heidegger. In his study of Heidegger, *Being-in-the-World,* philosopher Hubert Dreyfus compares Heidegger's description of the experience of derealization to Sartre's. Dreyfus writes: '... that in revealing itself as insignificant, the world does not cease to be a referential whole. It does not collapse into an unstructured, viscous mass as it does for Roquentin in Sartre's *Nausea.* Rather, the world collapses *away* from the anxious Dasein; it *withdraws*' (Dreyfus 1991: 179). Further, he quotes Heidegger who said that: 'Anxiety brings [Dasein] back from its absorption in the "world". Everyday familiarity collapses.' Thus, in derealization, the world withdraws and familiarity collapses; a precise description of what I experienced. From a Heideggerian perspective what I witnessed during my panic attack was a brief glimpse into the grounding of consensual reality by a process of pre-reflective meaning-giving by Dasein, what Dreyfus calls 'the worlding of the world' (Dreyfus 1991: 90).

Heidegger's well-known use of compound words such as being-in-the-world is meant to convey the sense that humans find themselves 'always already' in a meaningful world. We are not Cartesian 'subjects' or 'selves' who discover reality 'out there'; we 'constitute' reality in the act of perceiving it. That is because each of us live in a particular culture at a particular time in history where that culture's shared background beliefs, its 'horizon of intelligibility' defines what we come to know and live in as 'reality'. For example, I was born into a time and place in history where the existence of television as a comforting and available source of distraction and entertainment was a pre-given in the culture. Unless I had a special desire or need to encounter the television as a physical object made of wires and wood and glass, such as when the television breaks, there would be no reason or stimulus in my day to day life to experience the physical 'thingness' of my television. In my state of panic anxiety, however, that is precisely what I, without any reason, did experience. The terror attached to that experience, however, resides at a deeper level because what I also saw (or at least sensed) in that moment was that what lies beneath and behind the shared background intelligibility of my familiar everyday world, what constitutes the metaphysical foundation of all reality is...nothing.

10.9 Heidegger and primordial moods

Heidegger's description of derealization derives from his conception of the ontological status of moods in human existence. While generally neglected in the philosophical tradition, mood is a central organizing principle in Heidegger's philosophy. He views fundamental moods (*Grundstimmungen*) as essential ontological characteristics of human existence, equiprimordial with understanding and facticity in forming the background horizon of intelligibility of being-in-the-world. Thus fundamental moods are at work, so to speak, behind the scenes, contributing to the emergence of the world as 'always already' intelligible and meaningful. Philosopher Michael Zimmerman explains that 'Moods make it possible for entities to show themselves. Moods do not represent things; they open up a realm in which things can first be represented' (Zimmerman 1990: 114). Fundamental moods are always present but are not experienced as subjective emotions. As philosopher Klaus Held puts it: '[mood] is not a subjective state of mind; it is rather like an atmosphere in which the whole being of world is immersed' (Held 1993: 289). Heidegger distinguishes fundamental moods from everyday emotions like being upset, nervous, or unhappy; fundamental moods are much more influential and pervasive but at the same time, as Dreyfus says, 'often so pervasive as to be transparent' (Dreyfus 1991: 173). Fundamental moods are not available for causal examination or scientific analysis because, as Dreyfus points out: 'we cannot get behind our moods; we cannot get clear about them and we cannot get clear of them' (Dreyfus 1991: 173).

I am not proposing that any and all anxiety attacks are the direct experience of Heideggerian primordial anxiety. The experience of primordial anxiety is linked to the particular perceptive awareness of the nothingness at the core of existence. Held says: 'The fundamental temperament anxiety reveals to Dasein that, as being-in-the-world, it hovers over the abyss of the nothing' (Held 1993: 289). This nothingness is felt as a horrifying disconnection not just from objects but from people and society as well. Zimmerman points out that 'Anxiety...reveals the groundlessness of the anyone (socially conforming) self and its culture' (Zimmerman 1990: 24). These elements of arbitrariness, finiteness and groundlessness concealed from thematic awareness in everyday life are what I believe was disclosed to me by my brief encounter with primordial anxiety. Despite the depth and importance of this insight, however, I would not welcome another panic attack. Anxiety is an extremely uncomfortable state that cries for relief as anyone in the mental health profession knows. But if primordial anxiety is inherent to human existence and not the manifestation of a particular individual's faulty wiring or life trauma, then why aren't we all in a constant state of panic? According to Heidegger it is because we flee from it; we flee into the distractions of everyday life. As Zimmerman puts it: 'anxiety is such a disquieting mood that we spend most of our lives trying to keep it from overtaking us' (Zimmerman 1993: 244). This motivated fleeing is such a powerful element of existence that, Heidegger suggests, 'the everyday world is organized precisely to provide Dasein with ways to cover-up its unsettledness' (Dreyfus 1991: 182). At a superficial level this means that we keep ourselves busy, engaged in the tasks and diversions of what Heidegger called 'average everydayness'.

However, there is a more profound and disturbing consequence to the motivated fleeing from the unsettledness at the core of existence. That is the emergence and total domination of the previously discussed technological understanding of reality, *Gestell*. Only now we can see what lies behind, motivates and drives this dominating worldview. As Held describes it: 'In the enterprise of an all-encompassing, organized scientificotechnical management of Dasein (Gestell) all questions are viewed as tasks that are, in principle solvable' (Held 1993: 291). Thus, as Zimmerman points out: 'People living in... the technological world presuppose that nothing is concealed in their world, everything is present' (Zimmerman 1990: 121). In this worldview there is no disturbing unsettledness at the core of existence that lies concealed behind our immersion in everyday life, no incomprehensible mystery, only problems to be solved by the unstoppable technological progress of Western humanity. And where better to bear witness to this than in the field of psychiatry and its technological instantiation as biopsychiatry?

As previously discussed, the hegemony of biopsychiatry has thus far effectively muffled alternative perspectives despite a growing recognition of its dehumanizing impact (Kendler 2005; Schwartz and Wiggins 2002). Certainly there is little room or motivation in the biopsychiatric clinician's practice for an in-depth exploration of the philosophical and spiritual ramifications of an experience like derealization. Treat the disorder and the symptoms will remit. And would it not be antithetical (if not downright unethical and illegal) to propose that the suffering experienced in panic attacks or depression might somehow, as psychiatrist David Kaiser puts it, 'teach us something, deepen our experience, or point us to different possibilities' (Kaiser 1996: 3)? Yet that is exactly what I want to propose here. I am not arguing that we should abandon helpful treatments of painful emotional states or that appropriate medications cannot play a role, I am only asking that we broaden our understanding of what we might learn and how we might grow from our dysphoric experiences.

10.10 **Bored to tears?**

While primordial anxiety is often viewed as a transhistorical concept in Heidegger's philosophy, he also identified other fundamental moods as characteristic of particular epochs in the history of Being. Among the fundamental moods for the ancient Greeks were wonder and awe, for the Cartesian epoch, certainty, and for the technological epoch of Being, profound boredom (Zimmerman 1990: 115). This should come as no surprise because feelings of boredom abound in our culture, creating an unceasing demand for a vast array of distractions and novelties to keep us entertained. It is great for the economy! However, this superficial experience of feeling bored is not the same as the primordial mood of profound boredom. A primordial mood is a part of the background horizon of intelligibility of human existence, and, when directly experienced, is disclosive of the nature of that existence. Although primordial anxiety discloses the nothingness at the core of existence, profound boredom discloses a slightly different but equally unsettling aspect of reality, indifference. Philosopher Wooten Oudemans describes profound boredom as being 'left behind empty by all entities, including our situation, including ourselves. In this state of profound boredom, the indifference of all things, and of ourselves in their midst is revealed' (Oudemans 1994: 47). Similarly, Held says: 'Things no longer appeal to us in the fundamental mood of deep boredom; all beings as a whole including ourselves sink into an abysmal indifference' (Held 1993: 291). Put simply, what profound boredom discloses is that, despite our deeply held beliefs to the contrary, the universe is simply indifferent to our efforts to understand and control it. As Oudemans puts it: 'While expanding planetary needs are all taken care of, a needlessness with relation to the whole manifests itself' (Oudemans 1994: 48). Thus all of our grand projects, our accomplishments, our goals, our shared dreams of a utopian future, at some level, just do not matter. That is pretty grim; certainly not a state of mind that would be very pleasant to live in all of the time. How would anything matter to anyone? Why would we bother getting up out of bed to do anything? How would we feel there was any meaning or purpose to our lives? If these questions sound familiar to the clinician it is because they are the very questions typically asked by someone suffering from a melancholic major depression.

According to DSM IV (American Psychiatric Association 1994) the features of the melancholic subtype of depression include 'a loss of pleasure in all, or almost all activities and/or a loss of reactivity to usually pleasurable stimuli' along with other features including a 'distinct quality of depressed mood' (American Psychiatric Association 1994: 384), different from grief or even less severe periods of depression or sadness. What DSM IV is trying to capture here is a description of what Fink calls 'the quintessential depressive mood disorder' where the feelings of agony, helplessness and pain so dominate daily life that 'suicide becomes a logical solution' (Fink 2006: 34). Anyone who has experienced an episode of melancholic depression or who has been involved clinically in treating it can attest to the depth of the pain of this condition. How is melancholic depression linked to Heidegger's profound boredom? Oudemans describes Heidegger's conception of the experience of profound boredom this way: 'In profound boredom everything that is characteristic of 'us' is sucked away into indifference: name, status, profession, role, age and fate, mine and yours, all of this ceases to have a grip on us. We become an indifferent nobody' (Oudemans 1994: 49).

Oudemans is not a clinician describing the symptoms of melancholic depression. Yet his description of profound boredom is uncannily similar to how patients describe their suffering in this severe depression. For example, clinician and researcher Peter Whybrow in his book *A Mood Apart* describes melancholic depression in the words of one of his patients who says: 'I feel no more than those trees, frozen there in winter. There is no despair for there is no meaning. It is a state of nonbeing...of being condemned to life.'

And finally: 'As the ability to live recedes...only the idea of death itself gives hope' (Whybrow 1997: 23).

In his book *Darkness Visible*, author William Styron chronicles his own prolonged episode of melancholia. He says: 'To most of us who have experienced it, the horror of depression is so overwhelming as to be quite beyond expression...It kills in many instances because its anguish can no longer be borne' (Styron 1990: 20).

Putting together the philosophical description of profound boredom and these clinical descriptions of the lived experience of melancholia, it becomes clear why the outcome of this experience of depression is sometimes suicide. Put into a Heideggerian frame of reference, it could be said that during my one short-lived panic attack I was afforded a brief glimpse into the horror of the nothingness lying at the core of existence whereas, in melancholia, one must endure an unremitting face-to-face encounter with the terrifying indifference of all things that feels like it will never end.

There is, I believe, an inarguable heuristic value to Heidegger's ontology of fundamental moods in gaining a more comprehensive understanding of the lived-experience of panic anxiety and melancholic depression. However, is there any clinical applicability? Can these esoteric philosophical concepts somehow enhance and expand the practicing clinician's effectiveness in the treatment of depression and anxiety disorders? I believe they can.

As I have described elsewhere (Sinaikin 2003), my approach to patient care is pluralistic and pragmatic, grounded in a social constructionist and narrative perspective. From the social constructionist point of view, a clinician's understanding of the Heideggerian concept of *Gestell* and the resultant hegemony of biopsychiatry can be a valuable therapeutic tool. This is especially true when it would be helpful (as I think it usually is) to modify a patient's overly simplistic (and often overly optimistic) beliefs that complex emotional problems are scientifically proven to arise from 'chemical imbalances' in the brain and will be fully relieved by an appropriately chosen psychopharmacologic agent. Beyond that though, I believe that choosing a narrative interpretative framework rooted in Heidegger's concept of primordial moods has the potential do much more than simply dispel the myths of biopsychiatry.

William Styron's depression did not respond to pharmacologic treatment or psychotherapy. He believed he recovered primarily from the passage of time and his asylum in the psychiatric hospital. He also believed that the dogged insistence on a biopsychiatric narrative by his treating psychiatrist served only to increase his suffering and delay his recovery. This is how Styron describes his recovery in the last paragraph of his book: 'To those who have dwelt in depression's dark wood, and known its inexplicable agony, their return from the abyss is not unlike the ascent of the poet, trudging upward and upward out of hell's black depths and at last emerging into what he saw as "the shining world." There, whoever has been restored to health has almost always been restored to the capacity for serenity and joy, and this may be indemnity enough for having endured the despair beyond despair' (Styron 1990: 84).

There is a crucially important difference between Styron's statement and the explicitly stated goals of modern psychiatry. In the STAR*D study the successful outcome is defined as remission, 'the virtual absence of symptoms of depression'. Put another way, it is to restore the patient to the non-depressed emotional state that existed before the onset of depression. But look at Styron's statement. He is saying something completely different. He is saying that living through the excruciating experience of depression restored in him the capacity for serenity and joy, echoing Kaiser's previously mentioned idea that perhaps episodes of emotional pain can 'broaden our horizons or point us to different possibilities'.

Emotional and spiritual growth through depression is not a new or radical idea, only to medical model psychiatry. In her book *Healing through the Dark Emotions*, psychotherapist Miriam Greenspan traces the long history of humankind's relationship with the dark emotions of grief, fear, and despair (Greenspan 2003). She believes that despair is a natural and normal response to encountering the painful truths of human existence. 'Why do the innocent suffer? Why is there so much unnecessary cruelty and pain in the world? Does God exist? What am I here for?' What is deviant and bizarre to Greenspan is the very recent emergence of the idea that it is pathological to feel despair. She says: 'From the standpoint of almost every culture and time except this era in the United States, the psychiatric approach to despair would be seen as naïve or nutty. The idea that cheeriness is normal has a distinctly Brave New World feel' (Greenspan 2003: 124). In her book, this experienced psychotherapist outlines her ideas about how despair can transform to faith, grief to gratitude and fear to joy. She says: 'Enter this dark night of the soul, insists the voice of despair. Look at the world's pain without your usual protections. Descend to this place of near-annihilation. If you can bear your way through this night with patience, you will be moved to a muscular faith that has looked into the heart of darkness and emerged to affirm life' (Greenspan 2003: 121–122). This spiritual tone, also prominent in other successful (and culturally accepted) healing programs such as Alcoholics Anonymous, is heard in Heidegger's philosophy as well.

Interpreters of Heidegger's philosophy have expressed the view that there are significant parallels between his works and what are traditionally considered spiritual disciplines. Caputo analyzes the similarities between Heidegger and

Christian mysticism (Caputo 1986) whereas Zimmerman looks at the relationship to various sects of Zen Buddhism (Zimmerman 1993). These and many other authors and scholars are responding to ideas in both early and late Heidegger that something mysterious and wonderful might lay beyond an unflinching encounter with primordial moods, a mode of existence no longer grounded in boredom and anxiety, but grounded instead in the moods of awe and wonder. Awe and wonder about what? As Heidegger believes it was for the pre-Socratic Greeks (and hopes it can be for us even in the technological epoch of Being), wonder and awe about existence itself! This is a reference to a spiritual experience that is not easily described. Here are a few examples:

> In and through anxiety we experience the wonder of all wonders; that being is.
>
> (Caputo 1986: 20)
>
> ...wonder that a world worlds around us, that the entity is rather than nothing...so that we may encounter the extraordinary in the ordinary.
>
> (Zimmerman 1990: 153)
>
> ...a reservedness with respect to the world, reverence in the face of the wonder that there is something at all rather than nothing.
>
> (Held 1993: 295)
>
> ...when I have it I wonder at the existence of the world. And I am inclined to use such phrases as how extraordinary that anything exists.
>
> (Wittgenstein, as quoted in Dreyfus 1991: 188)

In the fundamental mood of wonder and awe the resultant state of mind and way of life has been characterized as a 'relaxed willfulness' (Held 1993: 292), an 'openness to the "Mystery"' (Caputo 1986: 187), an 'empty, open spontaneous way of being' (Dreyfus 1991: 321), and later by Heidegger as a state of releasement (*Gelassenheit*) where we 'let beings be' (Zimmerman 1993: 256). This may sound like New Age jargon to some but I believe it is an attempt to express in words the frame of mind associated with living a life less prone to frustration, anxiety, anger, boredom, and depression and, in Styron's words, encompassing a greater capacity for serenity and joy. In the 12 Step spiritual program of recovery, this state of mind is called an 'attitude of gratitude'.

What role can the clinician play in facilitating the transition from the experience of primordial anxiety and profound boredom in panic and melancholia to a state of wonder and awe? It is actually quite straightforward; narrate it that way for the patients. Present to them the possibility that although you will work to try to alleviate the pain of their depression and anxiety they should consider the opportunity afforded to them by these dysphoric states to see life anew, to grasp an understanding of human existence at a level usually concealed from us; or, to put it into the poetic language of the later Heidegger, 'To hearken to the silent call of the primordial mood' (Held 1993: 287). It may not register with or appeal to all patients but that is alright. It is worth a try if for no other reason than offering an alternative to clinicians and users under such pressure to surrender to 'the degenerative science of modernity [which] compels the entity to reveal those aspects of itself that are consistent with the power aims of scientific culture' (Zimmerman 1990: 182). For the clinician that means to make a diagnosis, write a prescription, give the patient a drug-company-generated educational pamphlet about their 'disorder', and make a follow-up appointment. For the users it means to fill out checklists and passively surrender control of treatment to the overly busy doctor sitting across from them. Or, as Dreyfus puts it in the poetic language of Heidegger: 'Dasein's only choice, then, is whether to keep silent so as to hear the call [of the primordial mood] or to try to drown it out by plunging into the noise of the everyday rat race' (Dreyfus 1991: 318).

10.11 **Conclusion**

In this paper I have formulated an alternative conceptualization of melancholic depression based on Heidegger's ontological category of primordial moods. Beyond that I have leveled a strong critique at the current practices of exclusionary biopsychiatry and have embraced and supported the concept of a postpsychiatry perspective. However, I believe that more needs to be said. I believe that it is time for clinical psychiatrists, as well as psychologists and therapists, to take a stand. The STAR*D study outcome makes it compellingly clear that something needs to change. Clinicians cannot just sit passively by as the research psychiatrists continue to launch one foundationally flawed drug study after another, affording the clinician and their patients little more useful information than the advertisements that glut our journals and papers. I believe that the STAR*D and CATIE studies could and should mark the beginning of the end of the era of the hegemony of biopsychiatry. As Greenspan sees it: 'What's needed is a way to rewrite our culture's story about depression to make it a story that allows not only for treatment with brain-altering chemicals, but also for a redemptive process of spiritual renewal and transformation' (Greenspan 2003: 125). Rewritten by whom? Lewis rightly bemoans the fact that 'It is difficult these days to find well-rounded and intellectually nuanced psychiatrists' (Lewis 2006: xiii). However, these are precisely the type of psychiatrist needed to spearhead the postpsychiatry movement because biopsychiatry is powerful and its dominant position will not easily yield. I suggest we can begin to plant the seeds of change by championing a curriculum change in our training programs. Of all the medical disciplines, psychiatry must broaden its horizons and realign itself with the humanities. As Lewis says, 'psychiatry (the quintessential human concern) cut off from the humanities and critical postdisciplinary programs is absurd' (Lewis 2006: 17).

A psychiatric residency is four years long. Surely some of that time can be devoted to the study of philosophy and other humanitarian disciplines so clearly crucial to the deepest understanding and optimal care of our patients (and ourselves).

References

American Psychiatric Association (1994) *Diagnostic and Statistical Manual of Mental Disorders*, 4th ed. (Washington, DC: American Psychiatric Association Press).

Bracken P. and Thomas P. (2005). *Postpsychiatry: Mental health in a postmodern world* (Oxford: Oxford University Press).

Caputo J. D. (1986). *The mystical element in Heidegger's thought* (New York: Fordham University Press).

Dreyfus H. L. (1991). *Being-in-the-World. A commentary on Heidegger's Being and Time, Division I* (Cambridge, MA: The MIT Press).

FDA News. (2005). FDA advisory of risk of birth defects with Paxil. 8 December. http://www.fda.gov/bbs/topics/NEWS/2005/NEW01270.html.

FDA Public Health Advisory. (2005). Deaths with antipsychotics in elderly patients with behavioral disturbances. 11 April. http://www.fda.gov/cder/advisory/antipsychotics.html

Fink M. (2006). Should the diagnosis of melancholia be revived? *Psychiatric Times*, **23**, 33–34.

Greenberg R. P. and Fisher S. (1997). Mood mending medicines: probing drug, psychotherapy and placebo solutions' in S. Fisher and R. P. Greenberg (eds.) *From Placebo to Panacea: Putting psychiatric drugs to the test* (New York: John Wiley and Sons), 115–173.

Greenspan M. (2003). *Healing through the Dark Emotions* (Boston, MA: Shambhala).

Heidegger, M. (1971) *The Question concerning Technology and Other Essays* (tr. W. Lovitt) (New York: Harper Textbooks).

Held, K. (1993) 'Fundamental moods and Heidegger's critique of contemporary culture' in J. Sallis (ed.) *Reading Heidegger: Commemorations* (Bloomington, Indiana: Indiana University Press), 286–307.

Kaiser D. (1996). Commentary: against biological psychiatry. *Psychiatric Times*, **13**, 1–7.

Kendler K. S. (2005). Toward a philosophical structure for psychiatry. *American Journal of Psychiatry*, **162**, 443–440.

Kutchins H. and Kirk S. (1997). *Making us Crazy: DSM: The psychiatric bible and the creation of mental disorders* (New York: Free Press).

Lewis B. (2006). *Moving beyond Prozac, DSM, and the New Psychiatry. The birth of postpsychiatry* (Ann Arbor, MI: The University of Michigan Press).

MacNeil J. S. (2006). Depression trial results: don't augment too early. *Clinical Psychiatry News*, **34**, 1–7.

Medical News Today. (2006). Landmark STAR*D depression study offers 'sobering' third round results. 2 July. http://www.medicalnewstoday.com/medicalnews.php?newsid=46265.

NIMH National Institute of Mental Health Press Release. (2006). Initial results help clinicians identify patients with treatment-resistant depression. January 1. http://www.nimh.gov/stard.cfm.

NIMH National Institute of Mental Health Press Release. (2006). Strategies help depressed patients become symptom free. 23 March. http://www.nimh.gov/stard.cfm.

NIMH National Institute of Mental Health Science Update. (2006). Switching to a third antidepressant may prove helpful to some treatment-resistant depressions. 1 July. http://www.nimh.gov/stard.cfm.

Oudemans T. C. W. (1994). 'Heidegger: reading against the grain' in T. Kisiel and J. Van Buren (eds.) *Reading Heidegger from the Start. Essays in his earliest thought* (Albany, NY: State University of New York Press), 35–55.

Pre-2006 Archives of the Alliance for Human Research Protection. (2005). Federal study finds no benefits of new antipsychotic drugs. 20 September. http://www.ahrp.org/infomail/05/09/20.php.

Sartre J.-P. (1949). *Nausea or the Diary of Antoine Roquentin* (tr. L. Alexander) (New York: New Directions).

Schwartz M. A. and Wiggins O. (2002). 'The hegemony of the DSM's' in J. Sadler (ed.) *Descriptions and Prescriptions* (Baltimore, MD: The Johns Hopkins University Press), 199–210.

Sinaikin P. (2003). Categorical diagnosis and a poetics of obligation. *Journal of Ethical Human Sciences and Services*, **5**, 141–148.

Splete H. (2005). VNS therapy is approved for severe depression. *Clinical Psychiatry News*, **33**, 1–7.

Styron W. (1990). *Darkness Visible. A memoir of madness* (New York: Vintage Books).

Whybrow P. C. (1997). *A Mood Apart. The thinker's guide to emotions and its disorders.* (New York: Harpers Collins).

Zimmerman M. E. (1990). *Heidegger's Confrontation with Modernity: Technology, politics, Art* (Bloomington, IN: Indiana University Press).

Zimmerman M. E. (1993). 'Heidegger, Buddhism and deep ecology' in C. Guignon (ed.) *The Cambridge Companion to Heidegger* (Cambridge: Cambridge University Press), 240–270.

Part 4

Technological instruments and psychiatry

Chapter 11

Psychiatric rehabilitation and the notion of technology in psychiatry

Abraham Rudnick

11.1 Introduction

Contemporary civilization is dependent for its survival on technology: for example, on electricity, on transportation, on computers, and so on. Furthermore, it may be argued that modern civilization is partly defined, or perhaps manifest, by technology. It is clear that contemporary medicine is largely technological, for better or worse. Although technology can facilitate more effective and efficient healthcare, it is commonly argued that technology de-humanizes medicine in general and psychiatry in particular, as it deals with patients as objects (of technical manipulation), rather than as subjects (or whole persons).

Technology can be simply—and arguably not too simplistically—construed as a set of tools, or more broadly, devices. Devices are the general case, consisting of tools, machines and automata. A tool is a device where man himself constitutes the source of energy and the source of information in operating the device, such as a knife or a screwdriver; a (classical) machine is a device that man operates by making use of external sources of energy outside himself, such as a windmill or a steam engine; and an automaton is a device that operates on the basis of its own information and thus controls itself, such as a thermostat or a computer (admittedly, even the most perfect computers are not complete automata, because they always operate on the basis of a certain program prepared by man) (Tondl 1974: 9–11).

Perhaps 'the most general characterization of technology can be given in the following way: technology is everything which man in his activity puts between himself and the objective world and its individual parts with the goal of transforming this world in accordance with his needs and intentions' (Tondl 1974: 5–6).[1] But this may be insufficient as a characterization of technology, for example, as related to psychiatry, which arguably addresses the subjective world while using technological devices of all sorts (physical, biochemical, and psychosocial in particular). Still, what stands out in this characterization of technology is that it views technology as a set of tools or devices that help a person or a group of persons achieve their goals (by overcoming problems that impede those goals), rather than as a set of tools or devices that fix problems independently of persons and their goals. Such a notion of technology is humanistic in that it posits persons and their goals, rather than problems or tools/devices, as the primary guide for decisions related to those persons.

Thus, perhaps it is not technology or the inevitable use of technology that may de-humanize medicine in general and psychiatry in particular, but rather the particular notion of technology that is used in medicine, particularly in psychiatry. The idea that a notion of technology can be more or less humanizing is not a standard one in contemporary philosophy. Many scholars claim that the notion of technology entails or at least implies a de-humanizing approach, as manifest in the technological mode of being (which is instrumentally oriented), and that this should be balanced by a humanizing approach, as manifest in the poietic mode of being (which is existentially oriented); indeed, recent writing in philosophy of psychiatry has endorsed this set of claims and elaborated extensively on it (Sadler 2005). In contrast, I argue here for a broadening of the notion of technology, as supported by common sense, according to which technology can be more or less humanizing, depending on factors such as the goal for which it is used and the way in which it is used; furthermore, I argue that the notion of technology can be more or less humanizing, as illustrated in this paper. This paper explores notions of technology used in psychiatry, and suggests an alternative and more humanizing notion of technology for psychiatry, one that is used in psychiatric rehabilitation.

It should be noted that it is taken here as a given that contemporary psychiatry de-humanizes its care recipients to an extent. The claim that contemporary psychiatry sometimes de-humanizes its care recipients has been forcefully argued by many and illustrated by involuntary commitment, forced treatment, and more. On a more mundane level, psychiatry more often assumes a paternalistic attitude towards patients. Such paternalism can be regarded as a necessary but insufficient condition of de-humanizing. The proposed remedies for this de-humanizing are myriad. For instance, some have argued that contemporary psychiatry should also be based on understanding of meanings rather than—as it is supposedly now—only on explanation of causes (Schwartz and Wiggins 1986). More radically, others have argued that contemporary psychiatry should be de-medicalized so that it addresses problems of living rather than psychiatric disorders—the latter claimed to be a 'myth' (Szasz 2001).

There may be additional causes of the de-humanization of psychiatry, such as the reductionism prevalent in contemporary psychiatry (Rudnick 1990, 2002*a*) and the mechanism prevalent in modern medicine in general (Rudnick 2000, 2002*b*), which may require additional remedies. Reductionism has many versions, but perhaps most simply it refers to the explaining of one category of phenomena fully by another category of phenomena; in contemporary psychiatry, the reductionism that is prevalent is that of explaining psychological abnormalities fully by biological abnormalities. Mechanism also has some versions, but perhaps most simply it refers to the explaining of phenomena fully by their components (and their interactions); in contemporary psychiatry, the mechanism that is prevalent is that of explaining abnormal behavior, experience, and cognition of persons fully by their abnormal brain structure and function. Clearly, reductionism and mechanism are related, although distinct, at least in contemporary psychiatry, where abnormal behavior, experience, and cognition of a person, which is a set of biopsychosocial phenomena, is explained by a biological component of the person—his or her presumably abnormal brain.

11.2 Technologies and notions of technology in psychiatry

Psychopharmacology refers to the use of psychotropic chemicals. Psychotropic chemicals modify mental phenomena such as emotion, cognition, and/or behavior, and include psychiatric medications, such as antipsychotics, antidepressants, mood stabilizers, and others; recreational drugs, such as opiates, amphetamines, hallucinogens, and others; and other substances that are used for other purposes, such as in laboratory experiments. Psychopharmacology may be the paradigmatic technology in contemporary psychiatry. It is probably the technology that is most used in clinical practice and in research—basic and clinical—in contemporary psychiatry. It is so well established that, for some time now, it has had its own journals, and perhaps more significantly (Kuhn 1970), its own widely accepted textbooks (Bloom and Kupfer 1995). Psychotropic medications are prescribed for psychiatric symptoms, with the assumption that these medications correct some underlying neurochemical imbalance. To illustrate, antipsychotics are prescribed for schizophrenia with the underlying hypothesis, still supported despite some contrary evidence (Kapur and Remington 2001), that they reduce dopaminergic hyperactivity in the mesolimibic system of the brain of the person with schizophrenia.

It is generally assumed that certain psychotropic medications are suitable for certain symptoms, independently of other—particularly psychosocial—features of the person with the disorder, such as his or her personality profile. For instance, a person diagnosed with schizophrenia will usually be prescribed an anti-psychotic medication, regardless of his or her personal features. The decision which antipsychotic medication to prescribe rests largely on differences in adverse effects and effectiveness for that patient in the past. These are clearly not indicators of a person, but rather of a biological organism in general. Moreover, if a psychiatric patient has a goal that conflicts with the goal of alleviating symptoms, such as finding meaning in life by being psychotic (Roberts 1991), the mainstream approach to psychopharmacology cannot accommodate that and would usually label that as non-compliance and may revert to treatment by force, as illustrated in community treatment orders. Thus, the person as a whole is not addressed by the notion of technology that is assumed by psychopharmacology, at least as commonly practiced. This implies a notion of psychopharmacological technology where the problem to be resolved by the technology is posited independently of the person with the problem, namely the patient with the symptom.

Psychotherapy is another well-known technology of psychiatry. Actually, there are many psychotherapies, some of which vary considerably—theoretically and practically—from others. Let us take as examples two rather different types of psychotherapy: psychoanalytic therapy and cognitive behavioral therapy (recognizing that each of these has distinct subtypes which differ considerably from each other, especially within psychoanalytic therapy).

Psychoanalytic interventions are recommended for disturbed experiences or behaviors, with the assumption that these interventions correct some underlying mental abnormality. It should be noted that mental abnormalities are viewed differently within different psychoanalytic theories. To illustrate, a more traditional psychoanalytic theory, such as the drive theory, as formulated by Freud, emphasizes conflict between postulated mental structures or functions, whereas a more novel psychoanalytic theory, such as self-psychology, as formulated by Kohut, emphasizes lack of postulated mental structures or functions (McWilliams 1994).

It is generally assumed that certain psychoanalytic interventions are suitable for certain experiences or behaviors, but (unlike psychopharmacology) this fit is considered to be dependent on other—particularly psychosocial—features of the person with the disorder, such as his or her developmental history. For instance, 'confrontation of grandiosity' (which is a psychoanalytic technique) may be appropriate for narcissistic clients who were raised adequately by their parents but not for clients who were seriously neglected during their childhood.

Yet the goal of psychoanalytic interventions is pre-determined, consisting of resolving the presumed abnormality (be it a conflict, an ego weakness, or some other presupposed psychoanalytic construct), and thus not determined by the client. Moreover, if the client denies the existence of such a presumed abnormality, it can be viewed as a sign of that abnormality (as denial is considered an unconscious defense mechanism), sometimes resulting in the upholding of the predetermined goal even if the client upholds a different—and possibly conflicting—goal.[2] This implies a notion of psychoanalytic technology where the problem to be resolved by the technology is posited independently of the person with the problem.

Cognitive behavioral interventions are offered for disrupted emotion, thought, and behavior, with the assumption that these interventions correct some underlying psychological impairment. It should be noted that psychological impairments are viewed differently within different cognitive behavioral approaches. To illustrate, a more cognitively oriented approach, as formulated by Beck, emphasizes distorted thought schemas, whereas a more behaviorally oriented approach, as formulated by Skinner, emphasizes maladaptive behavioral patterns (Hawton *et al.* 1989).

It is generally assumed that certain cognitive behavioral interventions are suitable for certain emotions, thoughts or behaviors, and (like psychoanalysis but unlike psychopharmacology) this fit is considered to be dependent on other—particularly psychosocial—features of the person with the disorder, such as his or her educational background. For instance, 'collaborative empiricism' (which is a cognitive behavioral technique) that addresses scientific evidence may be appropriate for clients with panic phenomena who are highly educated but not for clients with similar panic phenomena who are not educated. Yet the goal of cognitive behavioral interventions is pre-determined, consisting of resolving the presumed impairment (be it a distorted schema, a conditioned response, or some other presupposed cognitive behavioral construct), and thus not determined by the client. Furthermore, although cognitive behavioral therapy is considerably different from psychoanalysis, it seems to share with it the idea that the client may not be aware of his or her impairment, and to similarly attempt to uphold its predetermined goal even if the client persists in upholding a different—and possibly conflicting—goal. For instance, if a client is expressing a somatic complaint due to depression, cognitive behavioral therapy would typically attempt to address the client's presumed cognitive distortion, even if the client thought that the experience of pain should be addressed directly. This implies a notion of cognitive behavioral technology where the problem to be resolved by the technology is posited independently of the person with the problem.

11.3 The notion of technology in psychiatric rehabilitation

Psychiatric rehabilitation addresses psychiatric disability and handicap/lack of participation, which is the inability to perform activities and roles successfully, respectively, because of psychiatric impairments and their complications. The notions of disability and handicap are well established in general healthcare, and standardized by the World Health Organization (2001). Indeed, the notions of physical disability and handicap were a major inspiration for the construction of the notions of psychiatric disability and handicap, and following that, for the establishment of the field of psychiatric rehabilitation (Anthony *et al.* 2002). It should be noted that the notions of disability and handicap are subject to philosophical discussion and criticism (Edwards 1997, 1998; Nordenfeldt 1997, 1999), while continuing to prove useful in clinical practice and policy making.

Psychiatric rehabilitation is the set of (psychosocial) interventions—mainly involving enhancing and maintaining client skills and supports—aimed at assisting individuals to overcome their psychiatric disabilities and handicaps so that they can successfully perform activities and roles. Psychiatric rehabilitation comprises setting personal goals, assessing what are the challenges in achieving and maintaining them, planning interventions that can address those challenges, and implementing these interventions (Anthony *et al.* 2002). An example of the process of psychiatric rehabilitation is that of a person who has schizophrenia with typical working memory impairment and who wants to learn to cook. A pertinent challenge could be that the person may not be able to independently retain recipe information and act on it in a stepwise fashion. A plan to be implemented to address that challenge could be to use a memory aid such as a written recipe, where each step is written on a separate page and broken down further into sub-steps, and each step is taught repeatedly in an errorless fashion that has proven helpful in many areas of skills training in psychiatric rehabilitation (Kern *et al.* 2005).

The leading approach in psychiatric rehabilitation is client-centered; this is the view that the person with the psychiatric disability can (and should) choose the activities and roles, namely, the goals, to work on (Anthony *et al.* 2002). Of course, a more paternalistic model of psychiatric rehabilitation would presuppose the activities and roles to work on, independently of the person with the psychiatric disability, as is sometimes still the case, for example, with the activity of grooming (Liberman *et al.* 1993). Hence, the goal of client-centered psychiatric rehabilitation interventions, but not necessarily of all psychiatric rehabilitation interventions, is not presupposed but rather determined by the individual client, who chooses which activities and roles to work towards (admittedly, part of the clinical challenge is to clarify personal goals, particularly for severely cognitively impaired persons who may have difficulty in setting clear and realistic goals). This implies a notion of (client-centered) psychiatric rehabilitation technology where the problem to be resolved by the technology is not posited independently of the person with the problem, but rather according to his or her choice.

Of course, this raises the issue of free choice or autonomy of persons with severe psychiatric impairment, such as with schizophrenia. I take schizophrenia as a prime example involving severe psychiatric impairment as it is considered the most severe of psychiatric disorders, partly because it involves many psychiatric impairments, including definitional or core symptoms such as positive and negative symptoms, as well as co-morbid and cognitive impairments (American Psychiatric Association 2000). It is commonly claimed that such persons are not autonomous, at least not to the degree that so-called mentally normal persons are.[3] The claim that people with severe psychiatric impairments are deficient in their autonomy is commonly discussed and tested in the field of competence to consent to (or refuse) treatment or research, where it is widely agreed that competence or decisional capacity, as a paradigm of autonomy, is decision-specific, so that a person may be capable of deciding on a particular treatment but not on another; as a matter of fact, many individuals with severe psychiatric impairment such as schizophrenia are found to be competent in their decisions about most, if not all, of their treatment (Grisso and Appelbaum 1998). If so, the claim that persons with severe psychiatric impairment are not autonomous (to the extent that normal persons are), is false, at least as an unqualified generalization.

Furthermore, decisional capacity about the rehabilitation goals of activity and role achievement is usually less prone to impairment compared with decisional capacity about the treatment goals of symptom alleviation and relapse prevention. This is so partly because decisional capacity about treatment requires—among other things—insight (Grisso and Appelbaum 1998), which is commonly absent in severe psychiatric disorders such as schizophrenia (Amador and David 2004), whereas decisional capacity about rehabilitation requires—among other things—felt need (Anthony *et al.* 2002), which is commonly present even in severely mentally ill people.[4] Also, there is considerable variance in choice of activities and roles in the general population, so that it overlaps with the range of choice of activities and roles of people with severe psychiatric disorders; put simply, so-called normal people many times choose unusual activities and roles, perhaps no less than people with severe psychiatric disorders, as illustrated in criminal activities (which, by and large, are not more common in people with severe psychiatric disorders than in the general population). Of course, this is not to say that decisional capacity should not be assessed for psychiatric rehabilitation; indeed, relevant tools have been generated that can assess just that, such as readiness assessment (Anthony *et al.* 2002).

Hence, client choice directing interventions in psychiatric rehabilitation may be sound. This is so particularly if client choice is not directly induced by psychiatric impairment (such as delusional thinking) and if it is not expected to result in serious danger (Rudnick 2002*c*). To summarize, the notion of technology used in (client-centered) psychiatric rehabilitation primarily addresses the person with the problem and his or her choices, rather than primarily addressing the problem to be resolved by the technology independently of the person with that problem and his or her choices, as psychopharmacology and psychotherapy seem to do.

11.4 Conclusion

What can we learn from the notion of technology used in (client-centered) psychiatric rehabilitation? Perhaps the most important lesson is that the general characterization of technology cited in the introduction, particularly the part about technology being in accordance with man's needs and intentions, is relevant to psychiatric technology (with the addition that this characterization also applies to the modification of the subjective world). Specifically, as needs and intentions are arguably person-specific, it seems that the notion of technology used in (client-centered) psychiatric rehabilitation involves this general characterization of technology in that it addresses the person with the problem, rather than the problem independently of the person. The question then is whether other psychiatric technologies that do not commonly use such a notion of technology, such as psychopharmacology and psychotherapy, could use this humanizing notion of technology more frequently. However, that is a matter for a separate discussion.

Another lesson may be that there is something to learn from psychiatric rehabilitation for psychiatry in general, specifically the client-centered approach incorporated in its notion of technology. Although psychiatric rehabilitation has been around for more than three decades as an established evidence-based field, it is still not fully assimilated into mainstream psychiatry. This is particularly so in psychiatric education, which mostly emphasizes psychopharmacology and psychotherapy (Kay *et al.* 1999). As psychiatric education should presumably incorporate the client-centered approach as much as possible, it would benefit generally from emphasizing psychiatric rehabilitation (in addition to the benefit of facilitating a distinct clinical expertise through psychiatric rehabilitation training). Be that as it may, and controversial as this may sound, it appears that the notion of technology used in (client-centered) psychiatric rehabilitation is more humanizing than that used in psychopharmacology or even in psychotherapy.

Endnotes

1 It is interesting that a more recent philosophical characterization of technology is confined to material technology: 'First, we shall insist that a technology must have some concrete component, some material element, to count as a technology. And, second, a technology must enter into some set of praxes—'uses'—which humans may make of these components. And, third, we shall take as part of the definition, a *relation* between the technologies and the humans who use, design, make, or modify the technologies in question.' (Ihde 1993: 47). This may be too narrow, particularly for psychiatry, where some tools such as psychotherapy may not have much of a material component if at all. Current writings in philosophy of technology are no different (Scharff and Dusek 2003). I prefer to use the above definition of technology as suggested by Tondl, as it is more general, albeit older.

2 Much ink has been spilt over the argument that psychoanalysis is pseudoscientific because it uses self-reinforcing statements such as that denial of a problem is a sign of that problem. Perhaps most well known is Popper's argument that such statements are irrefutable (Popper 1959). Admittedly, Grunbaum argued for what he considered a more careful philosophical treatment of psychoanalysis, concluding that it is largely refuted rather than irrefutable (Grunbaum 1984).

3 Note that no one is fully autonomous, and autonomy fluctuates within any individual in relation to both internal conditions and external circumstances (Laor 1984).

4 The common presence of felt needs of patients with schizophrenia has been recognized for long. This is perhaps best illustrated in the double bookkeeping effect, where many schizophrenia patients, even when actively psychotic, for example, with messianic delusions, attend to their basic needs, such as feeding (Bleuler 1911/1950).

References

Amador X. and David A. (eds). (2004). *Insight and Psychosis: Awareness of illness in schizophrenia and related disorders* (Oxford: Oxford University Press).

American Psychiatric Association. (2000). *Diagnostic and Statistical Manual of Mental Disorders*, 4th edn, text—revised (Washington, DC, American Psychiatric Association).

Anthony W. A., Cohen M., Farkas M., and Gagne C. (2002). *Psychiatric Rehabilitation*, 2nd edn (Boston: Center for Psychiatric Rehabilitation).

Bleuler E. (1911/1950). *Dementia Praecox or the Group of Schizophrenias* (New York: International Universities Press).

Bloom F. E. and Kupfer D.J. (eds.) (1995). *Psychopharmacology: The fourth generation of progress* (New York: Raven).

Edwards S. D. (1997). Dismantling the disability/handicap distinction. *Journal of Medicine and Philosophy*, **22**, 589–606.

Edwards S. D. (1998). Nordenfelt's theory of disability. *Theoretical Medicine and Bioethics*, **19**, 89–100.

Grisso T. and Appelbaum P. S. (1998). *Assessing Competence to Consent to Treatment: A guide for physicians and other health professionals* (New York: Oxford University Press).

Grunbaum A. (1984). *The Foundations of Psychoanalysis: A philosophical critique* (Berkeley: University of California Press).

Hawton K., Salkovskis P. M., Kirk J., and Clark D. M. (1989). 'The development of principles of cognitive–behavioural treatments' in K. Hawton, P. M. Salkovskis, J. Kirk, and D. M. Clark (eds.) *Cognitive Behaviour Therapy for Psychiatric Problems: A practical guide* (Oxford: Oxford University Press), 1–12.

Ihde D. (1993). *Philosophy of Technology: An introduction* (New York: Paragon House), 47.

Kapur S. and Remington G. (2001). Dopamine D(2) receptors and their role in atypical antipsychotic action: still necessary and may even be sufficient. *Biological Psychiatry*, **50**, 873–883.

Kay J., Silberman E. K., and Pessar L. (eds.) (1999). *Handbook of Psychiatric Education and Faculty Development* (Washington, DC: American Psychiatric Association).

Kern R.S., Green M.F., Mitchell S., Kopelowicz A., Mintz J., and Liberman R. P. (2005). Extensions of errorless learning for social problem-solving deficits in schizophrenia. *American Journal of Psychiatry*, **162**, 513–519.

Kuhn T. (1970). *The Structure of Scientific Revolutions*, 2nd edn (Chicago: The University of Chicago Press).

Laor N. (1984). The autonomy of the mentally ill: a case-study in individualistic ethics. *Philosophy of the Social Sciences*, **14**, 289–302.

Liberman R. P., Wallace C. J., Blackwell G., Eckman T. A., Vaccaro J. V., and Kuehnel T. G. (1993). Innovations in skill training for people with serious mental illness: the UCLA social and independent living skills modules. *Innovations and Research*, **2**, 46–59.

McWilliams N. (1994). *Psychoanalytic Diagnosis: Understanding personality structure in the clinical process* (New York: Guilford).

Nordenfelt L. (1997). The importance of a disability/handicap distinction. *Journal of Medicine and Philosophy*, **22**, 607–622.

Nordenfelt L. (1999). On disability and illness: a reply to Edwards. *Theoretical Medicine and Bioethics*, **20**, 181–189.

Popper K. R. (1959). *The Logic of Scientific Discovery* (London: Hutchinson).

Roberts G. (1991). Delusional belief systems and meaning in life: a preferred reality? *British Journal of Psychiatry*, **159** (suppl. 14), 19–28.

Rudnick A. (1990). Towards a rationalization of biological psychiatry: a study in psychobiological epistemology. *Journal of Medicine and Philosophy*, **15**, 75–96.

Rudnick A. (2000). The ends of medical intervention and the demarcation of the normal from the pathological. *Journal of Medicine and Philosophy*, **25**, 569–580.

Rudnick A. (2002a). The molecular turn in psychiatry: a philosophical analysis. *Journal of Medicine and Philosophy*, **27**, 287–296.

Rudnick A. (2002b). The notion of health: a conceptual analysis. *Israel Medical Association Journal*, **4**, 83–85.

Rudnick A. (2002c). The goals of psychiatric rehabilitation: an ethical analysis. *Psychiatric Rehabilitation Journal*, **25**, 310–313.

Sadler J. Z. (2005). *Values and Psychiatric Diagnosis* (Oxford: Oxford University Press).

Scharff R. and Dusek V. (eds.) (2003). *Philosophy of Technology* (Oxford: Blackwell).

Schwartz M. A. and Wiggins O. P. (1986). Systems and the structuring of meaning: contributions to a biopsychosocial medicine. *American Journal of Psychiatry*, **143**, 1213–1221.

Szasz T. (2001). Mental illness: psychiatry's phlogiston. *Journal of Medical Ethics*, **27**, 297–301.

Tondl L. (1974). 'On the concepts of "technology" and "technological sciences"' in F. Rapp (ed.) *Contributions to a Philosophy of Technology: Studies in the structure of thinking in the technological sciences* (Dordrecht: Reidel), 1–18.

World Health Organization. (2001). *International Classification of Functioning, Disability and Health* (Geneva: World Health Organization).

Chapter 12

Drugs, not hugs: antidepressant medication trials and suicidality in children—a case history in the philosophy of science as an argument for the need for improved technology in psychiatry

Stuart L. Kaplan

12.1 Introduction

Technology has played a central role in the development of science. Who cannot be moved at imagining Galileo looking through the telescope he invented and built as he first viewed the moons of Jupiter? Shapin and Schaffer (1985) have described in detail the vacuum-creating machine built by Boyle, Boyle's development of the experimental method in science, and the disputations that arose between him and Hobbes from this technology. It was part of Boyle's genius to appreciate the value of a machine to tell us about the world as it is. The development of new technologies makes it possible for contemporary science to enhance our understanding 'of the real world as it really is' (Klee 1997).

I shall consider the technology of the double-blind psychopharmacological clinical trial by examining some of the methodological issues raised by a series of public hearings about the safety and efficacy of selective serotonin reuptake inhibitors (for example, fluoxetine (Prozac), and sertraline (Zoloft)) and other antidepressants in children and adolescents. I will show that some aspects of the technology used by psychiatry to study psychopharmacological agents are simple and error prone. This argues that psychiatry is greatly in need of more and improved technology, not less, as I believe some of my colleagues suggest in this book.

12.2 Overview of the hearings and the presented data

In the USA, a series of public hearings and news reports occurred between May 2003, and October 2004, on the safety and efficacy of antidepressants in children and adolescents. The story was covered closely by major newspapers and the professional trade-association press. The story had several aspects that helped it gain and hold the public's attention. Parents of children who had killed themselves while taking these agents testified in open committee hearings. There were several hints of scandalous behavior. One Food and Drug Administration (FDA) employee, Mosholder, had let it be known that his testimony against antidepressant agents in children and adolescents was being suppressed by his employers at the FDA, and he was not going to be allowed to testify at the hearings. Pharmaceutical companies had withheld medication trial results. They had been allowed to not report these studies, but their failure to report all of the trials was seen as less than full disclosure by the press and public. The results of the trials as disclosed at various hearings and investigations were riveting. Not only were antidepressants in general not effective in the treatment of children and adolescents, but they led to more suicidality. Finally an air of suspense developed with the drama of a courtroom trial based on the keen interest in what action the FDA would decide to take to address the problem (Rosack 2004*b*).

On 15 October 2004, the FDA issued a black-box warning on all antidepressants for children and adolescents. The warning stated that these agents could increase the risks of suicidal behaviors, and recommended that children taking these medications should be seen frequently during the first weeks of treatment with these agents. This date gives promise of becoming a minor landmark in the history of contemporary psychiatry. It has been called 'Black Friday' in reference to the black-box warning, the dismay of physicians who prescribed these agents, and the families of children who used them. In addition to the distress of practitioners and patients, this controversy and announcement continues to be a major inspiration for many studies about antidepressants and suicidality that continue to the present day. As I prepare this chapter in the summer of 2007, I note the *American Journal of Psychiatry* has an article (Libby *et al.* 2007) and an editorial (Pfeffer 2007) in the June 2007 issue, and three articles (Gibbons *et al.* 2007; Posner *et al.* 2007; Simon and Savarino 2007) in the July 2007 issue, about antidepressants and suicidality related to the 2004 black-box warning. I will briefly summarize some of the salient events in this long and complex chronology.

The controversy could be regarded as beginning in the USA over a year earlier, in May 2003, after the FDA received a data set from GlaxoSmithKline reporting a possible increase in suicidal events in patients taking paroxetine (Paxil). The FDA issued a public health advisory suggesting that Paxil not be given to depressed children and adolescents. The FDA requested data sets from all pharmaceutical companies that had been performing clinical trials with antidepressants in children and adolescents. In October 2003, after reviewing the data sets, the FDA found the descriptions of suicidal behavior described in some of the adverse event reports of the trials to lack credibility. They asked the Columbia University Departments of Psychiatry and Epidemiology to review the data and to suggest a classification scheme for suicidality. In February 2004, the first public hearings were held, and in March the FDA issued an advisory warning to monitor child and adolescent patients taking antidepressant medications carefully for suicide. Various reports were completed, and in September 2004 two congressional hearings were held.

Let us briefly examine some of the content presented at the hearings. Data from 23 double-blind pharmaceutical company sponsored trials and one National Institutes of Mental Health (NIMH)-sponsored trial, the Treatment of Adolescent Depression Study (TADS), were examined. There were 4,582 patients in the data set. The trials took place from 1983 to 2004. The trials studied the efficacy of antidepressant medications in several distinct disorders. Sixteen of the trials were for major depressive disorder, five were for obsessive compulsive disorder, two were for generalized anxiety disorder, and one was for social anxiety disorder. Medications studied included the selective serotonin reuptake inhibitors (SSRIs) citalopram (Celexa), fluoxetine (Prozac), fluvoxamine (Luvox), paroxetine (Paxil), and sertraline (Zoloft). Atypical antidepressants studied included buproprion (Wellbutrin), mirtazapine (Remeron), nefazodone (Serzone), and venlafaxine (Effexor). The trials were short term, lasting from four to sixteen weeks. The data were combined in a meta-analysis, which provides a means for combining and analyzing multiple studies as one. The data were primarily analyzed to provide a measure of the association between taking antidepressants and suicidality as well as measures of medication efficacy.

Patients enrolled in these trials were over 2.1 times more likely to have suicidal thoughts or behaviors if they received medication for depression than if they received a placebo agent. This finding would be due to chance only once in twenty thousand times. There were no completed acts of suicide (Leslie *et al.* 2005). Three of the fifteen trials for major depression demonstrated efficacy. The single NIMH-sponsored trial had the unique feature of having a psychotherapy component to the trial. Some of the depressed patients in the trial received cognitive behavioral treatment for depression. A portion of this subgroup received fluoxetine (Prozac) and a portion did not.

Fluoxetine (Prozac) was efficacious in the treatment of depression. Although cognitive therapy alone was helpful in 43% of the cases, it was not significantly different from placebo. Cognitive therapy was significantly more helpful with suicidality than was fluoxetine (Prozac) or placebo. Thus, based on the TADS data, the optimum treatment for depressed adolescents was cognitive therapy combined with fluoxetine (Prozac) (March *et al.* 2004).

12.3 **The double-blind trial**

To appreciate the primitive nature of the technology used in the study of pharmaceutical agents, we will take a more detailed examination of the performance of a form of the medication trial itself—the double-blind parallel groups placebo-controlled trial. This is the type of trial used in all of the studies considered in the hearings and it is the type of trial required by the FDA for approval of medication. Neither the patients nor the investigators know who has received the active agent and who has received the placebo—they are both 'blind.' Blinding is done so that the investigators and the patients will rate changes in symptoms free of the bias of knowing who has received the active drug.

In the double-blind parallel groups placebo-controlled trial, the active medication under study (experimental agent) and the placebo are randomly assigned to a group of patients with a specific disorder. The process of randomly assigning the drug serves to control a wide array of variables such as social class, education, severity of psychopathology, positive or negative life events that may occur over the trial, and an infinite number of additional variables that may have never been considered. The double-blind randomly assigned clinical trial is one of the few true experimental paradigms in clinical psychiatry and the social sciences. Most studies in clinical psychiatry and other social sciences are correlational. Unlike correlational designs, a randomized double-blind trial with a positive outcome provides a basis for causal statements: for example, the drug administered led to the improvement in the group of patients receiving it.

Despite the methodologic elegance and the high scientific status accorded to the placebo-controlled double-blind study, there are many criticisms of the validity of this methodology. First, it has been argued that the blind is easily broken (Fisher and Greenberg 1993). Because the placebo does not have side effects and the active agent often has telltale side effects, the patient and the investigator may be able to guess accurately when the subject is on the active agent. Regrettably, data about the frequency of breaking the blind by correctly guessing the active agent or placebo are typically not gathered and not reported in FDA-sponsored trials.

Although this critique has merit, it is not as devastating as it might first appear to be. Many patients who receive placebo report side effects similar to those already known to occur with the active agent. This is because the patients are presented with these side effects in detail in the informed consent document that precedes each trial. Some of the side effects in placebo recipients are severe enough to lead them to be removed from the trial. Investigators (those who actually see the patients and dispense medications) typically find it very difficult during the course of the trial to determine who is on a placebo and who is on an active agent. As a further argument against this critique, if investigators and patients could correctly guess who was on placebo and who was on active medication, the differences between active agent and placebo would not be as small as they are routinely found to be in studies of antidepressants in children and adolescents.

In the depression trials under discussion there was a large placebo response. This diminishes the differences between the responses of the group receiving the active agent and the group receiving the placebo. Before it will approve a drug, the FDA demands a statistically significant difference between active agent and placebo in two separate double-blind placebo-controlled trials. Very often the trials are not successful with antidepressants because of the substantial placebo response. Minimizing placebo response is a major objective in the performance of these trials. In an effort to minimize placebo response in depressed patients, investigators are asked to be matter of fact and to minimize expressions of warmth and concern.

12.4 **The economic context of the trials**

The clinical trials endeavor seems at times not to lead to Bacon's marketplace of ideas, but rather to the marketplace itself. To understand fully the antidepressant trials in children controversy, the economic context in which these studies took place must be acknowledged. Most of the studies in the FDA review were paid for by pharmaceutical companies. Although these companies embrace a variety of professional standards, their primary obligation is to increase shareholder returns (Relman 2007). Government regulation by the FDA is designed to enhance adherence to high standards of scientific integrity. Nevertheless, despite governmental oversight and regulation, economic greed lurks as a constant threat to the validity of trials. The amounts of money involved in conducting the studies and the enormous economic rewards for successful trial outcomes are constant forces threatening the integrity of the double-blind placebo-controlled trial. Although most of those who perform clinical trials are scrupulously honest, economic self-interest may operate to varying degrees from the highest levels of the pharmaceutical company down to the individual investigator.

According to the pharmaceutical industry, each new drug that is successfully brought to market costs $1.6 billion, including the cost of failed drugs (Relman 2007). When a new medication is introduced, it is protected by a patent. The patent is for seventeen years but the patent begins to run (expire) during the course of drug development and clinical trials. The monopoly that the pharmaceutical industry has on the medication is ticking toward expiration during the clinical trial period before the medication has been brought to market. The industry has an economic incentive to complete the trials as rapidly as possible to bring the medication to market for as long as possible and to reap the economic rewards of selling the drug under higher-priced patent protection.

The trials are usually conducted at sites all over the country. There may be more than thirty sites. The sites that perform clinical trials operate under a system of economic incentives. They are only paid by patient visit. They must enroll patients with the diagnosis and illness severity called for in the study protocol. There is some ambiguity in psychiatric diagnosis in general as well as ambiguity in the diagnosis of depression in particular. There is a strong economic incentive to enroll patients whose depression diagnosis is less certain than that called for in the protocol. Similarly, many studies of depression require the patient to remain at a high level of depression for several initial visits before the patient actually being administered the study medication. In the studies of depression reviewed at these hearings, patients were usually seen for about one to three sessions and were required to maintain a moderate level of severity before they were actually enrolled in the study. One study of this process reports that severity levels of illness decline abruptly after patients are enrolled (Landin *et al.* 2000). This has been taken to suggest that patients' severity ratings are inflated to a level that will insure their enrollment into the study. After the enrollment visit, severity scores decline to reflect more accurately the patients' actual ratings. Exaggerating the severity of the illness to meet the severity of illness called for in the protocol serves to allow the investigator to enroll more patients and thus earn more reimbursement from the pharmaceutical company.

In the early 1990s there was a dearth of information and studies about the response of depressed children and adolescents to SSRI medications. Adults seemed to respond to the medications. There was evidence that earlier versions of antidepressants, the tricyclic antidepressants, worked to some degree in adults but were completely ineffective in children and adolescents. There were almost no data-based studies in the published literature about experience with recently developed antidepressants in children and adolescents. There was a sense of urgency about developing some data about the use of newer antidepressants, as well as other frequently used but untested agents, in children and adolescents. The FDA developed incentives that promised six months' additional patent exclusivity to pharmaceutical companies who studied their adult-approved agents in children and adolescents. Extending drug patents of these drugs for six additional months was worth hundreds of millions of dollars to each pharmaceutical company. The companies did not have to demonstrate that the medication worked.

Most childhood antidepressant studies reviewed by the FDA were performed under this rule rather than to obtain FDA approval for the drug. It has been speculated that one reason the SSRIs failed to demonstrate that they were effective in children and adolescents was the lack of attention the studies received from the pharmaceutical companies (Rosack 2004*a*). The companies knew they were to be rewarded with an additional six months' exclusivity for simply conducting the trial rather than receiving a reward for the results or quality of the trial. The latter was the case when the trials were earlier performed in adults to garner FDA approval for marketing.

Only one childhood antidepressant study conducted in an attempt to gain a patent extension demonstrated that the drug (fluoxetine or Prozac) separated from placebo. It was a replication of an earlier Prozac study that also had demonstrated that the drug worked for children and adolescents. The original study and its replication were designed by Emslie. Both Emslie studies were done with exceptional attention to detail and exceptional diagnostic rigor (Emslie *et al.* 1997, 2002).

A third trial that was included in the FDA childhood antidepressant review and which demonstrated effectiveness of an SSRI (again this was Prozac) was the Treatment of Adolescent Depression Study (TADS), an NIMH sponsored trial authored by March (March *et al.* 2004).

Again, no other agent and no other trial covered in the FDA antidepressant review demonstrated effectiveness for depression. In other words, the drugs did not work for depression in children and adolescents.

12.5 **Public disclosure of failed trials**

One of the most egregious methodological or policy errors to come to public attention during the hearings was the absence of a requirement to have the results of all clinical trials become accessible to the public. As mentioned earlier, for a medication to be approved by the FDA, two double-blind trials in which the medication is statistically significantly better than placebo are required. The number of unsuccessful trials is irrelevant to the approval process. Ten unsuccessful trials may have preceded the two successful trials that form the basis of the FDA approval. That unsuccessful trials were not made public was heavily criticized.

Intuitively, a medication that works twice in a series of ten trials is less likely to work than a medication that works twice in a series of two trials. One trial in twenty will be successful by chance alone.

12.6 Additional criticisms of clinical trials

Many double-blind psychiatric pharmaceutical trials have been criticized on several additional grounds that are also applicable to these trials in the FDA antidepressant review. Trials for FDA approval usually require that patients only have the disorder under study. Because most psychiatric patients have more than one disorder, clinical trials patients are not a representative sample of the patients with the disorder in the community. In the childhood antidepressant studies, the studied depressed children and adolescents were not supposed to be suicidal at entry to the study. This requirement may have biased the sample studied as it renders the sample less like depressed children and adolescents in the community. Also, the study sample was required to be seriously depressed, which means the results might not be generalizeable to patients with milder forms of the illness. The studies were short term: 4–12 weeks. The short-term nature of the studies is not informative about longer treatment time lengths. Usually, the illness lasts longer and usually the medications are taken for a longer time than twelve weeks. Many side effects are rare and may take time to appear. There are relatively few patients in a study compared with the number of patients with the disorder in the general population. There were no completed suicides in the trials reviewed, but completed suicide is a relatively rare event and the size of the sample was too small to test for the incidence of suicide in the antidepressant treated samples. Sample sizes are too small to test for rare side effects in most clinical trials.

12.7 Suicidality

Perhaps the most salient feature of the FDA hearings and studies was the finding that antidepressant agents given to children and adolescents increased suicidal thoughts and behavior. Those who received the active agent were twice as likely to experience suicidal ideation and behavior than those who received the placebo.

The primitive technology used to assess suicidality during these studies best illustrates the thesis of this article: that psychiatry requires improved technology to function effectively. Evaluations for vulnerability to suicide or suicide risk are performed routinely in innumerable child and adolescent psychiatric patient visits every day. Evaluations for suicide risk are a routine part of the initial psychiatric evaluation of all child psychiatric outpatients and occur at all child psychiatric inpatient admissions and discharges. Given the clinical, legal, and economic consequences for an error in these evaluations, it could easily be imagined that the technology and competence for the evaluation of suicidality would be well developed. The FDA review of the material revealed a shameful amount of ineptitude in detecting and classifying suicide risk. Some examples will be given below.

Suicidality and other noteworthy difficulties that were spontaneously reported by the patients were classified as adverse events by the investigators. An adverse event in a clinical trial is a worsening in a patient's condition from baseline (before receipt of the drug or placebo). In accord with FDA and clinical trials methodology these events were described in writing and became part of the narrative of the patients' cases and were reported to the pharmaceutical company sponsoring the trial and the FDA as well. These events were classified by the investigator and then the pharmaceutical company as part of the reporting process; many adverse events that were obviously suicide attempts were not reported as such, and some events that were not suicide attempts were reported as suicide attempts. Two examples of the latter are classifying as a suicide attempt a 14-year-old girl who slapped herself in the face, and reporting a 10-year-old boy with suicidal ideation as a suicide attempt. Examples of the former include the reporting as a personality disorder without suicidality an episode in which a 10-year-old boy tried to hang himself, and the reporting of a patient who took eleven pills at one time and then went to school as a medication error, and classifying an intentional taking of six pills after an argument with the child's mother as an accidental overdose (Posner *et al.* 2007).

The FDA advisory panel asked the Columbia University Departments of Psychiatry and Epidemiology to develop a classification system of suicidality and to review the data from these studies to assess the classification of adverse events reported by the pharmaceutical companies that performed these trials. The request seemed to suggest that the pharmaceutical companies might be underreporting suicidality related to these agents. Columbia found that twelve events classified by the drug companies as suicidal were not suicidal and that twenty-six events not identified as suicidal by the drug companies were identified as possibly suicidal by the new methodology. The specific category of suicide attempt was reduced by 50% compared with the rate reported by the pharmaceutical company. Thus, the less rigorous approach of the pharmaceutical companies served to increase the number of events classified as suicide attempts. Presumably, this is the very opposite of the bias the pharmaceutical companies are assumed to have. It is in their obvious self-interest to minimize the number of suicide attempts associated with their medications. Yet they were actually overestimating the risk, according to the Columbia review panel.

12.8 **Suicide and epidemiology**

Epidemiology provides an alternative perspective on this problem. It is highly relevant because it raises the disturbing possibility that as an unintended consequence of the FDA hearings, black-box warnings on SSRIs may lead to an increase in completed suicides in children and adolescents.

Gibbons *et al.* (2007), in an introduction to their important study, reviewed some of the basic epidemiologic data about suicide. Completed suicide is rare in adolescence; among ages 15–19 its prevalence is 0.008%. Although completed suicide is rare in this age group, it is still the third cause of death in this age range in the USA and is the leading cause of death in this age range in many countries of the world.

Only 2% of adolescents who complete suicide have antidepressants in their blood. Ninety-eight per cent of the completed suicides are not taking antidepressant medicine at the time they kill themselves. This seems to undercut the allegation that antidepressants lead to suicide.

Olfson *et al.* (2003) note that a major national trend in suicide rates has been its decline over the past ten years. For decades, the rates of suicide in adolescents climbed relentlessly. In the mid-1990s it began to reverse and decline each year. One of the variables that may have been associated with the onset in the decline in suicide rates in adolescents was the increasing use of newer antidepressants. Other variables may have contributed to the decline such as the development of the catalytic converter (which lessened the lethality of carbon monoxide suicide attempts) and increased gun regulation (Olfson *et al.* 2003). If increasing use of newer antidepressants contributed to a decline in suicide rates, a decline in the use of the newer antidepressants in response to the FDA black-box warning might contribute to an increase in suicide rates.

In an epidemiological study of antidepressant use and suicide rates in American 10- to 19-year-olds, Olfson *et al.* (2003) combined data from a large pharmacy benefit management organization with national suicide data, census data, and other databases to examine the relation between antidepressant use and suicide rates in 1990 and a decade later in 2000. The data were analyzed in geographical units down to the zip code level. The authors examined the data for the relation between antidepressants and suicide rates over the two time points. Analyzing for change over the decade-long period, the use of SSRIs was strongly associated with a decrease in the suicide rate. A 1% increase in the use of antidepressants in the 15–19 age range resulted in a decrease of 0.23 suicides per 100,000 adolescents per year. This inverse relation was found in males and in individuals with lower family income. Tricyclic antidepressants, which have failed to show any efficacy in this age range for years, did not demonstrate a relation with suicide rates in this study. Also, in this study, the inverse relation between antidepressants and suicide rates could not be demonstrated in 10–14 year olds, although such a relation was later found in a related study by Gibbons *et al.* (2007). These epidemiological studies suggest that antidepressants decrease suicide rates rather than increase them. This seems contrary to the implications of the FDA review we are considering.

An important consideration in the FDA advisory of October 2004 was the relation between time of the initiation of SSRI treatment and the onset of suicidality. The trials' data seemed to suggest that subjects who became suicidal did so during the first four weeks of treatment with an SSRI. In the FDA warning, clinicians were advised to closely monitor SSRI patients for suicidality during the first four weeks of treatment. Simon and Savarino (2007) studied the relation between SSRI treatment initiation and suicidality. Their data set was mostly adults but did include children and adolescents. Also, unlike the childhood antidepressant studies reviewed by the FDA, inpatients as well as outpatients were studied. They examined suicide attempts and suicidal behavior that began within the six months that followed SSRI initiation or the three months that preceded it. In contrast to the clinical trials data, there was no increase in suicide in the first month after the initiation of antidepressant treatment. There was a marked increase in suicidal behavior during the month before the initiation of antidepressant treatment. The risk of suicidality in patients treated with the newer antidepressants reviewed by the FDA (34 per 100,000) was almost half that of older medications (51 per 100,000). Similarly, suicide attempts were much less in the newer antidepressants (76 per 100,000) compared with the older antidepressants (129 per 100,000 patients). The older medications were primarily tricyclics and trazodone. The study supports the concepts that suicidality is a part of the depressive illness and that the newer antidepressants are helpful in treating it. It contradicts the conclusions drawn by the FDA on the basis of clinical trials data.

After the FDA hearings and black-box warnings the prescription of antidepressants for children and adolescents measurably decreased (Daly 2005; Libby *et al.* 2007). I will not review these studies here. The decrease in antidepressant prescription might result in an increase in the adolescent suicide rate. There is no evidence of this so far, but the studies have yet to be done or to be reported.

12.9 Discussion

12.9.1 Technology as a value

The contribution of technology to Western science is inestimable. The development of the computer, atomic energy, space exploration, nuclear accelerators, reproductive technologies, and countless other technological innovations is responsible for many of the scientific advances that characterize our contemporary culture. Scientists advance their fields by using technology with great ingenuity, if not genius. To take a position against the use of technology in contemporary psychiatry verges on taking a position against science.

Science fluctuates in the regard with which it is held by the American public. In this current era of religious revival, reflected in the political power of religious fundamentalism in the USA, the public's regard for science as a worthy endeavor is relatively low (Moran 2007). The technology of stem-cell research and its promise to address a variety of illnesses has been substantially limited by religion-based US government fiat. Similarly, the recent effort to secure legal sanction to teach intelligent design as an alternative to Darwinian evolution is symptomatic of an excessive willingness to abandon the fruits of Western scientific rationality for more primitive modes of thought.

Technology has had some unwelcome consequences for Western society such as nuclear weapons, biological warfare, and global warming, but the use of technology in science and medical research is not in dispute. This does not mean that technology cannot be misunderstood or poorly used in research. With time, critical discussion, and further studies, early misunderstandings in the use and limitations of new technologies become appreciated.

Psychiatry and psychology themselves are not immune to irrational anti-scientific anti-technology strains of thought. Spiritual psychiatry and psychology are regular symposia at national professional mental health meetings and are offered without critical discussion. Many psychiatrists are ambivalent about the science supporting the field of psychiatry. Psychiatry is a clinical specialty and most of those who train in it are interested in learning how to take care of patients rather than performing research. Most psychiatrists after training engage in full-time clinical work. There is no nationwide requirement that psychiatry residents perform or participate in research during their residency training programs. In contrast, US psychiatry residents are required to be competent in the practice of psychoanalysis. Although psychoanalysis offers interesting insights about human behavior, and its status as a science has been subject to a considerable amount of philosophical scrutiny, currently it has little claim to scientific validity.

12.9.2 Clinical trials and the Boyle–Hobbes controversy

The Boyle–Hobbes controversy might enhance our understanding of the antidepressant clinical trials controversy. The clinical trial can be compared with

Boyle's vacuum machine. Boyle developed his vacuum machine in conjunction with the experimental method in the 1660s. The experimental method serves as the basis for contemporary science. Introduced in the mid-twentieth century, the double-blind trial remains the most rigorous experimental paradigm in contemporary clinical psychopharmacology. It is illuminating to compare the controversies of this relatively recent experimental technology with some of the controversies that surrounded the 400-year-old experimental technology of Boyles's vacuum machine. Boyle had an actual machine—the vacuum pump, whereas the double-blind clinical trial is simply a concept and a set of general instructions for studying treatments. Both the vacuum pump and the clinical trial are technological innovations. The vacuum machine and Boyle's experimental methods were sharply criticized by many. Noteworthy among his critics was Thomas Hobbes—best known today for his political philosophy.

Hobbes complained that although the experiments were supposed to be seen and verified by the public, they could only be seen by a few of Boyle's close associates. To understand the vacuum pump fully, a visit to Boyle's laboratory was a necessity. Boyle strongly wished to include the public, and published detailed descriptions of his experiments and detailed directions for how to build a vacuum pump. However, by physical necessity, access to the laboratory itself was limited. In contrast, Hobbes' work was more easily accessed. His work need only be read.

What was public about these antidepressant clinical trials? Most of these trials were not public. They were paid for and controlled by the pharmaceutical companies who released them at their own discretion.

Hobbs also complained that Boyle's experiments could not easily be replicated; the vacuum apparatus was the space shuttle of its day and could not be easily built to repeat and verify experiments. Similarly, a major problem today for clinical trials of antidepressants is their inability to be replicated; adult antidepressant studies that worked initially often fail to work on replication (Khan and Brown 2001).

Also, Hobbes noted that the technology was not perfect: the vacuum machine did not produce a complete vacuum. As already discussed, similar criticisms are routinely levied about the failure of the double-blind placebo-controlled study to detect significant differences between placebo and antidepressants in children. Despite the criticisms of the day, obviously, Boyle's vacuum machine and experimental method have become part of the accepted canon of Western science. Similarly, the clinical trial, though buffeted by a variety of trenchant criticisms, likely will remain the dominant technology for clinical psychopharmacology.

Hobbes and Boyle had different views of the roles of the State in science. Boyle, according to Shapin and Schaffer (1985), believed that the state would come to experimentalists with their problems and the experimentalists would do experiments to learn how to solve the problem. Hobbes believed that the state would develop natural philosophy in such a way to as to calm the populace and help maintain civic order. In the antidepressant clinical trial controversy, the state intervened to protect public health—a legitimate use of state power in a liberal democracy, most would concede. However, from the point of view of the Boyle–Hobbes controversy, the FDA and the congressional hearings had an aspect of the state intruding into the laboratory and challenging the way the experiments were performed. As Hobbes was an absolutist, and critical of the experimental method, this seems to be an intervention Hobbes might have relished.

12.10 **Conclusion**

This review of double-blind clinical trials to establish the safety and efficacy of newer antidepressants in children and adolescents has demonstrated substantial technical flaws in the endeavor. The meager and uncertain results of this major effort have left the clinicians and the patients they serve frustrated and confused about the safety and usefulness of antidepressants for depressed adolescents. The need for improved technological innovation is obvious.
Enhancing the double-blind clinical trial for the assessment of psychopharmacologic agents in childhood depression continues to challenge researchers. Clinicians and the public have a major stake in these efforts and should insist on continued public and fiscal support for these technologies.

References

Daly R. (2005). Drop in youth antidepressant prompts call for FDA monitoring. *Psychiatric News*, **40**, 18.

Emslie G. J., Rush A. J., Weinberg, J., *et al.* (1997). Fluoxetine in children and adolescents with depression. *Archives of General Psychiatry*, **54**, 1009–1015.

Emslie G. J., Heiligenstein J. H., Wagner K. D., *et al.* (2002). Fluoxetine for acute treatment of depression in children and adolescents: a placebo-controlled, randomized clinical trial. *Journal of the American Academy of Child and Adolescent Psychiatry*, **41**, 1205–1215.

Fisher S. and Greenberg R. (1993). How sound is the double-blind design for evaluating psychotropic drugs? *Journal of Nervous and Mental Disease*, **181**, 345–350.

Gibbons R. D., Hur K., Bhaumik D. K., and Mann J. J. (2007). The relationship between antidepressant prescription and rate of early adolescent suicide. *American Journal of Psychiatry*, **164**, 1044–1049.

Khan A. and Brown W. (2001). The placebo enigma in antidepressant clinical trials. *Journal of Clinical Psychopharmacology*, **21**, 123–125.

Klee R. (1997). *Introduction to the Philosophy of Science: Cutting nature at its seams* (New York, NY: Oxford University Press).

Landin R., DeBrota D. J., DeVries T.A., *et al.* (2000). The impact of restrictive entry criterion during the placebo lead-in period. *Biometrics*, **56**, 271–278.

Leslie L. K., Newman T. B., Chesney P. J., and Perrin J. M. (2005). The Food and Drug Administration's deliberations on antidepressant use in pediatric patients. *Pediatrics*, **116**, 195–204.

Libby A. M., Brent D. A., Morrato E. H., *et al.* (2007). Decline in treatment of pediatric depression after FDA advisory on risk of suicidality with SSRIs. *American Journal of Psychiatry*, **164**, 884–891.

March J., Siva S., Petrycki S., *et al.* (2004). Fluoxetine, cognitive–behavioral therapy, and their combination for adolescents with depression: treatment for adolescents with depression study (TADS) team. *Journal of the American Medical Association*, **292**, 807–820.

Moran M. (2007). Science can't thrive in ivory tower. *Psychiatric News*, **42**(13), 24–25.

Olfson M., Shaffer D., Marcus S. C., and Greenberg T. (2003). Relationship between antidepressant treatment and suicide in adolescents. *Archives of General Psychiatry*, **60**, 978–982.

Pfeffer C. (2007). The FDA pediatric advisories and changes in diagnosis and treatment of pediatric depression. *American Journal of Psychiatry*, **164**, 843–846.

Posner K., Oquendo M.A., Gould M., *et al.* (2007). Columbia classification algorithm of suicide assessment (C-CASA): Classification of suicidal events in the FDA's pediatric suicidal risk analysis of antidepressants. *American Journal of Psychiatry*, **164**, 1035–1043.

Relman A. (2007). Book review of R. Epstein (2007) *Overdose: How excessive government regulation stifles pharmaceutical innovation* Yale University Press. *The New Republic*, **237**, 36–42.

Rosack J. (2004*a*). Clinical trials controversy spotlights flawed system. *Psychiatric News*, **39**(14), 1–13.

Rosack J. (2004*b*). Congress hammers FDA over handling of SSRIs. *Psychiatric News*, **39**(20), 1–3.

Shapin S. and Schaffer S. (1985). *Leviathan and the Air Pump: Hobbes Boyle and the experimental life* (Princeton, NJ: Princeton University Press).

Simon G. E. and Savarino J. (2007). Suicide attempts among patients starting depression treatment with medications or psychotherapy. *American Journal of Psychiatry*, **164**, 1029–1034.

Chapter 13

Philosophical considerations of an Internet-enabled telephone and computer psychiatric symptom monitoring system: maintaining the balance between subjectivity and objectivity in research

Karen Iseminger and Dale Theobald

13.1 Introduction

This chapter concerns a philosophical investigation of a technology-driven assessment of psychiatric symptoms of cancer patients in Indiana. Its purpose is to articulate the unobserved and unappreciated philosophical aspects of this technology-based evaluation of cancer patients' lives. After some introductory comments about the need for research addressing symptom management for cancer patients, we will briefly describe community cancer care (CCC) and research we are conducting to investigate ways to lessen the symptom burden of cancer patients, including a description of how technology can assist researchers in obtaining data. We will discuss how philosophy assists in describing the depth of reflection required to represent patients' experiences more accurately. Finally, we will offer two pragmatic examples of ways in which we can honor these philosophical concerns by incorporating qualitative data into our research and employing a nurse care manager, who takes an existential approach in assisting patients to add meaningful personal expression of their experiences to the numerical representation of their quality of life. Our discussion will show that although patient-reported outcomes (PROs) are necessary to test the effectiveness of treatment and to understand conditions, they remain insufficient to assess fully the existential concerns that patients may have. Our primary concern is that technology may fail to capture information crucial to medical treatment on a practical level; and on a philosophical level, it may objectify patients and their lived experience with cancer, thereby reducing their humanity.

In recent years, because of improvements in early detection and medical treatment, cancer survival rate are improving and patients are living longer. As a result, we have seen increased focus on psychiatric symptom management as a crucial adjunct to medical treatment. Symptom management efforts typically focus on reducing symptom burden and improving patients' quality of life by relieving symptoms, providing much needed emotional support, and easing distress caused from disease and its treatment. By maintaining their ordinary daily activities, patients are often more likely to maintain optimism and improve their cooperation with medical treatment. Symptom management is essential for the patient at all stages of treatment. Researchers and clinicians are working to move symptom-focused assessments and interventions earlier in the care process for cancer patients. These supportive care interventions also focus on providing support to the patient's family throughout the course of the illness. Ameliorating symptoms improves their lived experience, freeing them to focus their energy on getting well.

Throughout this chapter, we will use the term 'quality of life' to indicate both a type of research as well as the general notion of patient's well-being. When used to indicate a type of research, it will be capitalized (QOL), and it will be written as 'quality of life' when used descriptively. One working definition of quality of life is as follows: 'quality of life is described as individuals' overall satisfaction with life and the general state of personal well-being. Six dimensions relevant to this definition include: cognitive, social, physical, emotional, personal productivity and intimacy' (Shumaker 1990). The terminology used in the professional community of cancer providers differs from that which one might expect in the psychiatric community. The National Comprehensive Cancer Network (NCCN) has set standards for the care of oncology patients' distress. They chose the term distress because it causes fewer stigmas than other psychiatric terms. They define distress as a multifactor, unpleasant emotional experience of a psychological (cognitive, behavioral, emotional), social, or spiritual nature that may interfere with the ability to cope effectively with cancer, its physical symptoms, and its treatment. Distress extends along a continuum, ranging from common, normal feelings of vulnerability, sadness, and fears, to problems that can become disabling, such as depression, anxiety, panic, social isolation, and existential and spiritual crisis. We emphasize existential and spiritual crises because, to our knowledge, this category of distress has not been addressed in traditional symptom management research. The need to evaluate and care for the existential needs of patients requires us as researchers to delve deeper than traditional symptomatology, to investigate observable signs that indicate patients' existential and spiritual status. With this admonishment to evaluate and care for the existential needs of the patient, it behoves oncologists to research phenomena beyond traditional symptomatology, to include existential aspects of cancer care.

At this time, most published research on symptom reduction is exclusively quantitative in nature. Researchers spend great energy on validation and standardization of forced-choice inventories. The motivation of the scientific community is sincere, with their goal to improve patients' quality of life by managing their psychiatric symptoms. Nonetheless, we believe that the potential to misidentify crucial symptoms is inherent in any system that automates symptom assessment by reducing it to a mechanical, forced-choice process instead of one that works individually with each client in a more personal way.

From a scientific perspective, this reduction of patient interaction in a more automated system adds efficiency and cost effectiveness. Researchers argue that quantitative measures yield data that are reproducible and predictive of outcomes and therefore have more validity and usability. From a philosophical perspective, we must consider whether this process somehow reduces patients in a way that diminishes their humanity. We examine the process of symptom assessment and investigate how to gain valid information from patients while honoring and preserving their humanity. Although PROs are necessary to conduct randomized research regarding symptoms, we hold that we must redefine PROs to include qualitative reports that accurately reflect the human experience of (in this case) cancer. Further, we can view PROs and QOL research as an avenue for the application of philosophy to healthcare, forming a framework for the appreciation of existence, especially when an alien cancer has challenged existence. An understanding of the philosophical basis of QOL can positively influence all facets of traditional medical and psychosocial research: its design, conduct, report, and interpretation. The inclusion of philosophical inquiry in the scientific process deepens our understanding of patients' needs and forges an important alliance with traditional medical and psychosocial research.

13.2 The Community Cancer Care quality of life program: research strategies for symptom management

CCC partners with hospitals to provide cancer patients with care and programming. CCC has formed partnerships with more than 20 hospitals in Indiana, providing state-of-the-art oncology care for rural populations in underserved hospitals as well as urban locations. One of the unique features of

CCC is the provision of psychiatric supportive care to many of these clinics. This enables patients to receive treatment close to their home without having to travel to larger cities for treatment. Since the early 1990s, the program has actively pursued a quality of life/symptom management clinical and research agenda. After completing a series of investigations of outcomes studies for targeted symptoms, practice and research focus has turned toward finding a technology-based solution for integrating regular symptom assessment and feedback in our diverse, community-based cancer practices.

Increased awareness of the range of symptoms experienced by cancer patients and its effects on the success of medical treatment highlights the need to measure the frequency, severity, and progress in alleviating those symptoms. Recent literature has documented the effectiveness of interventions for symptom management in cancer patients in both the acute treatment setting and in palliative settings such as in hospices (Chang and Ingham 2003; Cleeland and Reyes-Gibby 2002; National Institutes of Health 2003). Accordingly, CCC is an evidenced-based practice, basing policy and procedure as much as possible on this research.

CCC has been conducting investigation of the effectiveness of a computer-automated system that uses the technologies of both the touch-tone telephone and the Internet to enable patients to provide home-based ratings of their symptoms between office visits with their oncologist and oncology nurses. Results so far have indicated that technology for assessing cancer patients' psychiatric symptoms balances the anticipated philosophical problems with some surprising benefits such as empowering patients by giving them a voice in their treatment. By gathering information about specific symptoms, we can individualize patients' care. In this way, CCC strives to avoid objectifying patients, thus limiting the potential risk of harm that using technology poses.

In the next section, we will describe research programs being conducted by CCC.

13.3 Technology applied to symptom management

Multiple epidemiologic studies have demonstrated the comorbidity of pain and depression (Kroenke 2003; Kroenke and Price 1993; Kroenke *et al.* 1994, 1997; Jackson *et al.* 1998). A critical review of 169 published research reports found a high co-occurrence rate of pain and depression, averaging in the thirty to fifty per cent range (Bair *et al.* 2003). Studies also demonstrated that comorbid pain adversely affects depression, health status, work functioning, and other clinical outcomes. Comorbid depression has a similar effect in patients with pain (*ibid.*; Gallagher and Verma 1999; Gupta 1986;). Cost-effectiveness analyses from many trials have suggested that improving primary care depression management is a good value (Goldman *et al.* 1991; Kaplan and Anderson 1988; Valenstein *et al.* 2001).

In summary, these data indicate that pain associated with chronic or debilitating disease, more than merely a symptom, is a subjective correlate of a physiological process that can negatively interact with medical treatment and exacerbate the course of the disease. As well, life-threatening disease, incumbent pain, and feelings of helplessness caused by a patient's sense that an alien disease is invading their body often cause psychiatric symptoms or exacerbate pre-existing psychiatric disorders that in turn also worsen the plight of the patient.

All these factors contribute to higher cost of treatment, which, in its turn, can increase the stress experienced by the patient and the patient's family. Increased stress, like pain, also contributes to exacerbation of both psychiatric symptoms and the target physical disease. In addition to providing significant long-range cost-effectiveness benefits, beginning the process of physical and psychiatric symptom management as soon as possible after diagnosis is crucial to prevent impairment of QOL in general and in health-related quality of life in particular.

Consequently, we can expect that research designed to develop cost-effective, easily accessible systems to identify psychiatric symptoms known to impair quality of life would assist in early identification and treatment. In turn, we can expect this to have salubrious effects on the course of treatment for the target disease. The most salient symptoms we wish to target include pain, correlates of depression, and behavioral measures, from which we can infer that the patients and their families enjoy an increased sense of empowerment. So with the ultimate goal of improving patients' lived experience and survival rates, our initial task is to develop the symptom identification and management system so conceived.

After completing a series of investigations of outcomes studies for targeted symptoms, CCC has turned its research focus toward finding a technology-based solution for integrating regular symptom assessment and feedback in our diverse, community-based cancer practices. Paper and pencil reporting systems have problems with access and potentially prohibitive cost to deal with labor-intensive tabulation, interpretation, and communication of results. Given the practical limitations of paper and pencil reporting systems, CCC and Interactive Performance Technologies Inc. are collaborating on an evaluation of the feasibility of automating symptom screening and feedback across a state-wide cancer outreach network using the cancer 'Symptom

Monitor' (CSM). CSM is a computer-automated system that uses an innovative software application integrating interactive voice response (IVR) telephone technology and Internet-connected computers enabling patients to provide home-based ratings of their symptoms between office visits with their oncologist and oncology nurses. Using data collected in this way, the patient care team easily, conveniently, and quickly assesses and regularly monitors symptoms patients are experiencing and how the symptoms are interfering with their daily activities. Obtaining real-time results allows the team to address symptoms in a timely manner.

The Symptom Monitor uses the MD Anderson Symptom Inventory (MDASI). The MDASI uses a series of questions designed to monitor thirteen core symptoms patients may experience. The instrument includes six questions addressing how those symptoms interfere with patients' daily activities. Multi-symptom self-reports are recorded, stored in a database, and reported simultaneously by facsimile and email to the office where the individual patient receives treatment. The database enables us to establish norms and standards for outcome evaluations.

Members of the care team at each outreach location receive orientation to the MDASI and the automated system. At six-monthly intervals, the care team at each clinic is offered a focus group session at a convenient time to review their experience with the CSM. During these sessions, investigators ask participants to complete brief objective and qualitative assessments focusing on the utility of the CSM to identify areas of symptom concern, promoting clinical interventions, assisting in communication with patients, and identifying areas of need. We also elicit less structured qualitative feedback. So far, data reflect excellent acceptance of the technology by nursing staff (Theobald *et al.* 2004).

In traditional treatment settings, symptoms are frequently either unrecognized or under-treated. Four common barriers to treatment include under detection, inadequate initial treatment, failure to monitor treatment compliance and symptom response, and failure to adjust treatment in patients not responding to, or intolerant of, the initial course of therapy. With early detection based on CSM, nurse-delivered care management models proven effective for depression in primary care have considerable potential for depression and pain care for cancer patients. With our automated system, however, reliable identification of clinically significant symptoms supports more effective, early treatment. For example, when a Likert scale rating for fatigue, pain, or nausea and vomiting exceeds a preset cut point, we send team members a summary of the National Comprehensive Cancer Network (NCCN) clinical guideline for that symptom incorporated into the faxed back report.

Similarly, pain and depression are two of the most prevalent and treatable cancer-related symptoms, each present in twenty to thirty per cent of oncology patients. Preliminary research done by CCC demonstrated that healthcare teams often failed to recognize clinically significant psychiatric symptoms (McDonald *et al.* 1999; Passik *et al.* 1998).

13.4 **Philosophical issues raised by technologically assessed psychiatric and oncology symptoms**

Although psychosocial research has been used in clinical trials, the relevance of philosophy to that endeavor has not been adequately established. Our philosophical exploration is founded on the work of Martin Buber and Emmanuel Levinas' consideration of the existential tenets of alienation and subjectivity as they apply to cancer patients' experience with a technology-based system to assess their psychiatric needs. We consider Buber's conceptualization of 'Thou,' a being whose unique presence responds to individuality and, accordingly, resists reductionistic measures requisite for a technology-driven process, and Levinas' emphasis on ethics as it relates to existentialism. Building upon this conceptual challenge, we address technology using Jürgen Habermas' arguments as a cornerstone of this discussion

Martin Buber holds that vital to understanding our humanity, is the distinction between the I–it relationship and the I–Thou relationship (Buber 1958). To be considered valid, traditional scientific research requires precisely stated operational definitions that can be tested under the rubric of randomized design with observable, independently verifiable outcome measures such as toxicity levels, morbidity, and mortality statistics—objective reality. We may come to know objects (I–it relationships) on many levels through objective, scientific analysis—positivistic reduction being therein inevitable—with each dimension suggestion different ways of acting on the object that might cause predictable results we could agree benefit us in some way. This sort of research, for example, might develop less-invasive surgical techniques or new surgical instruments. An individual's perspectives, feelings, beliefs, and desires, although produced by the nervous system and crucial to a sense of well-being, are internal mental events not objectively verifiable by independent observers—subjective reality.

But when our 'object of inquiry,' is not an 'it,' but a 'Thou,' if we presume to effect benefit to human beings' lived experience (I–Thou relationships), then we must acknowledge and remain mindful that to come to know, even in a limited way, another human being's subjective experience requires respectful human dialogue. Our patient's subjective experience of self is not directly available to us to study as we would examine a rock or an atom.

As Levinas reminds us, our existence is centered in solitude, separateness from others. We must escape that solitude to connect with others, to form social contracts. With the first connection being between infant and mother, we progress from close family and caretaker relationships, through close community (usually school), and finally to larger social circles we define as society and the world. Buber teaches us that the way in which we engage in this social dialogue defines our existence just as much as our personal identity influences the nature of the social relationships into which we enter. Of primary importance is that for healthcare providers to engage in effective treatment (a social dialogue with our patient), we must give them a voice with which to express their presence and the tools with which they can leave that solitude.

Cancer, or any major or chronic disease, can lead to feelings of alienation. Persons so afflicted might come to view themselves as battling an invading force alone, or as someone about to leave the company of the living, frozen, as it were, in some place between the company of the living and the dead, a place in which they stand alone. Cancer patients commonly complain about the disruption and fragmentation of their daily lives that they experience after diagnosis and subsequent medical treatment of their disease. All of their usual activities and relationships suffer as their primary focus shifts to doctor's appointments, check-ups, medical treatments that might include chemotherapy, radiation, or surgery, and the side effects of those treatments. The focus switches from what they usually do, who they truly are, and their identity-defining social relationships to a never-ending stream of interactions with machinery, drugs, surgeries, and other medical treatments.

Doctors have often been criticized for treating the disease instead of the patient (Dr Smith might be called 'to see the Kaposi's sarcoma in room 318' instead of 'John Smith'). Exigencies of modern medical practice leave little time for personal interaction between healthcare providers and patients. Patients with appointments to see their doctor about one symptom are often asked to make another appointment if they have a collateral or new concern, because health insurance companies sometimes only allow the physician to see (bill for) 'the presenting compliant.' They are not allowed to address 'other concerns' in the same visit because it creates medical billing code confusion!

In summary, to provide ethical treatment of psychiatric symptoms experienced by oncology patients, the work of Buber and Levinas convincingly argues not only the morality of, but also the necessity of, entering into a personal dialogue centered within, and driven by patients' subjective expression of their lived experience. With that duty acknowledged, we next consider some aspects of communication by which we can engage in such a dialogue.

As analyzed by Habermas, communicative action is the fundamental vehicle by which individuals enter into this dialogue, in ever-widening human spheres to form unions, families, social groups, societies, and cultures. *Lebenswelt* (life-world) is the saturation of communicative action by tradition and routinized way of doing daily activities. Conduct happens within this pre-established set of forms of life. From the beginning of time, the needs of individuals, societies, and cultures have driven individual action to determine the direction of technology development. Technology is not neutral. Over time, as technology has permeated the fabric of our daily lives at all levels of human interaction, the action of societies and cultures and individual personality has become articulated by the lifeworld as much as these entities drive the further development of technology. Technological development transforms what it is to be human.

In the context of identifying, monitoring, and managing psychiatric correlates of cancer, the task of assessing the ethics and morality of technology to accomplish the task is complex. Preliminary analysis indicates that the IVR system has been demonstrated to assess effectively and efficiently psychiatric symptoms that frequently go undiagnosed or under-treated in older venues using traditional interview techniques. The system, therefore, ostensibly meets feasibility and cost-effectiveness criteria—the means apparently achieve the desired ends. Once so determined, we must turn our attention to ethical issues relative to the objectifying aspects of using technology for symptom management and the question whether emergent phenomena such as mental states can be adequately measured to form valid data for scientific analysis.

Using our present research as a specific example of these more general issues, we question whether replacing personal diagnostic and monitoring interviews with automated data collection systems—replacing person-to-person interactions with a person-to-machine interaction—further complicates the patient's lived cancer experience. We contend that such a process reduces patients' humanity to something less, which we term a 'reductionistic insult.' We question whether developing operational definitions of mental states adequate to form the basis of valid data analysis can also sufficiently tap the emergent qualities of those states.

In a traditional setting, we presume that in addition to gathering information during an in-person interview, the personal transaction ('hand holding') itself can alleviate some of the patient's concerns. On the other hand, sometimes conversation is difficult. Patients may not have adequate language to describe their symptoms. Some symptoms such as alienation, known to be problematic in oncology patients, create a psychological chasm between patient and healthcare team members. Our investigation must be multifaceted.

Does the automated system with structured questions provide privacy to put patients at ease and suggest to them appropriate words to express their distress? Does the impersonal technology rob patients of the compassionate interaction that ordinarily provides them comfort? Does reducing their deepest angst to electronic impulses somehow also reduce their humanity? How can we promote the benefits and curtail the detriments of such a technology?

We need to create a service delivery system adequate to meet the needs of our patients, and test the efficacy of treatment. On the other hand, we need to find some balance between those needs and our duty to honor the humanity of our patients. Our goal, then, is to investigate whether our automated systems, by comparison with traditional quantitative data collection systems, cause cancer patients to feel more dehumanized—whether by these methods patients experience greater philosophical insult than that caused by traditional data collection systems. We want to evaluate whether the technology could be adding another level of psychological distance between the researcher and the patient.

The purpose of PRO is to provide an avenue for scientific analysis of subjective experience—arguably eliminating the 'scientific' nature of the inquiry according to strict positivist thinking, but essential, in our view, to deal with human beings as the object of inquiry. We view PRO research as an improvement over standard scientific research that discounts any subjective experience as beyond measure. However, we caution that researchers must remain sensitive to the need for PRO data collection methods to obtain as accurate information as possible. Some of the risks in this process are easy to identify. For example, if our questionnaire asks about thirteen symptoms thought by us to be significant, how are the results compromised if the patient does not think of his or her symptoms in the terms we used on the questionnaire? How is our ability to treat compromised if the patient is experiencing a symptom such as 'inability to describe feelings,' or 'detachment,' causing the patient to be apathetic towards answering the questions? Other issues are more complex. Underestimating patients' lifeworld by relying too heavily on a technological approach to symptom monitoring, can further alienate them. Applying Habermas' discussion to PROs, the integration of qualitative and quantitative research methodologies enhances our ability to understand some greater truth of experience.

13.5 Epistemological approach to knowledge gained by technology-driven symptom management systems

We have seen that typical QOL data collection, using objective scientific methods, may fail to elicit meaningful information about patients' lived experience.

The form of the questions, the preconceived, researcher-driven alternative answers, and the delivery method can all impose an unnatural form of reality on patients that fails to capture what the patients might have wanted to express had they been approached personally and in a different way. Researchers represent these data as objective reality, without acknowledging the subjective aspects of knowledge. What we know is integrally related to how we come to know it. Philosophical objections to the method of inquiry make equally suspect any claims about knowledge gained by these methods. Although conclusions from standard quality of life measures offer the scientific community valuable information, we cannot say that these data fully represent patients' truth. Epistemology, the study of the nature and scope of knowledge and the reliability of claims to knowledge, can shed more light on these issues.

In clinical medicine, the difference between objective measures (signs) and subjective measures (symptoms) is significant. For example, an objective investigator can observe, measure, and document an irregularly shaped lesion on the left buttocks of a 65-year-old female, who lives alone. However, the subjective evidence of some diseases, something felt by the patient, may not be directly observable to others; for example, the same 65-year-old woman reports sensations of tingling or pain radiating down her leg.

In the strictest application of positivist scientific method, we would only give weight to objective measures, because we cannot independently corroborate the self-report of 'tingling' or 'pain.' In the case offered, however, had the patient not experienced the symptoms of tingling or pain, she might never have thought to seek treatment until cure was no longer possible.

Obviously, we must find some balance between the benefits of knowledge gained from a positivist approach to medical research and a holistic approach that values subjective expression of lived experience. To assist patients to emerge from solitude and to rectify their alienation, the best way to truth is through relational knowing—gathering evidence of the patient's lived experience through a personal relationship expressed in terms of interpersonal dialogue based first in the patient's center, not driven by the researcher's preconceived notions of what we will find. Using only a technologically based symptom management system, what would we make of a questionnaire not completed? Another with only blanks? Others not submitted at all?

In her masterpiece *Middlemarch*, George Eliot (1956) observes, 'If we had a keen vision and feeling of all ordinary human life, it would be like hearing the grass grow and the squirrel's heart beat, and we should die of that roar which lies on the other side of silence' (Belenky 1986). Accordingly, Joanne Hall and Patricia Stevens admonish healthcare professionals to learn to see beyond and behind what we have traditionally been socialized to believe is there (Hall and Stevens 1996).

The medical care management team must be most sensitive to the roar behind the silence. Blanks on an objective questionnaire do not mean 'nothing to report.' We can only fully understand this silence in the context of the patient's wider life. We cannot fully appreciate the meaning of a symptom unless we also elicit the context in which the symptom arises. Pain in the hips reported by a patient who sat throughout the day on a sofa may have significantly different meaning from pain reported by a patient after climbing a mountain trail. Pain reported at a score of 3 on a scale of 10 may mean something very different as reported by an habitually stoic patient who has become accustomed to many physical hardships compared with the same 3 reported by a patient for whom this is the first experience with physically painful experiences. So PROs can provide needed voice for entire groups of patients to let their needs be known about their healthcare and for them to tell us about their lives, but only insofar as the method aims to capture contextual components of the data and incorporates ways of coming to hear them in a relational setting.

Lorraine Code (1983) describes importance of this sort of contextual knowledge by appealing for 'thicker' descriptions of knowledge, noting that traditional theories of knowledge are based upon 'thin' descriptions and an 'impoverished explanatory scope' that does not consider the life processes in individuals and among knowers. Objective surveys that ignore subjective data are thin, lacking contextual clues necessary to discover crucial information. She holds, 'there is no knowledge without knowers, no knowledge without context.' Our licorice parable emphasizes the importance of asking about individuals' unique lived experience as opposed to merely subjecting them to our preconceived standardized, 'objective' measures.

A normative epistemic approach necessitates pluralistic approaches to acquiring knowledge. Until recently, we have seen a disparity between objective quantitative research (questionnaires with numbers) and the qualitative research (analysis of texts of patient recorded interviews). We advocate a mixed methodology of quantitative and qualitative approaches to capture a fuller, more accurate, and philosophically sound picture of the oncology patient's lived experience. Thomas Kuhn documents and follows metaphysical and epistemological considerations of this paradigm shift in his works on the structure of scientific revolutions (Kuhn, 1996). These approaches adopt a phenomenological approach to data collection, paying explicit and special attention to patient-reported outcomes to assess the content of their consciousness. Using these qualitative methodologies allows patients to supply evidence of their own understanding of and meanings associated with the disease, their symptoms, their treatment, as well as their own sense of health and well-being. This system of research is starkly different from traditional quality of life studies.

In the next section of this chapter, we offer some suggestions about how to develop such a mixed methodology, a pluralistic endeavor, which provides enhanced strategies for the acquisition of deeper knowledge and decreasing objectification of patients. We encourage researchers to be open to asking new questions or using new techniques that might unearth results they might not have hypothesized using more traditional, positivistic methods.

13.6 Pragmatic applications of philosophy to a mixed methodology of objective and qualitative research inquiry

Thus far, we have endorsed a technology-based symptom management system with the proviso that it be augmented with methods to elicit qualitative, subjective measures of patients' lived experience. We have argued that health-care providers/researchers have a duty to expand their intentional acts of consciousness toward the subjective otherness of the patient. In this section, after describing some qualitative research techniques, we will describe some ways CCC is conducting this sort of qualitative inquiry.

Although completely capturing subjective experience in a research paradigm is impossible, we encourage scholars to attempt to do so by integrating qualitative research with more traditional quantitative research. CCC uses qualitative data gleaned from focus group analysis within the larger quantitative study of cancer patients reporting of symptoms. These focus groups conduct interviews, which use group interaction to produce data and insights that would be less accessible without the interaction found in a group (Morgan1997).

We assign patients and care team members to focus groups composed of six to ten participants. Patient-only groups allow more detailed discussion of psychiatric and physical symptoms than questionnaires typically allow. We also encourage the patients to articulate their feelings and their pragmatic experiences with using the CSM. Care team member groups, composed of nurses and physicians, focus on how the team uses the data once they receive it in the clinic. We attempt to ascertain patients, physicians, and nurses' perceptions of the advantages, disadvantages, and issues associated with the symptom monitoring system. We examine closely whether the severity alert feedback component captures data that is an accurate representation of the acuity of the patient's needs. Through this process, we hope to gain deeper insight from the users' perspective, not generally achieved in quantitative analysis.

We hypothesize that these additional methods of research are necessary to mitigate potential philosophical damages potentially caused by traditional quality of life research and symptom management research. We struck on this component of our proposed paradigm somewhat unexpectedly. Heretofore, we had been advocates of honoring the subjective experience of patients primarily via some form of formalized qualitative research. However, we discovered an additional mechanism for championing subjectivity as we participated in Kurt Kroenke's INCPAD trial. The trial uses a model of care previously found to be a successful method for augmenting care within a research protocol. Although Dr Kroenke probably did not have philosophy in mind when he wrote the protocol, we were able to suggest that the nurses' conversations with the research participants allowed a more complete 'knowing' of the patient, in a manner that Levinas, Buber, or Habermas could endorse.

The three-component model, used in the INCPAD trial, allows the nurse care manager to expand upon scores within the PRO with unique subjective accounts of the complex issues ordinarily condensed in technology. The nurse care manager's institution discusses patients' objective symptom monitoring reports with them to ascertain any discrepancies between patients' subjective report of experience and the data collected with the objective instruments. In addition, they hold a care conference to discuss cases so that the entire group of providers learns the significance of the patients' numerical scores.

During one of those care conferences, listening to a nurse describe the information she got, when I thought, 'Aha! This is exactly what I have been saying for years!' Thus, the weekly care conference allows us to examine what the numbers mean and enhances our ability to individualize care at a deeper level of knowing. It combines quantitative PROs with subjective accounts from patients, which are richer and deeper in their descriptions of 'what is really going on here.' On a practical level, the care conference used in this way lessens the objectifying nature of the research and technology.

Contrast the following paragraphs with a technologic representation of depression as a score of '19' with the following two narratives obtained from a nurse care manager, who did routine follow-up on scores. 'I've had drastic changes in my life…like eliminating my job, dealing with the fistula, and now the colostomy.' She had to quit teaching school after a seventeen-year teaching career. She states 'I was so disappointed about this.' She reports feeling 'tired of all this.' She has a history of a fistula and reports being homebound for six months, before recent surgery for colostomy. 'Now I'm having to adjust to the changes since the colostomy.' She reports significant fatigue and decreased strength and states 'it just doesn't seem like I'm bouncing back as well this time.' She has concerns about intimacy with her husband since the colostomy was done. She also voices disappointment for her family and states 'I didn't get to go to my son's recent college graduation, and I'm concerned about not being as involved in my daughter's senior year of high school as I'd like to be.'

A second patient also reports low mood in vivid terms. He states 'I think I'd be better off dead, and I've thought this way about every day this week.' He denies any plan or intent. He states 'I wouldn't do anything because I don't want to put my family through anything more than I have to.' He states 'I feel like such a burden.'

The potential to gain this sort of enriched information about patients' lived experience forms the foundation for us to advocate that the home-based symptom monitoring should be paired with a nurse care manager. Looking at patients' responses to the symptom monitoring and calculating scores is easy. However, only looking at a patient's 'numbers' is not enough. Having someone personally talk with a patient before making any attempt to treat their reported symptoms is crucial. For instance, a pain score could be elevated due to anything from a recent invasive procedure, to an impending infection, or only an extra long hike in the woods over the weekend. Clarifying the symptom and getting a description of its onset and nature provides a much more meaningful view than simply looking at the score as a measure of a symptom's severity.

Hearing the description in the patient's words is powerful. Every person's view of severity differs. A score of 10 to one person may only be a score of 4 to another. Yet, when you discuss the patient's pain to which he or she assigned a score of 4, you may discover that it interferes with their life more than the pain scored as a 10 might interfere with the other patient's life. Listening to the patient validates them and reassures them that someone is interested in them as a whole and not in just their 'numbers.' Also, we have observed that some patients feel safer and are more likely to share honestly with a person over the telephone they might withhold complaints to avoid disappointing their physician or other medical staff, whom they see in person.

13.7 **Summary and conclusions**

In this chapter we have identified philosophical theories that inform an enhanced understanding of quality of life and PROs. We have examined the ways these theories can improve medical research and evidence-based treatment.

In particular, we have presented qualitative research in one of our studies and the use of the nurse care manager in another study as two examples of ways in which CCC attempts to appreciate the philosophical issues inherent in research endeavors. Attention to these sorts of philosophical concerns increases our appreciation of the phenomenological and existential components of the patient experience, which in turn facilitates better service to oncology clients.

References

Bair M. J., Robinson R. L., Katon W., and Kroenke K. (2003). Depression and pain comorbidity: a literature review. *Archives of Internal Medicine*, **163**, 2433–2445.

Belenky M. F. (1986). *Women's Ways of Knowing* (New York: Basic Books).

Buber M. (1958). *I and Thou* (New York: Scribner).

Chang, V. T. and Ingham J. (2003). Symptom control. *Cancer Investigation*, **21**, 564–578.

Cleeland C. S. and Reyes-Gibby C. C. (2002). When is it justified to treat symptoms? Measuring symptom burden. *Oncology*, **16** (Suppl.), 64–70.

Code, L. (1983). Father and son: a case study in epistemic responsibility. *The Monist*, **66**, 274.

Eliot, G. (1956). *Middlemarch.* (Boston: Houghton Mifflin), quoted in M. F. Belenky (1986). *Women's Ways of Knowing: The development of self, voice, and mind* (New York: Basic Books), 3.

Gallagher R. M. and Verma S. (1999). Managing pain and comorbid depression: a public health challenge. *Seminars in Clinical Neuropsychiatry*, **4**, 203–220.

Goldman L., Weinstein M. C., Goldman P. A., and Williams L. W. (1991). Cost-effectiveness of HMG-CoA reductase inhibition for primary and secondary prevention of coronary heart disease. *Journal of the American Medical Association*, **265**, 1145–1151.

Gupta M. A. (1986). Is chronic pain a variant of depressive illness? A critical review. *Canadian Journal of Psychiatry*, **31**, 241–248.

Hall J. and Stevens P. (1996). Rigor in feminist research. *Advances in Nursing Science*, **13**, 6–29.

Jackson J. L., O'Malley P. G., and Kroenke K. (1998). Clinical predictors of mental disorders among medical outpatients: validation of the 'S4' model. *Psychosomatics*, **39**, 431–436.

Kaplan R. M. and Anderson J. P. (1988). A general health policy model: update and applications. *Health Service Research*, **23**, 203–235.

Kroenke K. (2003). The interface between physical and psychological symptoms. *Primary Care Companion to the Journal of Clinical Psychiatry*, **5** (Suppl. 7), 11–18.

Kroenke K., Jackson J. L., and Chamberlin J. (1997). Depressive and anxiety disorders in patients presenting with physical complaints: clinical predictors and outcome. *American Journal of Medicine*, **103**, 339–347.

Kroenke K. and Price R. K. (1993). Symptoms in the community: prevalence, classification, and psychiatric comorbidity. *Archives of Internal Medicine*, **153**, 2474–2480.

Kroenke K., Spitzer R. L., Williams J. B. W. *et al.* (1994). Physical symptoms in primary care: predictors of psychiatric disorders and functional impairment. *Archives of Family Medicine*, **3**, 774–779.

Kuhn T. (1996). *The Structure of Scientific Revolutions*. (Chicago: University of Chicago Press).

Levinas, E. (1985). *Ethics and Infinity* (Pittsburgh, PA: Duquesne University Press).

McDonald M., Passik S. D., Dugan W. M., Rosenfeld B., Theobald D. E., and Edgerton S. (1999). Nurses' recognition of depression in their patients with cancer. *Oncology Nursing Forum*, **26**, 593–599.

Morgan D. (1997). *Focus Groups as Qualitative Research*. (Thousand Oakes, CA: Sage Publications).

National Institutes of Health. (2003). State-of-the-science conference statement: symptom management in cancer: pain, depression, and fatigue. *Journal of the National Cancer Institute*, **95**, 1110–1117.

Passik S. D., Dugan W. M., McDonald M., Rosenfeld B., Theobald D. E., and Edgerton S. (1998). Oncologists' recognition of depression in their patients with cancer. *Journal of Clinical Oncology*, **16**, 1594–1600.

Shumaker A., Anderson R., and Czajkowski S. (1990). 'Psychological tests and scales' in B Spilker (ed.) *Quality of Life Assessments in Clinical Trials* (New York: Raven Press).

Theobald D. E., Butler D., Coburn J. *et al.* (2004). IVR-based cancer symptom assessment: nurses' expectations and perceived barriers [abstract] (New Orleans, LA: American Society of Clinical Oncology).

Valenstein M., Vijan S., Zeber J. E., Boehm K., and Buttar A. (2001). The cost-utility of screening for depression in primary care. *Annals of Internal Medicine*, **134**, 345–360.

Chapter 14

The assessment of emotional awareness: can technology make a contribution?

Robert S. Kruger

14.1 Introduction

This paper attempts to address two related issues: (1) how well individuals can tell what emotions they and others are feeling; and (2) whether or not it is possible to measure this in a meaningful way that is clinically relevant. It is a tenet of folk psychology that emotions are private and privileged knowledge such that only the actor experiencing the emotion truly knows what it is. However, recent research on the communication of emotional expressions through non-verbal behavior and on 'mind reading' in autistic children leads to the conclusion that emotions may be publicly observed. Moreover, it is commonplace in psychotherapy that patients often experience difficulty in identifying their emotions. Accordingly, they may be said to be unconscious of their emotions to varying degrees. More recent research on the expression of emotion suggests that individuals also vary in their abilities to identify emotions in others. Being able to empathize is crucial for the establishment of attachments to others and, therefore, for psychological well-being. Accordingly, a deficit in one's capacity to identify and understand what others feel bodes poorly for one's mental health. The current widespread availability of videotaping has made possible the development of simple and easy to use assessment tools to measure how well children and adults can identify emotions in others and draw inferences from affective behavioral displays. This paper explores two such instruments and their potential use in clinical practice. Finally, I offer some thoughts on the educational implications of training children in emotional recognition and inferential thinking about emotions.

14.2 **Knowing the emotions of another**

Psychotherapists take it as a given that human beings are a social species. Indeed, psychotherapy itself is a type of social conversation designed to enhance self-awareness and, with it, effect changes in behavior and point of view. However, what does it mean to say that humans are social? At the very least this assumption implies that we typically interact with one another in certain ways and simultaneously engage in a particular type of cognitive activity which has been variously labeled 'mind reading' (Baron-Cohen *et al.*, 2000). Mind reading is the activity of discerning the emotions, desires, beliefs, and intentions of another based upon the interpretation of his/her non-verbal behavior and prosodic variations while integrating these with the semantic content of the speech of the agent. This is accomplished through a conversation, which includes both listening and questioning. Human beings, quite unlike other species, can communicate conflicting messages by using different communication channels in opposing ways. Thus, one type of message can be displayed through non-verbal and prosodic behavior while a different, even contradictory, message can be conveyed semantically. In such cases, human observers usually give weight to the non-verbal and prosodic data while dismissing the semantic message. Therefore, to a significant degree, we determine what others feel and want by observing and evaluating their non-verbal displays, which include facial expressions, gestures, movements, and prosody.

14.3 **The development of mind reading**

Quite early in their development, infants learn the art of reading minds. Research by Nelson (1985) has shown that by the age of five months infants can distinguish certain facial expressions such as a smile and a frown. This capacity clearly has adaptive and survival value for the infant insofar as smiles from caretakers signal acceptance and probable nurturing behavior while frowns are signals of displeasure. Clearly, behavior eliciting smiles is much more likely to result in caretaking and attachment behavior than is behavior eliciting negative affect. Research on the development of social referencing has demonstrated that babies learn to use their mothers' facial expressions as indicators of the relative safety of possible courses of action (Klinnert *et al.* 1983). Moreover, visually inspecting the mother's facial expression allows the child to decide how to act under conditions of uncertainty (Astington 1993: 40–48). Social referencing evolves naturally into the capacity for joint attention (Scaife and Bruner 1975) which forms the basis for reciprocal communication. The baby learns to look in the direction where the mother points. Subsequently, the child learns to follow the mother's gaze and to take an interest in the object or situation at which the mother is looking. The baby eventually learns to point and then look at something s/he wishes the mother to see (Butterworth 1991).

The emergence of these looking and pointing behaviors marks the development of the infant as a social being. Researchers such as Schaffer (1984) and Trevarthen (1980) have noted the infant's next social step: reciprocal turn-taking which generally occurs at about nine months.

From this type of social reciprocity, it is a short developmental jump to beginning to identify the emotional states of others. With the identification of affect, the child can begin the slow process of entering the social world of other actors and begin to grasp their intentions. Eventually, human infants begin to comprehend that other actors have minds and that these minds can be understood (i.e., read) by the ways others express emotions, articulate plans, and act deliberately. Moreover, they begin to learn how to weave their own thinking, wanting, and planned acting into the flow of the behavior of others who are important to them and can influence their lives. At a certain point in development, a child also understands the concept of duplicity. That is, an actor can express a particular intention or desire for the specific purpose of being misleading to other actors who are observers of his/her behavior.

14.4 **Mind-reading failures**

Unfortunately, some children do not develop the skills of social referencing, joint attention, gaze alternation, and reciprocal turn-taking which are the foundation of social perception and mind reading. Such children are, in Simon Baron-Cohen's felicitous phrase, 'mindblind.' Thus, studies of autistic individuals have revealed that the abilities to discern the emotions, wishes, and intentions of others as well as to coordinate one's behavior in synchrony with them during social interaction do not naturally evolve as do those of developmentally typical children raised in normal family environments (Baron-Cohen 1995).

Individuals who fail to acquire the skills requisite to interpret the actions and intentions of others may be taught these skills through intensive early intervention in the form of specialized therapies utilizing play, communication games, and movement (Greenspan and Weider 1998). It is clear that such skills are fundamental to successful social life and are the foundation of being able to communicate effectively with others.

However, not all persons who lack the skills necessary to conduct their lives in a social world are autistic. To varying degrees, some individuals may fail to develop the capacities to perceive and parse the meaning of those behaviors through which others communicate their emotions and intentions. These people are certainly 'mindblind' to some extent but perhaps not to the extreme of having autism. Rather, there appears to be a spectrum of capability with regard to being able both to identify significant non-verbal and vocal behaviors and, most importantly, to attribute meaning accurately to these behaviors. Attributing meaning accurately generally implies that an observer has discerned the actor's understanding of the social context in which s/he acts and has correctly read that actor's intentions towards other actors in that context. Some of us do this rather well, some less well, and some not at all. As a rule, those in the latter category are viewed as pathological (e.g., suffering from autism or Asperger syndrome) whereas those who are simply less competent are generally described as either insensitive or socially impaired.

14.5 **Understanding intentionality**

Those individuals who are inept or deficient in identifying what types of non-verbal and vocal behaviors are worthy of one's attention are also usually equally poor at attributing meaning to those cues, namely, in reading minds. As Baron-Cohen (1995) suggests, they are also less successful in achieving what Daniel Dennett (1987) has called the Intentional Stance. Borrowing from Daniel Dennett, they have not been successful in developing and using an intentional stance as a framework for interpreting the behavior of other persons.

Dennett has argued that there are three types of framework by which we try to make sense of the behavior of persons or objects. The first is the physical stance, which describes the physical qualities or characteristics of an object but offers little insight into the possible reasons for its behaving as it does. The framework of the physical stance explains how things come about and attempts to explain systems as a result of features of their physical make-up. Yet, as Baron-Cohen (1995: 22) observes:

> ...Attempting to understand the behavior of a person or of any kind of animal by adopting the Physical Stance would be a non-starter, in view of the state of our knowledge: we would need to know about the millions of different physiological (brain) states that give rise to different behaviors in order to understand animal or human behavior in purely physical terms.

In Dennett's classificatory scheme, a second approach to explanation is the design stance. This framework provides functional explanations (i.e., elucidation of actions in terms of their putative functions or purposes). Accordingly, expositions of behaviors in terms of their possible functions gives some insight into the reasons why an object or feature of an object is designed as it is (e.g., alarm clocks are designed to wake us up and, if set properly, will go off at a certain time irrespective of how they are physically made). The design stance is useful when we do not know about the underlying physical makeup of an object. The design stance works well, as Baron-Cohen (1995: 23–24) notes,

> ...when we wish to explain a system composed entirely of observable and operational parts...But adopting the Design Stance toward understanding the behavior of people or animals would not get one very far, since people and animals have few external, operational parts for which one could work out a functional or design description.

Alternatively, we ordinarily adopt what Dennett calls the intentional stance to explain the behavior of ourselves and others. This perspective derives from the work of Brentano (1874) and other phenomenologists in which the term 'intentional' implies 'aboutness' insofar as human mental states are always about something, that is, have a designated or identifiable focus. This focus may be comprised of objects and events in the world or non-existent things such as unicorns (Astington, 1993, 22). The intentional stance is the perspective within which we 'treat the object or animal or person as a rational agent. We infer its beliefs and desires and predict that it will act to fulfill its desires in the light of its beliefs.' (Astington 1993: 20.) This perspective is the basis for mind reading in Baron-Cohen's sense and is known as 'folk psychology.' As Dennett (1987: 48) points out:

> We use folk psychology all the time, to explain and predict each other's behavior; we attribute beliefs and desires to each other with confidence—and quite unselfconsciously—and spend a substantial portion of our waking lives formulating the world—not excluding ourselves—in these terms.

14.6 **Developing empathy**

Baron-Cohen (1995) asserts that there are four basic components which are necessary to develop skills requisite for competent mindreading. He calls these: (1) the intentionality detector; (2) the eye direction detector; (3) the shared attention mechanism; and (4) the theory of mind mechanism. He suggests that if a child is to develop the ability to view other persons from a social perspective and successfully interact with them within a social context, the child must be capable of at least attributing intentionality to people, identifying when others are watching something, taking an interest in what they are watching, communicating that interest, and, finally, developing a framework for inferring the full range of mental states of other agents from observing their behavior. Observing means, in this case, looking at and listening to other individuals.

The construction of a theory of mind, or folk psychology, evolves quite early in humans. Alan Leslie (1991) notes that this emerges as early as age two when children first begin to pretend and to engage in imaginative play. Leslie argues that the significance of early pretend play is that it constitutes the initial indication that children understand another's mental state (Leslie 1987). As a child engages in imaginative play, s/he assumes the role of another. This requires some degree of understanding of the role, the expectations of others regarding that role, and what adults would call empathy for those who play the role on the part of the actor assuming the role. Astington points out that 'This must be so if they can coordinate their pretending with that of another person, because they have to link their actions to what the other person is pretending, not what he or she is actually doing' (Astington 1993: 56).

Leslie was interested in how children acquire a theory of mind and the accompanying ability to understand the mentality of others. He wondered why two-year-olds are not confused by pretense. To explain this he postulated that human perceptual and cognitive functioning has evolved sufficiently to allow us 'to form correct representations, that is, true beliefs about the world…' (Astington 1993: 56). Leslie designated these correct representations of the world as primary representations. Such mental representations are crucial to an individual actor's ability to coordinate her/his social behavior with that of other actors in either a real or imagined situation.

However, our cognition is not limited to beliefs about the world as delineated by Leslie's primary representations. We also have what Leslie called secondary representations, or ideas about our own and others' mental states including beliefs, hopes, fears, desires, intentions, and pretenses (Astington 1993: 57). Leslie went on to identify these secondary representations as *metarepresentations* to indicate their higher-order logical quality. It is our capacity for forming metarepresentations that makes it possible for us to construct a theory of mind. Moreover, it is the relative deficit in metarepresentational thinking which characterizes autistic spectrum disorders and separates individuals on the autistic spectrum from those who may be capable of metarepresentational thinking but are socially insensitive because they either do not accurately identify non-verbal and vocal cues in the behavior of other actors or because they do identify such behaviors but assign inaccurate meanings to them (e.g., a paranoid individual who pays scrupulous attention to the non-verbal and vocal cues of others with whom s/he comes into contact but mistakenly attributes a signification of malevolent intent to these cues).

14.7 **Measuring competence at mind reading**

As noted previously, autistic children are not the only individuals who display deficient metarepresentational thinking, especially when it comes to interpreting the emotional responses either of oneself or, especially, other persons.

As stated previously, accurately identifying and representing what others feel encompasses a set of skills that varies in accomplishment among human beings. Moreover, successful identification of others' emotions is a highly valued competence as much of the recent popular writing on 'emotional intelligence' attests. For practicing clinicians, two important questions about the ability to identify and interpret emotions arise:

1. What is required to be good (i.e., accurate) at inferring the emotional states of others?

and

2. How could we measure such abilities?

If we reflect on how we know what others feel, it becomes apparent that non-verbal behavior is the fundamental vehicle that provides evidence to answer these queries (Ekman and Rosenberg 1998). Thus, facial expressions, gestures, posture, and prosody tell us what words alone may not. Moreover, the former may contradict the latter, leading to the common lament of the individual with Asperger syndrome that people rarely say what they mean or mean what they say.

Fortunately, with the widespread advent of videotaping, we now have some good, user-friendly technology and measures that allow us to quantify how well children and adults can identify emotional expression in others and how well they can attribute meaning accurately to such data. I shall briefly discuss two of these.

The Child and Adolescent Social Perception Measure (CASP) was developed by Joyce Magill-Evans and her research team at the University of Alberta (Magill-Evans *et al.* 1996). It is a test that provides data on how well a child can observe the behavior of peers interacting in typical social situations, identify the relevant non-verbal and prosodic cues from which to interpret the emotional states of the actors, and, based on those non-verbal and prosodic cues alone, both accurately interpret the emotions of the actors and arrive at a clear formulation of what is taking place among them (i.e., construct a plausible storyline about the actions displayed). By means of an audio filter, the verbal content of the actors' dialogue is masked so that an observer cannot tell what an actor is actually saying although the prosodic variations (i.e., vocal tonality) in each actor's voice are preserved.

Thus, based on their observations only of the actors' non-verbal behavior and prosody, a child is asked to identify what is going on in the scene (i.e., to create a narrative that makes sense about it), what the individuals s/he observes might be feeling, and what sorts of behavioral cues s/he have used as a basis for his/her attributions about each actor's emotionality. A basic underlying assumption of the test is that we use non-verbal displays and prosody far more than the verbal content of speech to interpret the emotions and intentions of others, that is, to mind read. Ethologists who study the natural history of various species have known for some time that careful observation of animals in their natural habitats yields valuable information about the purpose(s) of an animal's behavior pattern, that is, an animal's intentions, as well as about the animal's emotional state. These techniques have been previously applied to the study of children's behavior (Blurton Jones 1972). However, previous ethological studies generally failed to recognize that children themselves vary considerably in their skills at observing, identifying, and interpreting the behavior of others. Recent studies of children with autism, Asperger syndrome, and non-verbal learning disabilities have documented that some children are deficient in their ability to identify relevant non-verbal and prosodic social cues in the behavior of others. Accordingly, such children have difficulty in attributing accurate emotionality and intentionality to other agents. With advent of the CASP, we now have a way to measure how well children can mind read because Magill-Evans has provided a comprehensive scoring system for evaluating a child's responses to the filmed scenes on the CASP and has conveniently provided standardization data to allow a comparison between a given child's performance on the test and those of age- and gender-matched peers. Fortunately, comparison measures are separated by gender because, not surprisingly, pre-adolescent and adolescent girls are far more adept than boys on the tasks of the CASP.

The Awareness of Social Inference Test (TASIT) was developed in 2002 by Skye McDonald (McDonald *et al.* 2002) and his team at the University of New South Wales in Australia. It is designed for use with adults. The TASIT consists of three parts: emotion evaluation, minimal social inference, and enriched social inference. Unlike the CASP, the TASIT makes use of both verbal and non-verbal information to determine how well an observer can interpret others' emotions and intentions.

Part 1 of the TASIT, the emotion evaluation test, is based on the work of Ekman (1973), which has identified six basic emotions which are common across all cultures: happiness, sadness, anger, fear, revulsion (disgust), and surprise. In this test, 28 vignettes, portrayed by professional adult actors, are designed to illustrate these six basic emotions. The subject is asked to identify the label which best describes the actor's dominant emotion in the vignette and s/he is given a card with these printed on it as a reminder.

Part 2 of the TASIT, minimal social inference, requires the subject to determine 'the speaker's meaning and intentions based upon the dialogue, emotional expression and other paralinguistic cues of each of the participants. There is *no* external or additional information provided to the viewer to assist in making this interpretation.' (McDonald *et al.* 2002: 6.) There are two types of exchange covering three types of situation: sincere exchanges, sarcastic exchanges involving simple sarcasm, and sarcastic exchanges involving paradoxical sarcasm.

Part 3 of the TASIT, enriched social inference, uses a different series of vignettes all of which contain a message that is literally untrue. Half of these, as in part 2, are sarcastic exchanges in which the speaker states a message opposite to the one intended but states it in such a way that the meaning is clear to normal observers. The other half of the exchanges uses the same scripts as the sarcasm vignettes but, in each one, the speaker is lying. In some cases the lies are 'white' lies whereas in others they are 'sympathetic' lies, that is, spoken to make to make the individual towards whom they are directed feel better. The information provided to the viewer in part 3 is enriched because additional evidence is provided about either the true state of affairs or the true beliefs of the speaker (McDonald *et al.* 2002).

In parts 2 and 3, viewers are asked four different questions to determine how well they understood the intent and emotion of the actors in the scenes. These questions get to the heart of how adept viewers are at mind reading:

1. What are the speakers' intentions (i.e., what do they intend to do to their partners in the scenes)?
2. Do the speakers want the literal or non-literal meaning of their messages to believed (i.e., what are they actually saying)?
3. What are the speakers' knowledge and beliefs about the situation (i.e., what do they think)?
4. What are the speakers' emotions (i.e., what do they feel)?

Normative data are provided for parts 1, 2, and 3, allowing the evaluator to determine how well an adult subject is able to perform a series of complex social interpretive tasks.

14.8 **Conclusion**

In conclusions both the CASP and the TASIT, using videotape technology, provide the clinician with a practical means of evaluating how well individual children and adults can engage in some of the fundamental tasks of mind reading. Although neither test is designed to provide conclusive evidence of a specific psychiatric disorder, both may be quite helpful as part of an assessment battery. Moreover, discussing the types of error a subject makes with him or her after giving either test may have some clinical usefulness in terms of heightening self-awareness and/or teaching mind reading skills. By identifying the areas of social perception and attribution of affect in which an individual is weak, the clinician can target the therapy to begin to improve those skills. Additionally, there are now quite useful technological tools for children on CDs and DVDs to teach them the elementary skills of mind reading and to assist them in refining those skills (University of Cambridge 2004).

Clearly, the development of these types of skill is the foundation of most, if not all, successful social interaction in contemporary cultures. One could also argue that acquiring the skills of mind reading is fundamental not only to the understanding of others in one's social milieu, but to understanding oneself as well.

References

Astington J. W. (1993). *The Child's Discovery of the Mind* (Cambridge, MA: Harvard University Press).

Baron-Cohen S. (1995). *Mindblindness* (Cambridge, MA: MIT Press).

Baron-Cohen S., Tager-Flusberg H., and Cohen D. (eds.) (2000). *Understanding Other Minds* (New York: Oxford University Press).

Blurton Jones N. (ed.) (1972). *Ethological Studies of Child Behaviour*. (Cambridge: Cambridge University Press).

Brentano F. (1874). *Psychology from an Empirical Standpoint* (O. Kraus, ed.) (1970) (London: Routledge and Kegan Paul).

Butterworth G. (1991). 'The ontogeny and phylogeny of joint visual attention' in A. Whiten (ed.) *Natural Theories of Mind: Evolution, development and simulation of everyday mindreading* (Oxford: Basil Blackwell), 223–232.

Dennett D. (1987). *The Intentional Stance* (Cambridge, MA: MIT Press).

Ekman P. (1973). 'Cross cultural studies of facial expression' in P. Ekman (ed.) *Darwin and Facial Expression: A century of research in review* (New York: Academic Press), 169–222.

Ekman P. and Rosenberg E. (1998). *What the Face Reveals: Basic and applied studies of spontaneous expression using the facial action coding system* (Oxford: Oxford University Press).

Greenspan S. and Weider S. (1998). *The Child with Special Needs* (Reading, MA: Perseus Books).

Klinnert M. D., Campos J. J., Sorce J. F., Emde R. N., & Svenjda M. (1983). 'Emotions as behavior regulators: social referencing in infancy' in R. Plutchik and H. Kellerman (eds.) *Emotion: Theory, research, and experience*, vol. 2, *Emotions in Early Development* (New York: Academic Press), 57–86.

Leslie A. (1987). Pretence and representation: the origins of 'theory of mind.' *Psychological Review*, **94**, 412–426.

Leslie A. (1991). 'The theory of mind impairment in autism: evidence for a modular mechanism of development?' in A. Whiten (ed.) *Natural Theories of Mind* (Oxford: Blackwell), 63–78.

Magill-Evans J., Koning C., Cameron-Sadava A., and Manyk K. (1996). *Manual for the Child and Adolescent Social Perception Measure* (Edmonton: University of Alberta).

McDonald S., Flanagan S., and Rollins J. (2002). *The Awareness of Social Inference Test* (Bury St. Edmunds, Suffolk, UK: Thames Valley Test Company Limited).

Nelson C.A. (1985). 'The perception and recognition of facial expressions in infancy' in T. M. Field and N. A. Fox (eds.) *Social Perception in Infants* (Norwood, NJ: Ablex), 101–125.

Scaife M. and Bruner J. S. (1975). The capacity for joint visual attention in the infant. *Nature*, **253**, 265–266.

Schaffer H. R. (1984). *The Child's Entry into a Social World* (London: Academic Press).

Trevarthen C. (1980) 'The foundations of intersubjectivity: development of interpersonal and cooperative understanding in infants' in D. R. Olson (ed.) *The Social Foundations of Language and Thought* (New York: Norton), 316–342.

University of Cambridge (2004). *Mind Reading* [CD set] (London: Jessica Kingsley).

Part 5

Ethical issues in technology and psychiatry

Chapter 15

Thinking about the repair manual: technique and technology in psychiatry[1]

Jennifer Radden

> ...we are close to seeing the patient as something broken which can be fixed with a correct use of the psychiatric repair manual
>
> (Phillips 2002: 77)

15.1 Introduction

When applied to the psychiatrist, the technical expert model contains particular limitations and hazards. In addition to the traits shared by all ethical purveyors of technical and, increasingly technological, expertise, it is argued here, the practitioner in psychiatry will need to possess moral virtue—and virtues. And to the extent that advances in technology have blinded the profession to that long-recognized truth, they are dangerous and misleading. What follows falls into three parts. First, the technical/technological expert model is explained and explored. Second, it is shown how the technical/technological expert model occludes and betrays some of what is central to ethical psychiatric practice. Finally, examples illustrating the moral psychology of the virtuous practitioner in psychiatry indicate what the technical/technological expert model leaves out.

A disclaimer is required at the outset of this discussion: these assertions apply to psychiatry as practiced with patients suffering severe conditions such as major depression, manic-depression, obsessive–compulsive and schizophrenic disorders. The treatment of less severe disorders may require a different analysis, and will likely prove more hospitable to the technical/technological expert model outlined here.

15.2 Professional as technical/technological expert

A fast transformation of the identities of many professionals can be observed today, and it is nowhere more notable than in medicine, psychiatry's closest kin and disciplinary home. (Some of these changes within medicine were anticipated as early as the 1980s (Benatar 1987; Churchill 1989; Dyer 1988; Emanuel and Emanuel 1992; Frank and Frank 1991; May 1983, 1994; Veatch 1991).) This transformation is attributable in part to the burgeoning technological capabilities and focus found throughout medicine. Technology is altering all practice, and all doctors' identities, both the way they see themselves, and the way others see them. One, if not the, prevailing model, has become that of physician as purveyor of technical expertise derived, immediately or ultimately, from technology.

Many factors seem to have prompted and nourished the model of healthcare outlined here. As well as burgeoning technological capabilities and focus, these include managed medical care delivery systems, themselves the products of business and management models; the increased patient access to medical information and to fellow sufferers through the Internet and other media; and a more egalitarian understanding of the doctor-patient relationship both engendering, and engendered by, increased empowerment of the consumers of medical services.

Factors such as these affect every medical specialty, of course, but in varying degrees and different ways. Where psychiatric care is provided those with severe mental disorder, technological capabilities and focus include rapidly increasing availability of, and extensive reliance on, psychopharmacology, for example, as well as the use of interventions such as electroshock therapy and, more recently, functional magnetic resonance imaging and other scanning devices. Managed care delivery systems challenge psychiatric practice in distinct and striking ways, such as the demands they impose on the confidentiality and privacy vital to effective practice (Alarcon 2000; Meyer and McLaughlin 1998; Morrein 1990; Schlesinger *et al.* 2000; Swick 1998; Wahl 1999). The mass media and the Internet affect psychiatry powerfully. Psychiatric symptom descriptions have always been couched in intelligible lay language and the anonymity and access afforded by the Internet combine to foster communications about psychiatric disorders—by their sufferers, and by others—in ways unimagined even twenty years ago (Charland 2004; Elliott 2000; Showalter 1997). And, a final example, the more egalitarian understanding of the relationship between doctor and patient, together with increased empowerment of the consumers of psychiatric services, is particularly influential today, when movements made up of consumers of mental healthcare—such as 'Service User,' 'Survivor,' 'Mad Pride', and 'Recovery' groups – regularly voice their own perspective on these matters. It is worth noting that these groups too, often adopt the model of the psychiatrist as the purveyor of technical/technological expertise, and themselves as consumers or clients, rather than patients (Barham and Hayward 1995; Barker *et al.* 1999; Bracken and Thomas 2005; Davidson 2003; Neugeboren 1999; Read and Reynolds 1996).

15.3 **Implications for ethics**

The changes just noted have also affected the ethics and codes of conduct governing psychiatric (and indeed, all medical), practice. Practitioners are to a great extent now seen—and increasingly seem to see themselves—on analogy with other professionals offering expertise and special skills to their clients, and they are guided by professional's ethics (Cruess and Cruess 1997; Luhrmann 2000; Swick 1998, 2000, 2001; Wear 2004).[2] At the same time, however, the term 'professional' has come to be used more loosely in common parlance, so that it often includes groups that used to be distinguished as non-professionals, such as those practicing trades and crafts. Today, not only doctors and lawyers but anyone with marketable technical and or technological expertise ranks as a 'professional'—engineers and accountants, as well as dental hygienists, computer programmers, electricians, and plumbers, to name a few.

These developments, including this blurring of the distinction between traditional professions, trades, and crafts, have not been without positive effects. Such changes perhaps better allowed recognition of the commonalities shared by all purveyors, even the most modest, of technical/technological expertise. They have exposed the ethical dimensions of the relationship between those offering skilled professional services and the consumer of those services, and revealed the basis of what is often referred to as acting 'professionally,' in the sense of acting ethically. Emphasis on these commonalities in applied ethics has given rise to a great deal of valuable analysis of 'professional ethics'—the rules of conduct and principles governing the interaction between *any* kind of professional expert and client (Agich 1980; Bayles 1981; Dyer; 1988; 1999; Kronman 1987; Moore and Sparrow 1990; Oakley and Cocking 2001; Postema 1980).

The broad model of the relationship between professional purveyor of expertise and the recipient of those services is in many ways an attractive one, moreover. It portrays a bond of mutual advantage. It presupposes a shared respect and understanding between the two parties. It is a relationship that depends on trust. And it is one that upholds the fundamentally egalitarian and enormously appealing notion that the consumer is an autonomous agent, endowed with social power roughly equal to that of the expert, and able to use it. The expert's knowledge and skill are commodities like any other commodities, for which consumers are in a position to negotiate a fair exchange.[3]

Summing up then, several qualities we value seem to be integral to this model. These qualities can be expressed or described in the language of principles, of rules of conduct, or, as would be appropriate for a virtue ethics framework, traits of character. The principles of mutuality, equality, trust, and autonomy correspond to the character traits of mutual respect, egalitarianism, trustworthiness, and self-reliance. In our culture at least, these are all desirable and honored ideals and attributes.

As a professional ethics for the purveyors of many areas of technical/technological expertise—whether we call them 'professionals' or not—for the plumber, the engineer, and the dental hygienist—this works well and is likely sufficient. An ethical professional is one who is trustworthy in the sense of being able to be relied upon to respect the contractual agreement entered into. This can be called 'contractual' trustworthiness. (An additional, richer kind of trustworthiness that goes beyond this minimal 'contractual' kind will be distinguished later in this paper and it, too, is called for in practitioners of mental healthcare, I shall insist.)

To deserve the honorific 'professional', any of these technical experts must abide by the basic principles of reliability and fair dealing: they must respect contractual agreements, avoid conflicts of interest, and so on. Adherence to professional ethics so understood will likely be ethically sufficient, and all that is asked of these purveyors of expertise. And the achievement of that minimal standard will warrant our saying the person acted 'professionally,' regardless of his moral character otherwise understood. Because this concept of the ethical professional is a minimal one, there will be no inherent contradiction in saying 'He always acted professionally' of a person about whom we might also be able to say 'He beats his wife,' or 'He cheats on his taxes'—or at least, 'I know nothing about his moral character.'

As outlined thus far, ethical professionalism may well be sufficient to govern many expert/client relationships, even including some within other medical specialties (anesthesiology, and maybe surgery, for example). These values of equality, autonomy, and contractual fair dealing are the principles undergirding most contemporary biomedical ethics today, moreover (see, for example, American Medical Association 2000; Beauchamp and Childress 2001; Doukas 2003). In fact, it may be the enormous influence of this model within biomedical ethics that allows psychiatrists (also medically trained, and identified) and their patients, to alike embrace this model so unquestioningly (see, for example, Bloch *et al.* 1999).

However, despite the belief of many practitioners themselves and of many consumers of their services that such a conception of professional or practitioner is sufficient, this ethics remains insufficient for mental healthcare. Often—not always—psychiatric practice is different, and so, then, must be psychiatric ethics. The model of the ethical purveyor of technical/technological expertise is not only insufficient—because more virtue, and additional virtues, seem to be called for by the mental healthcare setting. It is in certain respects misleading and inappropriate. To put the case in the strongest terms, it may be said that the technical/technological expert model occludes and betrays some of what is most central to ethical psychiatric practice. The contrast drawn thus far emphasizes the difference between the professionalism of the technical/technological expert delivering services to clients on the one hand, and the ethical healer whose character virtues go beyond the minimal ethical demands, on the other. This depiction is somewhat oversimplified, because some contemporary discussions portray professionalism as a *remedy* against the dangerous influence of the consumer model (see Cruess and Cruess 1997, Swick 2000). These differences are more definitional than substantive, however. Deriving as it does from contemporary usage, the 'professionalism' described thus far captures the minimal requirements for ethical professional conduct. In using a richer conception of professionalism, these other discussions introduce something closer to the virtue ethics approach put forward in the last part of this paper.

15.4 The model of technical/technological expert is misleading and inapplicable

The charge that the model of technical/technological expert is misleading and often inapplicable can be demonstrated by pointing to core tenets of the model that are belied by features commonly found where people receive psychiatric care for severe mental illness. There may be more, but five such features are described here. They are its presumption that (1) the consumer acts with full agency, and (2) enjoys rough social equality with the expert, with whom (3) purposes and understandings are also shared; that the relationship is (4) governed by a contract nullified when either party violates its terms, and finally (5) incidental to the effectiveness of the transaction beyond the maintenance of basic 'contractual' trust.

(1) The model presupposes that the consumer of technical/technological services acts freely, knowingly, and with full agency. She is an autonomous person, understanding her options and their implications, able to examine these in light of her long-term goals and interests, and choosing the services best suited to her ends.

In psychiatry, however, the patient often has compromised autonomy. It is not merely that most patients have this status. It is that almost all those with a psychiatric history have stretches of compromised autonomy during that history (Dunn 1998; Edwards 1997; McHugh and Slavney 1983, 1998). If only temporarily and partially, psychiatric patients are at times deprived of the very capabilities required for the exercise of autonomous decision and action: their sense of matters concerning their immediate and long-term self interest; their reasoning ability, their insight into their own condition, their self-control, their personal and psychic integration, their capacity to communicate their concerns and needs to others, and their perceptions of other people's responses. These incapacities are rarely permanent or total. Moreover, this assessment in no way detracts from the courage, persistence, ingenuity, and frequent effectiveness with which those suffering severe mental disorders endure, and manage, their symptoms. Nevertheless, these obstacles to autonomous functioning are, at one point or another, an aspect of almost all severely ill mental patients' lives and experience.

(2) The model presupposes that a rough social equality pertains between the purveyor of technical/technological services and the consumer of those services. Part of this resides in the power each has in relation to what the other wants.

In the psychiatric setting, however, the practitioner has exceptional, some would say unprecedented, power over the patient; and the patient, for the most part, has exceptional social powerlessness and consequent vulnerability (Bloch *et al.* 1999; Bloch and Green 2006; McHugh and Slavney 1983, 1998). The explanation for these imbalances are several and well known. The social power attributed to the psychiatrist rests in his or her medical authority, and his or her status as arbiter over norms central to our culture's value system, especially those governing rationality, capability, and happiness (Bloch *et al.* 1999; Edwards 1997). Emblematic of this status is the fact that the psychiatrist, and often he or she alone, is empowered to involuntarily seclude and treat individuals who have committed no crimes and only pose a vague (and unverifiable) threat to themselves or to others. In addition, the relative social powerlessness of the consumer derives from his or her sometimes compromised autonomy, noted earlier. It derives from the stigma and shame associated with mental disorder and the discriminatory practices still denying basic social and occupational opportunities to those with psychiatric histories (Dain 1999; Fabrega 1990, 1991; Bracken and Thomas 2005). And it lies in the vulnerabilities to exploitation that come with many of the symptoms of mental disorder, as well as the economic and political marginalization to which these patients are so often subject, and the innumerable and varied sequelae of that marginalization (Davidson 2003; Bracken and Thomas 2005).

So the roughly even playing field presupposed in the model of the relationship between the purveyor and consumer of technical/technological services is not reliably, and perhaps not even commonly, met with in psychiatric practice.

(3) The model presupposes a certain mutuality of purpose and understanding between the purveyor of technical/technological services and the consumer of those services. There is frequently agreement over what the consumer's problem is, and how the technical/technological services are likely to resolve or assuage that problem. When not immediately apparent, this agreement is usually discussed and established at initial contact, and is presupposed in subsequent dealings and throughout the course of the relationship.

Between the psychiatrist and patient, such mutuality of purpose and understanding is sometimes never achieved at all, is often incomplete, and is a shifting and unsteady basis for subsequent dealings. Instead of a mutual understanding established at the initial contact, such understanding is often hard-won through the therapeutic engagement, and is judged an achievement of that process rather than a presupposition for it. Such fundamentals as whether there is a problem, what the problem is, what treatment responses are appropriate and the nature of the roles of each participant, are typically established only after lengthy negotiation and therapeutic intervention. Moreover, frequently, at least, such agreements have to be re-established with shifts in the patient's symptoms or life experience.

Quite typically, for example, the patient has to be urged to seek help by others (or by the courts); he or she will misidentify the condition (for example, attributing it to a problem outside rather than within herself), or they will resist its treatment. Quite typically also, the patient will challenge central ingredients of the practitioner's role, such as the practitioner's motives, legitimacy, authority, and or knowledge.

(4) In a relationship between consumer and purveyor of technical/technological services, as in any contract, the presumption is that if one party violates the terms of the agreement, the other party's obligations are nullified. If X refuses to pay, or in some other way fails to adhere to the initial agreement, then the service can be withdrawn.

In the relationship between the psychiatrist and her patient this expunging of any obligation does not as readily occur, it has been pointed out (Frank and Frank 1991). If the patient violates the contract and that violation endangers his or others' welfare, for example, then the psychiatrist's responsibility continues regardless of the dissolution of the contractual agreement. This feature encourages Jerome and Julia Frank to speak of the relationship between the psychiatrist and patient, as others have done, in terms of its fiduciary nature. It is an engagement 'based not so much on bargaining guided by considerations of self-interest as on trust' (Frank and Frank 1991: 180–181). That is, the practitioner is *entrusted with the patient's care*. This calls for not merely the 'contractual' trustworthiness involved in being able to be relied upon to keep the terms of the contract, but a fuller, deeper, 'fiduciary' trustworthiness, where a commitment to care for the patient is embedded in her moral character.

Fifth and finally, once a level of basic, 'contractual' trust is established, the relationship between purveyor and consumer of technical/technological services is incidental to the effectiveness of the transaction. The technical/technological skill and effectiveness of the professional expert is the fundamental measure by which we judge a successful professional dealing, on this model. An appealing manner, or an upright character, in the expert might add to the ease of the interaction or the subsequent satisfaction of the consumer, it is true. However, the primary criterion for assessing the outcome of the exchange will be pragmatic: was it effective?

In contrast to much, although not all, of the rest of medical practice, the person, or *persona*, of the practitioner in psychiatry is often portrayed as entering into the healing power of the therapeutic alliance between practitioner and patient (American Psychiatric Association 2001). Because therapeutic effectiveness is widely seen to depend on it, the practitioner's person, persona, or self is usually understood as a *sine qua non* of the therapeutic engagement (Dawes 1994; Moerman 2002; Rogers 1957). Others have portrayed it as not only necessary but sufficient for healing (Frank and Frank 1991). Either way, the relationship itself, created, fostered, maintained, and protected by the practitioner, is recognized to play an important causal role in the transaction.

Again, the importance of the relationship between psychiatrist and patient is different, in both emphasis and causal assumptions, from that implied in the model of consumer and purveyor of technical/technological expertise. Indeed, the effective technological approach to human problems, it has been pointed out, serves to expunge both the individuality and personhood of the practitioner; as James Phillips puts it, the 'technical reason' approach results in treatment in which 'the practitioner assumes the qualities of an unthinking robot' (Phillips 2002: 78).

In addition to this ability to harness the healing power of interpersonal relationship, the psychiatrist's technical skills include many common to other purveyors of technical/technological expertise—knowledge, observation, and diagnostic acumen, for example. What distinguishes the psychiatrist's technique, however, is her extensive use of the therapeutic relationship to achieve healing, sometimes alone (in psychotherapy) and at other times in combination with other treatments.

It is important to know how to construe this unusual exercise. One supposition, for example, is that just as the surgeon wields her scalpel or the plumber his spanner, the psychiatrist wields herself, or *persona*. The practitioner's self, or *persona*, *is* her technical tool or device in this case.

The way the practitioner skillfully monitors her self-presentation or *persona* during the therapeutic encounter does seem to have some parallels with a person's skillful use of a tool. And some such perspective might be thought to capture the self-monitoring, art, and skill, required of the practitioner in creating and cultivating such a relationship. However, although not entirely wrong, this picture is incomplete, and the analogy deeply misleading. The way in which the psychiatrist's *persona* or self enters into the therapeutic alliance cannot be merely as a tool or device. For an effective therapeutic relationship or alliance, the patient must believe the practitioner's regard, respect, interest, and concern are genuine, not feigned responses used to bring about some effect. If this engagement were understood in such terms by the patient, the therapeutic alliance would fail. To be effective, the self or *persona* of the practitioner must be seen *as another person*, not as the instrument of another person. The relationship must be experienced as a natural and real exchange. Carl Rogers recognized this point with his emphasis on the genuineness and transparency he identified as 'congruence' between inner states and their outward expression, required of practitioners engaging in therapeutic relationships (Rogers 1957).

15.5 **What is left out?**

Thus far, efforts have been directed toward demonstrating factors apparently preventing the ready subsumption of psychiatric practice under the technical/technological expertise model, and showing the way that model—for all that it appears to be an attractive professional identity for many in the field—leaves out and distorts the practice of psychiatry with the severe mentally ill.

A brief sketch of one alternative model provides a final illustration of these weaknesses and omissions in the model of practitioner as purveyor of technical/technological expertise. This alternative view emphasizes the need for additional virtue—and special virtues—in the character of those practicing in this field, and a few examples best suggest that need. (1) A group as vulnerable to exploitation as psychiatric patients might require exceptional forbearance and discipline on the part of the psychiatrist. (2) Disorders so frequently affecting what their sufferers (and those around them) conceive to be their core selves or identities—autonomy, mood, and reasoning capabilities—will likely call for extra moral seriousness and effort. (3) Symptoms as regularly attractive as those of mental disorders such as mania encourage complex and ambivalent attitudes in the persons experiencing them, and these attitudes likely demand additional attentiveness, sensitivity, and vigilance on the part of practitioners. (4) Because mental disorder remains deeply controversial, and is subject to misunderstanding and stigma, the intimate, personal, and private details regularly explored in treatment will demand extra care over confidentiality. (5) Disorders so dependent on the communication of symptoms and, at the same time, apt to interfere with communicative capabilities, will require great patience, penetration, and understanding from the practitioner. (6) The moral significance of the healing project undertaken—involving cherished cultural norms (of sanity, rationality, and autonomy) and often global, deep-rooted self transformation—would seem to demand unusual traits in the practitioner. As arbiter over our society's central values of autonomy, rationality, and happiness, the psychiatrist is 'moralist' (Rieff) as well as healer. This role would seem to call for judgment, gravitas, and perhaps integrity, beyond the ordinary. (7) Psychiatrists are vested by society with the power of restraining and treating adults against their wishes not only for the sake of others' safety but also for the sake of their own. This power seems similarly to call for a special degree of moral integrity in those who exercise it.

This is no more than a sketch. Yet it is consonant with much traditional thinking about medical practice that has been lost sight of in recent times. In a set of ideas long predating modern day biomedical ethics, it has been emphasized that not only skill but character and character virtues are required of the good doctor (Churchill 1989; Drane 1988; May 1983; Pellegrino and Thomasma 1993). From the time of Hippocrates, as James Drane puts it: '…Patients were expected to trust their physicians and to follow their advice because 'doctors were persons of *excellent character*.' Indeed, superior moral development was considered to be 'more important than following rules and regulations' (Drane 1995: 6–7, emphasis added). Emphasis on the character of the practitioner in psychiatry allows us to recognize some of the additional traits that set the ethical psychiatrist apart from the ethical purveyors of any other technical/technological expertise.

Almost certainly some (if not all) of these traits will also be called for in other medical settings as well. Without excluding these other practices, however, the present discussion is limited to the provision of psychiatric care for those suffering serious mental disorder, where the point can be made with particular force because of features such as those noted in (1)–(7) above.

Nor can an exhaustive depiction of the character of the ethical psychiatrist be furnished in what follows. Instead, focus is on a small group of traits or virtues arguably required in the character of the practitioner: sensitivity, warmth, emotional intelligence, restraint or self-control, and trustworthiness.

Some of these virtues are role constituted, specific to the psychiatric setting. Sensitivity, warmth, and emotional intelligence are none of them traits always considered moral virtues in everyday encounters. They are useful personal strengths, or even Aristotelian 'prudential' virtues, rather than moral virtues. (For a discussion of their usefulness, see Peterson and Seligman (2004).) Because they appear to be ingredients necessary for a successful therapeutic alliance, however, these traits become something more, and something closer to moral virtues for the practitioner, to be acquired and fostered within the practice setting.[4]

At other times, what is demanded is a greater degree of traits or strengths of character regarded as moral virtues in all settings. Restraint (also described as self-control), is an example of one of these character traits. Because psychiatric practice allows many opportunities for unethical behavior—it occurs in a private setting, significant power imbalances often separate practitioner and patient inviting the possibility of exploitation, the exchanges involve matters that are especially private, emotional, and personal for the patient, and so on—it arguably calls for a greater degree of restraint on the part of the practitioner than do many other professional settings. (Consider, for instance, that without conveying personal rejection, losing the patient's trust, or otherwise damaging or jeopardizing the therapeutic relationship, practitioners sometimes have to repel open seductiveness from patients in settings of the utmost privacy.)

Like restraint, trustworthiness is another character trait or virtue called for in every imaginable human setting, as Annette Baier and other philosophers have emphasized (see Baier 1985, 1992; Potter 2002). Moreover, it is one required in some degree, as we saw earlier, when any client receives technical/technological services from any expert. Both parties to the contract must trust one another to adhere to it. The client trusts the expert for reliability, honesty, accuracy, and fair dealing, and the expert trusts the client to, among other things, pay the bill. These contractual forms of trust will also apply when the practitioner offers psychiatric services, of course. However, trustworthiness in the character of the practitioner in that setting has special force. When the relationship is a more fiduciary one, a greater degree—or additional kind—of trustworthiness is demanded. For reasons centering around the patient's special vulnerability, enumerated earlier, the patient entrusts himself to the practitioner's care more wholly. And the ethical practitioner will live up to that added, deeper 'fiduciary' trust.

15.6 **Conclusion**

For all its initial appeal and undeniable popularity, the model of the professional as a purveyor of technical/technological services to a client has limitations. Moreover, it is one ill suited to the setting in which practitioners provide care to those suffering severe mental illness. (To greater and lesser degrees, for some of the same, and perhaps some different reasons, the model may be ill suited to other medical settings as well. That claim, however, must await a separate analysis.)

Rather than embodying what is central to ethical psychiatric practice, the model serves to occlude and betray it. This conclusion was reached first by first examining the presuppositions of that model and its mismatch with psychiatric care; and second, by noting some of the reasons why psychiatry might call for additional virtue, and virtues, in its practitioners, and noting some of the particular moral psychology and character virtues so called for. Sensitivity, warmth, emotional intelligence, and restraint exceeding the ordinary, together with trustworthiness that goes beyond the reliability of any honorable contractor, were offered as illustrations of such a moral psychology.

Endnotes

1 This paper grew out of one entitled 'Technology and virtues' which John Sadler and I presented at the Annual Meeting of the Association for the Advancement of Philosophy and Psychiatry in May 2005, and again at the American Philosophical Association in December of that year, where the respondent was Bradley Lewis. I am deeply indebted to both Sadler and Lewis, and to members of the audience at those meetings, for suggestions, examples, and clarifications.

2 These trends have not gone entirely unchallenged. See Wear (2004).

3 That the values and priorities that emerge when professional and business goals are merged are genuinely incompatible, is not denied here, and indeed must be acknowledged. See Swick (1998, 2001).

4 The process by which morally neutral traits are transformed by professional roles into moral virtues reflects a form of role morality. For a further explication of this reasoning see Freedman (1978), Oakley and Cocking (2001), and Radden (2002, 2006).

References

Agich G. J. (1980). Professionalism and ethics in health care. *Journal of Medicine and Philosophy*, **5**, 186–199.

Alarcon R. D. (2000). 'Culture and ethics of managed care in the United States' in A. Okasha, J. Aboleda-Florez, and N. Sartorius (eds.) *Ethics, Culture and Psychiatry: International perspectives* (Washington, DC: American Psychiatric Association), 83–102.

American Medical Association. (2000). *Principles of Medical Ethics. Code of Medical Ethics: Current opinions and annotations*, 2000–2001 edn. (Washington, DC: American Medical Press).

American Psychiatric Association. (2001). *The Principles of Medical Ethics: With annotations especially applicable to psychiatry* (Washington, DC: American Psychiatric Association).

Baier A. (1985). What do women want in a moral theory? *Noûs*, **19**, 53–63

Baier A. (1992). 'Trust' in B. Grethe (ed.) *The Tanner Lectures on Human Values*, vol. 13 (Salt Lake City: University of Utah Press).

Barham P. and Hayward R. (1995). *Relocating Madness* (London: Free Association Books).

Barker P., Campbell P. and Davidson B. (eds.) (1999). *From the Ashes of Experience, Reflections on Madness, Survival, Growth* (London: Macmillan).

Bayles M. (1981). *Professional Ethics* (Belmont, CA: Wadsworth).

Beauchamp T. and Childress J. (2001). *Principles of Biomedical Ethics*, 5th edn. (New York: Oxford University Press).

Benatar S. R. (1987). The changing doctor-patient relationship and the new medical ethics. *South African Journal of Continuing Medical Education*, **5**, 27–33.

Bloch S., Chodoff P., and Green S. (eds.) (1999). *Psychiatric Ethics* (Oxford: Oxford University Press).

Bloch S. and Green S. (2006). An ethical framework for psychiatry. *British Journal of Psychiatry*, **188**, 7–12.

Bracken P. and Thomas P. (2005). *Postpsychiatry: Mental health in a postmodern world.* (London: Oxford University Press).

Charland L. (2004). A madness for identity: psychiatric labels, consumer autonomy, and the perils of the internet. *Philosophy, Psychiatry & Psychology*, **11**, 335–349.

Churchill L. (1989). Reviving a distinctive medical ethics. *Hastings Center Report*, **19**, 28–34.

Cruess R. L. and Cruess S. R. (1997). Teaching medicine as a profession in the service of healing. *Academic Medicine*, **72**, 941–52.

Dain N. (1999). Reflections on antipsychiatry and stigma in the history of American psychiatry. *American Journal of Psychiatry*, **45**, 1010–1015.

Davidson L. (2003). *Living outside Mental Illness: Qualitative studies of recovery in schizophrenia* (New York: New York University Press).

Dawes R. (1994). *House of Cards: Psychology and psychotherapy built on myth* (New York: The Free Press).

Doukas D. (2003). Where is the virtue in professionalism? *Cambridge Quarterly of Healthcare Ethics* **12**, 147–154.

Drane J. (1988). *Becoming a Good Doctor: The place of virtue and character in medical ethics* (Kansas City: Sheed and Ward).

Drane J. (1995). *Psychiatric Ethics*, 2nd edn. (London: Polity Press).

Dunn C. (1998). *Ethical Issues in Mental Illness* (Aldershot; Brookfield: Avebury/Ashgate).

Dyer A. (1988). *Ethics and Psychiatry: Toward professional definition* (Washington, DC: American Psychiatric Press).

Dyer A. (1999). 'Psychiatry as a profession' in S. Bloch, P. Chodoff, and S. Green (eds.) *Psychiatric Ethics*, 3rd edn. (Oxford: Oxford University Press).

Edwards R. (ed.) (1997) *Ethics of Psychiatry: Insanity, rational autonomy, and mental health care* 2nd edn. (New York: Prometheus Books).

Elliott C. (2000) A new way to be mad? *The Atlantic Monthly*, December, 72–84.

Emanual L. and Emanual E. (1992). Four models of the physician–patient relationship. *Journal of the American Medical Association*, 267, 2221–2226.

Fabrega H. Jr (1990). Psychiatric stigma in the classical and medieval period: a review of the literature. *Comprehensive Psychiatry*, **31**, 289–306.

Fabrega H. Jr (1991). The culture and history of psychiatric stigma in early modern and modern Western societies: a review of recent literature. *Comprehensive Psychiatry* **32**, 97–119.

Frank J. and Frank B. (1991). *Persuasion and Healing* 3rd edn. (Baltimore, MD: Johns Hopkins University Press).

Freedman B. (1978). A meta-ethics for professional morality. *Ethics*, 89, 1–19.

Kronman A. T. (1987). Living in the law. *University of Chicago Law Review*, **54**, 835–876.

Luhrmann T. (2000). *Of Two Minds: The growing disorder in American psychiatry* (New York: Knopf).

May W. (1983). *The Physician's Covenant: Images of the healer in medical ethics* (Philadelphia: The Westminster Press).

May W. (1994). 'The virtues in a professional setting' in K. W. M. Fulford, G. Gillett and J. M. Soskice (eds.) *Medicine and Moral Reasoning* (Cambridge: Cambridge University Press), 75–90.

McHugh P. and Slavney P. (1983). *The Perspectives of Psychiatry* (Baltimore, MD: Johns Hopkins Press).

McHugh P. and Slavney P. (1998). *The Perspectives of Psychiatry*, 2nd edn. (Baltimore, MD: Johns Hopkins Press).

Meyer R. and McLaughlan C. (1998). *Between Mind, Brain, and Managed Care: The now and future world of academic psychiatry* (Washington, DC: American Psychiatric Press).

Moerman D. (2002). *Meaning, Medicine and the 'Placebo Effect'* (Cambridge: Cambridge University Press).

Moore M. and Sparrow M. (1990). *Ethics in Government: The moral challenge of public leadership* (Englewood Cliffs, NJ: Prentice-Hall).

Morrein E. H. (1990). The new economics of medicine: special changes to psychiatry. *Journal of Medicine and Philosophy*, **15**, 97–119.

Neugeboren J. (1999). *Transforming Madness: New lives for people living with mental illness.* (Berkeley, CA: University of California Press).

Oakley J. and Cocking D. (2001). *Virtue Ethics and Professional Roles* (Cambridge: Cambridge University Press).

Pellegrino E. and Thomasma D. (1993). *The Virtues of Medical Practice* (New York: Oxford University Press).

Peterson C. and Seligman M. (2004). *Character Strengths and Virtues: A handbook and classification* (Oxford and New York: Oxford University Press).

Phillips J. (2002). 'Technical reason in the DSM-IV: an unacknowledged value' in J. Z. Sadler (ed.) *Prescriptions and Descriptions: Values, mental disorders, and the DSMs* (Baltimore, MD: Johns Hopkins University Press), 76–95.

Postema G. (1980). Moral responsibility in professional ethics. *New York University Law Review*, **55**, 63.

Potter N. N. (2002). *How Can I be trusted? A virtue theory of trustworthiness* (New York: Rowman & Littlefield).

Radden J. (2002). Notes towards a professional ethics for psychiatry. *Australian & New Zealand Journal of Psychiatry*, **36**, 52–59.

Radden J. (2006). 'Virtue ethics as professional ethics: the case of psychiatry' in R. Walker and P. J. Ivanhoe (eds.) *Working Virtue* (Oxford and New York: Oxford University Press).

Read J. and Reynolds J. (eds.) (1996). *Speaking our Minds: An anthology* (London: Macmillan Press).

Rogers C. (1957). The necessary and sufficient conditions of therapeutic personality change. *Journal of Consulting Psychology*, **21**, 95–103.

Schlesinger M., Wynia M., and Cummins D. (2000). Some distinctive features of the impact of managed care on psychiatry. *Harvard Review of Psychiatry*, **8**, 216–230.

Showalter E. (1997). *Hystories: Hysterical epidemics and modern culture* (New York: Columbia University Press).

Swick H. M. (1998). Academic medicine must deal with the clash of business and professional values. *Academic Medicine*, **73**, 751–755.

Swick H. M. (2000). Toward a normative definition of medical professionalism. *Academic Medicine*, **75**, 612–616.

Swick H. M. (2001). Professionalism: a key to weathering the storm. *Obstetrics & Gynecology*, **98**, 156–161.

Veatch R. M. (1991). *The Patient–Physician Relation: The patient as partner, Part 2* (Bloomington, IN: Indiana University Press).

Wahl O. (1999). *Telling is Risky Business: Mental health consumers confront stigma* (Rutgers, NJ: Rutgers University Press).

Wear D. (2004). The professionalism movement: can we pause? *American Journal of Bioethics*, **4**, 1–10.

Chapter 16

Beyond repugnance: human enhancement and the President's Council on Bioethics

Michael A. Cerullo

16.1 Introduction

Modern neuroscience has given us more insight into the brain than many ever thought possible. Discoveries in neuroscience will continue to expand. I am interested in the possible applications of these biotechnologies toward human enhancement, particularly for what Peter Kramer has called 'cosmetic psychopharmacology,' the ability to alter mood and personality in those without mental illness (Kramer 1993). My interest and enthusiasm for these technologies naturally led me into discussions of their ethical implications. Exploring these issues further, I found that much of the opposition to human enhancement was based on political and religious ideology rather than on scientific evidence or sound ethical argument (Annas and Elias 2004; Blackburn 2004; Danforth 2005; Groopman 2002; Pinker 2002; Turner 2004). My foray into the ethics of human enhancement recently culminated in the reading of *Beyond Therapy: Biotechnology and the pursuit of happiness*, a report of the President's Council on Bioethics (2003). This document only increased my concern that serious policy decisions about biotechnology were being dictated, to a significant extent, by a political–religious coalition representing a religious fundamentalist ideology (Annas and Elias 2004; Blackburn 2004; Danforth 2005; Groopman 2002; Pinker 2002).

One goal of this paper is to review the arguments presented in *Beyond Therapy* and to demonstrate their logical fallacies and foundation in political–religious ideology. A second goal is to present an alternative approach to evaluating controversial biotechnological using the principles approach, the method of applied ethical reasoning adopted by most bioethicists (Beauchamp and Childress 1994; Buchanan *et al.* 2000; Edge and Groves 1999; Gruenberg 2000). This method requires understanding and application of the basic ethical principles of autonomy, beneficence, nonmaleficence, and justice. The optimal ethical decision is made, in theory, by considering the impact of a given course of action on each of these (sometimes) competing principles (Beauchamp and Childress 1994; Buchanan *et al.* 2000; Edge and Groves 1999), and there is precedent for this approach regarding the evaluation of biotechnologies (Davis 2004; Edge and Groves 1999; Harris 2004). I do not expect to resolve these complicated ethical issues. Instead, my goal is to demonstrate that sound ethical evaluations of biotechnology can be made, that the positions of those who favor the application of biotechnologies should be represented in any public debate on the issue, and that discourse can and should proceed without recourse to ideology. Although in this chapter I am focusing on the debate provoked in the US by the President's Council on Bioethics, I intend my argument to be applicable to any discussion of the ethics of human enhancement technologies.

As will be demonstrated, the authors of *Beyond Therapy* did not take the principles approach to ethical analysis in arguing their positions. There is no statement, analysis, or discussion of major ethical principles (nor did the council adopt an alternative method of ethical analysis such as a case, care, or virtue-based approach). Rather, a series of ideological pronouncements is made. This lack of focus on ethical principles makes it difficult to find focused arguments in *Beyond Therapy*, but certain themes appear repeatedly. Before discussing these specific arguments, it is helpful to review the history behind *Beyond Therapy*.

16.2 **The President's Council on Bioethics**

The President's Council on Bioethics was created by executive order number 12975, issued by George W. Bush on November 2001 (Bush 2001). The Council has 18 members appointed by the President. Its goal is to advise the President, legislature, and public about the potential use and abuse of biotechnologies. The specific goals of the Council were:

(1) to undertake fundamental inquiry into the human and moral significance of developments in biomedical and behavioral science and technology;

(2) to explore specific ethical and policy questions related to these developments;

(3) to provide a forum for a national discussion of bioethical issues;

(4) to facilitate a greater understanding of bioethical issues; and

(5) to explore possibilities for useful international collaboration on bioethical issues.

The Council has so far issued four publications discussing their findings and recommendations. Two of the publications concern stem cells (President's Council on Bioethics 2004*a*, *b*) and another relates to human cloning (President's Council on Bioethics 2002). *Beyond Therapy* (2003) is the Council's only publication that attempts to examine the issues surrounding human enhancement, and is the focus of this paper.

There are four major topics discussed in *Beyond Therapy*: the use of enhancement technology in children; physical enhancement; life extension; and cosmetic psychopharmacology. My main concern is with cosmetic psychopharmacology, but I will briefly touch on the topic of physical enhancement because the arguments used by the council against these forms of enhancement parallel their arguments for mental enhancement. First, however, I emphasize the importance of a fair and sound discussion of the ethics of biotechnologies. The precedent that has been established for biotechnologies by the current administration—and which the Council implicitly and sometimes directly supports—is to enact through legislation or by other means broad bans on such technologies (e.g., President Bush's decision on 9 August 2001 to withhold federal funding for stem-cell research). In a liberal democracy such as the USA, proposed limitations on personal autonomy, free speech, behavior, and economics—even if supported by a majority of citizens—must be evaluated against the principles of justice and beneficence. If the activity to be limited or banned has clear and obvious potential to cure disease and relieve suffering, such as the case with stem cells, the latter 'balancing act' is even more critical to the public welfare. Thus, in the present case, it is imperative that it can be demonstrated—from sound ethical analysis and the application of standards of objectivity, validity, and fairness—that the alleged potential harm imposed by new biotechnologies (necessitating a ban on these activities) outweighs their potential good. I will argue that the Council's version of the alleged harm imposed by new biotechnologies has no basis in science, medical biotechnology, or medical ethics, but is rooted in ideology.

Before discussing the topics reviewed in *Beyond Therapy*, it is useful to note the basic errors of logic that recur in that document. First, the Council does not provide a reasonable representation of the arguments of the opposition. Instead, various 'straw men' are created and then torn down. A classic example of this is repeated five times in *Beyond Therapy* and is what I call the *Brave New World* argument. Recall that in the book *Brave New World* (Huxley 1932), a futuristic human society is described that has used technology to clone people of different castes who live in a superficial world without meaningful human relationships. These citizens of the future take a drug called Soma that leaves them euphoric and submissive. The authors of *Beyond Therapy* imply that those who support new biotechnologies also support the creation of such a future society:

> Not everyone likes the idea of "remaking Eden" or of "man-playing God." Not everyone agrees that this prophesied new world will be better than our own. Some suspect it could rather resemble the humanly diminished world portrayed in Aldous Huxley"s Novel *Brave New World*, whose technologically enhanced inhabitants live cheerfully, without disappointment or regret, "enjoying" flat, empty lives devoid of love and longing, filled only with trivial pursuits and shallow attachments.
>
> (President's Council on Bioethics 2003: 8)

This is not, in fact, what supporters of biotechnology either support or desire. However, without the inclusion of a position statement from supporters of biotechnology, the Council is free to present this false assumption as fact. Annas and Elias (2004) have countered the *Brave New World* argument with the *1984* (Orwell 1949) argument, and I would add *The Handmaid's Tale* argument (Atwood 1985; another dystopian novel, where the dystopia is caused by those opposed to technology and change). Such trading of dystopian science fiction, while perhaps emotionally satisfying, serves no purpose in a serious debate about these ethical issues.

Another example of faulty reasoning is that many of the arguments in *Beyond Therapy* depend on a political–religious consensus of metaphysical and/or religious beliefs and values. Such assumptions are not falsifiable or evidence-based, but are taken 'on faith,' rendering them useless as counter-arguments to the position of those who do not share this belief. This form of reasoning is even more problematic when combined with what Leon Kass, chairperson of the Council, has referred to as the 'wisdom of repugnance.' Kass summarizes his argument as follows:

> To pollution and perversion the fitting response can only be horror and revulsion: and conversely, generalized horror and revulsion are prima facie evidence of foulness and violation. The burden of moral argument must fall entirely on those who want to declare the widespread repugnance of humankind to be mere timidity or superstition.
>
> (Kass 1997: 21)

Kass goes on to list many of his sources of 'horror and revulsion': the reproductive rights of single women; assisted reproduction; extramarital sex; birth control; abortion; feminism; homosexuality and gay rights; and analytic philosophy (Kass 1997: 17–18). Arguments against biotechnology that depend on such 'prima facie' repugnance (an incorrect generalization; one need only see Rowe versus Wade as evidence to the contrary) are themselves dependent on the assumption that such reactions of repugnance reflect another of Kass's unsupportable constructs, 'the emotional expression of deep wisdom.' (Kass 1997: 20). Again, these assumptions are neither universal nor evidence-based. Nevertheless, the Argument from Repugnance is used extensively in *Beyond Therapy*.

16.3 **Physical enhancement**

Beyond Therapy discusses the use of biotechnology to enhance the physical performance of adults in the chapter entitled 'Superior Performance.' Muscle growth technology is discussed at length in this chapter in a section entitled 'Muscles and Their Meaning.' There are two main lines of argument cautioning against muscle enhancement. The first focuses on how these technologies will affect athletes and sports in the USA:

> The runner on steroids or with genetically enhanced muscles is still, of course, a human being who runs. But the doer of the deed is, arguably, less obviously *himself* and less obviously *human* than his unaltered counterpart. He may be faster, but he may also be on the way to becoming 'more cheetah' than man, or more like the horses we breed for the racetrack than a self-willing, self-directing, human agent. He does the deed (running), and his resulting time may be measurably superior. But he is also (or increasingly) the passive recipient of outside agents that are at least partly responsible for his achievements.
>
> (President's Council on Bioethics 2003: 165, italics in the original)

It is challenging to evaluate the Council's odd statement that the runner will become 'less obviously human' and 'more cheetah.' If meant literally[1], this is a very naïve scientific statement, as the major focus of muscle enhancement technology in humans does not require animal muscle tissue or DNA (Sweeney 2004). Even if meant metaphorically, it is a weak and inconsistent position. This example illustrates the use of moralizing disguised as argument and the lack of scientific rigor, which is repeated throughout *Beyond Therapy*.

Another argument repeated throughout all sections of beyond therapy is that if any kind of enhancement is allowed through biotechnology, the first steps toward a dark dystopia—worse than the one in *Brave New World*—will have been taken. This argument is clearly illustrated in the following remark at the end of the chapter:

> We might lose sight of the difference between real and false excellence, and eventually not care. And in the process, the very ends we desire might become divorced from any idea of what is humanly superior, and therefore humanly worth seeking or admiring. We would become a society of spectators, and our activities a mere spectacle. Or a society of parasites, needing and taking, but never doing or acting. Worst of all, we would be in danger of turning our would-be heroes into slaves, persons who exist only to entertain us and meet our standards and whose freedom to pursue human excellence has been shackled by the need to perform–and conform–for our amusement and applause.
>
> (President's Council on Bioethics 2003: 177–178)

Unfortunately, there is no empirical evidence or sound ethical argument offered that would lead us to expect such a consequence. Using the principles approach we can evaluate whether the risks of the enhancement of our physical or mental abilities are so great with regard to creating a dystopia that we should abandon all efforts in this endeavor. In fact, human enhancement technologies have great potential to directly benefit society in specific, verifiable ways (Goldspink 2004; Roubenoff and Hughes 2000; Wagner *et al.* 2002). Although it is possible that muscle enhancement will be abused by athletes to the detriment of sports as currently defined (similar to the issue with steroids, see Sweeney (2004)), many more people with sarcopenia associated with aging or degenerative muscular disorders stand to benefit from the technology. Further, the protection of our society from some ill-defined and unsupported doomsday notion—for which no evidence is offered or, perhaps, even possible to generate in order to estimate risk—is clearly outweighed by the direct application of muscle growth technology to chronic disabling illnesses. The risks of such technology spiraling out of control can and should be the subject of further empirical, ethical, and philosophical study. The serious research that has been done so far does not suggest that physical enhancement technology will naturally lead to a doomsday scenario (Bostrom 2002).

16.4 **Cosmetic psychopharmacology**

Cosmetic psychopharmacology, specifically as envisioned by Peter Kramer (1993), is discussed in the chapter 'Happy Souls' in *Beyond Therapy*. Kramer defined cosmetic psychopharmacology as using pharmaceuticals to improve mood and personality in individuals *without* any diagnosed psychiatric illness (1993). The chapter is heavily influenced by the arguments in Kramer's book, *Listening to Prozac* (1993). Kramer is cited several times and was invited to present his position on cosmetic psychopharmacology to the Council (Kramer 2002). Early in the chapter, the Council expresses the following concern about cosmetic psychopharmacology:

> By directly inducing changes in our subjective experience, the new psychotropic drugs create the possibility of severing the link between feelings of happiness and our actions and experiences in the world. Who would need better children, superior performance, or more youthful bodies if medication could provide the pleasure and sense of well-being that is the goal of so many of our aspirations.
>
> (President's Council on Bioethics 2003: 233)

Unfortunately (and amazingly), this statement entirely misses the most important point raised by Kramer. We already *have (and always have had)* drugs that sever this link, including substances like cocaine, methamphetamine, 'psychedelic' mushrooms, heroin, LSD, and ecstasy. This is not to mention the most prevalent, dangerous, costly (to society), and *legal* drug of this type: alcohol. Kramer's book was interesting because it revealed that it may be possible to enhance mood and change personality *without* severing this link. He suggested Prozac may be the first drug to do this, and showed how it raised fascinating philosophical questions about the nature of 'self' and 'personality.' Instead of exploring these interesting questions from a sound ethical framework, the authors of *Beyond Therapy* compare selective serotonin-reuptake inhibiting drugs (SSRIs)—the current standard of care for mood disorders—with ecstasy and SOMA (the drug in *Brave New World*). That this is not a fair comparison should have been obvious to the Council. SSRIs are not 'mood brighteners' or 'happy pills'; rather, they are a class of *medications* that are used to *treat clinical diseases, including depression and anxiety disorders* (Kelsey and Nemeroff 2000). There is a clear diagnostic nosology supporting these mental illnesses and an overwhelming amount of evidence supporting the efficacy of SSRIs in treating these diseases (Rush 2000). SSRIs are also superior to the older classes of anti-depressants and have greatly expanded the number of people who can be treated safely and effectively (Kelsey and Nemeroff 2000). There is no clinical or scientific evidence that these compounds make people 'happy' (Bonne *et al.* 1999; Gelfin *et al.* 1998), nor do mental health professionals see them as 'artificial mood brighteners' in any sense (the *Diagnostic and Statistical Manual IV* of the American Psychiatric Association (2000) does not contain the word 'happy'). These medicines are not euphoria-inducing, do not change personalities, and do not suppress other emotions (the Council mistakenly assumes that these medicines inhibit the experience of grief; President's Council on Bioethics 2003: 289–295). Rather, they restore the patient to a *disease-free level of functioning*. Contrary to what the Council believes, therefore, these drugs actually restore people to their 'true' (non-depressed) selves, rather than creating artificial selves. A decade after Kramer's book, it is clear that the SSRIs are not a form of cosmetic psychopharmacology, and recent claims to the contrary by ethicists (Elliot and Chambers 2005) have been criticized by psychiatrists in major medical journals (Epstein 2004; Markowitz 2005).

In *Beyond Therapy*, one of the cases discussed by Kramer in *Listening to Prozac* is presented to illustrate the potential problems with cosmetic psychopharmacology. This is the case of Sally, a patient of Dr Kramer's. Before Sally met Dr. Kramer, she described herself in the following way:

> I am forty-one years old. I feel angry and hurt most of the time. I feel like my spirit has been shattered and fragmented with each piece having been trampled on and bruised. I am very, very anxious. I am afraid of everything, even centipedes and roaches. I keep thinking something very, very bad is going to happen to me, some

> great misfortune, or that I'll become handicapped and have to depend on people to take care of me. I don't know who I am, because that person stopped growing at the age of four, and it makes me very sad.
>
> (Kramer 1993: 145–146)

After being placed on Prozac, Sally's mood improved, she became less anxious and much more outgoing. She got promoted at work after 18 years, was able to start dating, and eventually got married. In a section entitled 'Living Truly,' shortly after discussing the case of Sally, the Council asks:

> To what extent is the happiness of the happy person attributable to the drug and to what extent is it 'her own?' To what extent are drug-induced psychic states connected with or disconnected from life as really lived? Surely, for Sally and others who benefit greatly from mood-brightening drugs, the drugs are not the direct cause of their happiness. Sally's happiness has much to do with her new husband and her new job, her new attachments and new achievements, though she would likely have not have sought or found them without taking Prozac. The drug itself did not make her happy; it merely enabled her *to do and experience* the many things that make her happy. But now imaging being Sally's husband: Just *to whom* am I married? Would I love Sally if she stopped taking Prozac and relapsed into timidity and hopelessness? Would Sally love me? Would Sally be Sally?
>
> (President's Council on Bioethics 2003: 285, italics in original).

The first set of remarks seems to acknowledge that Prozac has not altered Sally's personality but merely treated her depression and anxiety. The latter remarks seem to suggest otherwise.[2] Yet, these last remarks are not backed by empirical or philosophical argument and are inconsistent in their applicability to other forms of 'changes to self.' For example, for Sally's husband, the question must also be asked if he would still love 'Sally' if she went blind from diabetes, became psychotic, had an amputated arm reattached, or had a pituitary tumor that made her sexually unresponsive. Which 'Sally' is it: the sighted one or the blind one? What if the sexual unresponsiveness could be reversed, what of 'Sally' then? The Council provides no reasons why the return of major depression, anxiety, or social inhibition should be treated any differently from these other self-altering medical conditions and treatments. Again, without these distinctions their arguments have no obvious merit.

Even if we assume that Kramer is correct in suggesting that, in cases like Sally's, Prozac is actually treating social inhibition and temperament more than any underlying anxiety or depressive disorder, thereby qualifying as cosmetic psychopharmacology, the Council's arguments would remain invalid. Clearly Sally was suffering severely before treatment, and taking Prozac led to subjective and objective benefits in her mood level and overall functioning. Whether Prozac is treating anxiety or social inhibition, the effect is the same and unlike the effects of drugs of abuse. The Council does not justify why they believe Sally's symptoms must fit completely and neatly into one of the current syndromes that define mental illness as understood today (an impossible requirement, in any event). The concept of mental illness has evolved along with our ability to understand and treat mental disorders; there is no reason to think this will not continue. The Council also questions the authenticity of Sally's experience, but they provide no good empirical or ethical arguments to support this claim. It is clear from Kramer's description of the case that Sally has not suffered any severing of the link between her feelings of 'happiness' and her actions and experiences in the world. In fact, Sally describes her new state as more like herself than before, and unlike someone intoxicated by alcohol, we have every reason to believe her.

Using the principles approach to ethical analysis, it is clear that the benefits of Prozac are great in this case and the risks of side effects are minor and were taken into consideration by both Sally and Dr Kramer before starting treatment. The fact that the symptoms of depressive or anxiety disorders overlap with Sally's experience of herself (and resulting behavior) does not justify withholding an effective treatment for Sally's suffering. Of course, we should also consider the general effects of using such medications. The Council argues that such cases can have negative effects on our society:

> The medicalization of psychic pain, however necessary as a path to providing much needed relief for the sick, indicates (whether intended or not) a great advance for biological reductionism against the citadel of mind and soul, a march that knows no natural stopping place, and that at each point along the advance threatens to reduce further the dignity of our inner life – or at least our self understanding of it.
>
> (President's Council on Bioethics 2003: 296)

This argument literally suggests that Sally's (and others') autonomy and well-being should be sacrificed to some amorphous potential of these drugs to reduce the 'dignity' of others' 'inner' lives (or at least others' 'self understanding' of the 'dignity' of their 'inner' lives). When this argument is worded using the principles approach to ethical analysis, its flaws are obvious. In fact, there is every reason to believe that Sally's treatment would benefit society by allowing her to be more productive at work and more successful in interpersonal relationships. The successive improvements in medications developed to treat mental illness provide strong reasons to continue with this form of technology and to expect future benefits. Any risks of technology spiraling out of control can also be assessed as discussed previously (Bostrom 2002).

Finally, it is worth applying the principles approach to ethical analysis towards pharmaceuticals of the future that may allow *true* cosmetic psychopharmacology. The first relevant principle involves autonomy and will be discussed in light of a hypothetical, yet realistic, example. Assume that a chemical compound, call it Extravertia, is developed that alters the introversion–extraversion dimension of personality (Costa and McCrae 1992). People who score very low on the extraversion domain of a given personality assessment (i.e., those whose personalities are defined, in part, by a lack of gregariousness and social assertiveness and a high level of introversion and self-consciousness) can take Extravertia and transform their temperament. Those taking Extravertia would find themselves becoming comfortable in large groups of people, seeking social stimulation, speaking out in meetings, volunteering to be project leaders at work, widening their circles of friends, initiating conversations with people they have just met, and chatting at parties rather than retreating to a corner. Regarding autonomy, the first question that must be asked is whether this is any different from getting hair or breast implants, face lifts, or tummy tucks (and the presumed, indirect emotional/psychological benefits of those procedures)? Is it any different from taking a Dale Carnegie course and becoming a more affable person, having a religious conversion and becoming more altruistic, or reading *The Road Less Traveled* and becoming a less impatient and more 'spiritually centered' person? Is it any different from psychotherapy with a shy person that is transformative regarding social assertiveness? These cosmetic, 'self-help,' and therapeutic procedures are pursued routinely in the USA by people with no diagnosable medical or psychiatric condition. Perhaps one difference is that cosmetic psychopharmacology seems to affect manifestations of 'self' directly, rather than indirectly in the case of cosmetic surgery or through an effort of 'will' in self-help or psychotherapy. Yet there are clear benefits to individuals from cosmetic surgery, self-help, psychotherapy, and cosmetic psychopharmacology. To limit the autonomy of these individuals, real risks must be shown.

Assuming that Extravertia does not sever the link between 'happiness' and our experiences of the world, it is necessary in our discussion of autonomy to determine if extraversion is a relative or absolute trait. A simple example of an absolute trait would be health. Increasing an individual's health benefits everyone (ethically, it meets the principle of beneficence). If increases in extraversion provide absolute gains to those who undertake the enhancement, then Extravertia will provide a benefit to individuals and society. On the other hand, if extraversion is a relative trait like height, then making everyone more extraverted may only shift the desired goal (i.e., average extraverts would be redefined as normal) while committing resources that could have, potentially, been better used by society. The principle of autonomy, however, dictates that, within obvious limits, one is free to put one's resources into whatever one can afford (e.g., it is challenging to find any societal benefit accrued from a person spending several thousand dollars for larger breasts, but there are no governmental or legal restrictions placed on persons who desire this change, short of having the money to pay for it). Although the question of whether extraversion is a relative or absolute trait is an empirical one, for this example suppose that it is a relative trait. Before banning a compound like Extravertia, we would still need real evidence that the potential harms of altering the introversion–extraversion dimension of personality, *using a cosmetic psychopharmacologic compound*, outweigh the limits such a ban would place on autonomy. Learning from our experience with cosmetic surgery, it is not clear that everyone will decide to alter their temperament. Even if most people decided to become more outgoing, it is difficult to articulate any real threat from a huge number of extroverted people. (This is not to ignore, however, concerns about the potential usefulness of a balance in different personality types. Rather, it is difficult to determine how seriously to take such concerns.)

The second important ethical principle regarding cosmetic psychopharmacology is justice, reflected in concerns about the potential unequal distribution of cosmetic psychopharmacologic compounds based on income. However, there is no reason to think that these compounds would be any more expensive than Prozac, in which case nearly everyone who wanted them could take them. Yet, even if these compounds were prohibitively expensive, it would have to be argued that the suffering caused to the have-nots outweighs the benefits generated by these enhancements and the autonomous decision to acquire them. In our capitalist economy, those with money enjoy many 'enhancements' (to self and quality of life as experienced by the self) others cannot afford, such as expensive vacations, psychotherapists, cosmetic surgery, self-help seminars, nutrition consultants and personal trainers, better education and food, enhanced living conditions, enhanced healthcare access, etc. Our society has decided that these differences do not create enough injustice to override concerns about autonomy and beneficence. Yet even if this balance were to be tipped in the favor of justice, there are potential options to address these concerns, including making these cosmetic 'luxuries' more affordable through the supply–demand exigencies of capitalism (e.g., the 2005 Hyundai Tucson SUV costs about $17,000, whereas the 2005 Cadillac Escalade SUV costs about $54,000).

Finally, I shall address the challenge that the ethical approach above sets no imaginable limits on cosmetic psychopharmacology. In fact, I readily agree that this position sets no arbitrary limits. That is the core feature of the position: There are no easy answers to questions involving technology and power we cannot currently imagine. As history has shown us, strong reactionary positions against new technologies are no defense against disaster. Instead, each step in the evolution of cosmetic psychopharmacology will have to be evaluated using our best rational and ethical judgment. It is also worth reflecting that the abandonment of technology also entails risk, so in the end we have a choice. With each technology, we need to evaluate if and how it should be used. Any decision, whether for or against technology, will have a great impact on human well-being. Therefore there is no room in such debates for dogma and ignorance of the empirical evidence.

16.5 Conclusion

My goal in writing this chapter was not to resolve the complicated debates about the use of biotechnology in human enhancement. Instead, it was to voice concerns about the ideologically based and logically flawed method of the President's Council on Bioethics in addressing these issues, and to demonstrate that there are many strong ethical arguments that favor the use of cosmetic psychopharmacology. These arguments should be addressed by the President's Council or any other group that opposes cosmetic psychopharmacology. Those who wish to ban potentially useful technologies must provide strong arguments and clear reasoning that the potential harms outweigh the potential benefits. If one group of ethical principles is given more weight in these debates, this position must be clearly stated and defended. Religious and/or political dogma cannot be used alone to support arguments.

A national discussion of these controversial topics, giving fair treatment to all the viewpoints, would be a great achievement. Unfortunately, the President's Council on Bioethics has not proven to be such a forum. History suggests that democratic societies can and do cope with new technologies. Biotechnology can lead to benefits that promote all of the major ethical principles (e.g., public health measures), in addition to benefits that require more of a balancing act (e.g., the ever-growing expense of healthcare). Supporting the democratic resolution of these issues by attempting to balance fairly the ethical principles of justice, autonomy, beneficence, and nonmaleficence is the best defense we have in preventing a *Brave New World*.

Acknowledgments

I thank John Chibnall and Neil Scheurich for their comments on drafts of this manuscript.

Endnotes

1 This section from *Beyond Therapy* supports a literal interpretation: 'As embodied agents of our innermost will, muscles not only work our purposes in the world, but make manifest the deep qualities of our character and dispositions and intentions, our self-discipline, self-development, and self-image. We are highly attentive to posture and motion in others, and muscular actions make possible the communication and cooperative coordination essential for society.' (President's Council on Bioethics 2003: 129)

2 Immediately after this quote, Prozac is again compared to ecstasy and SOMA; subsequently, the Council states that Prozac is different from ecstasy and that the authenticity of Sally's experience is not being questioned: 'SSRIs do not *completely* sever how one feels from how one lives' (President's Council on Bioethics 2003: 295, italics added). Despite the multiple contradictions, it is clear that the authors compare Prozac to drugs of abuse.

References

American Psychiatric Association (2000). *Diagnostic and statistical manual of mental disorders*. 4th ed. rev. (Washington, DC: American Psychiatric Association).

Annas G. J. and Elias S. (2004). Politics, morals and embryos: can bioethics in the United States rise above politics? *Nature*, **431**, 19–20.

Atwood M. (1985). *The Handmaid's Tale* (Toronto, Ontario: McClelland and Stewart).

Beauchamp T. L. and Childress J. F. (1994). *Principles of Biomedical Ethics*, 4th edn. (New York: Oxford University Press).

Blackburn E. (2004). Bioethics and the political distortion of biomedical science. *New England Journal of Medicine*, **350**, 1379–1380.

Bonne O., *et al.* (1999). Clinical doses of fluoxetine and cerebral blood flow in healthy volunteers. *Psychopharmacology*, **143**, 24–28.

Bostrom N. (2002). Existential risks: analyzing human extinction scenarios and related hazards. *Journal of Evolution and Technology* **9**.

Buchanan A., *et al.* (2000). *From Chance to Choice: Genetics and justice* (New York: Cambridge University Press).

Bush G. W. (2001). Executive order: creation of the President's Council on Bioethics. Available at www.whitehouse.gov/news/releases/2001/11/20011128-13.html. Accessed 6 May 2005.

Costa P. T. and McCrae R. R. (1992). *NEO PI-R Professional Manual* (Lutz, FL: Psychological Assessment Resources).

Danforth J. (2005). In the name of politics. *New York Times*, March 30, 17.

Davis J. (2004). Collective suttee: is it unjust to develop life extension if it will not be possible to provide it to everyone? *Annals of the New York Academy of Sciences* **1019**, 535–541.

Edge R. S. and Groves J. R. (1999). *Ethics of Health Care* (Ontario: Delmar).

Elliot C. and Chambers T. (eds.) (2004). *Prozac as a Way of Life* (Chapel Hill, NC: University of North Carolina Press).

Epstein M. (2004). Review of *Prozac as a Way of Life*, by Carl Elliot and Tod Chambers (eds.). *New England Journal of Medicine* **351**, 2777.

Gelfin Y., Gorfine M., and Lerer B. (1998). Effect of clinical doses of fluoxetine on psychological variables in healthy volunteers. *American Journal of Psychiatry*, **155**, 290–292.

Goldspink G. (2004). Age-related muscle loss and progressive dysfunction in mechanosensitive growth factor signaling. *Annals of the New York Academy of Sciences*, **1019**, 294–298.

Groopman J. (2002). Holding cell: why the cloning decision was wrong. *New Republic* **227**, 5 August, 14–16.

Gruenberg P. (2000). 'Ethics in psychiatry' in B. J. Sadock and V. A. Sadock (eds.) *Kaplan & Sadock's Comprehensive Textbook of Psychiatry* (Philadelphia, PA: Lippincott Williams and Wilkins), 3290–3300.

Harris J. (2004). Immortal ethics. *Annals of the New York Academy of Sciences* **1019**, 527–534.

Huxley A. (1932). *Brave New World* (London: Chatto and Windus).

Kass L. (1997). The wisdom of repugnance. *New Republic* **216**, 2 June, 17–27.

Kelsey J. E. and Nemeroff C. B. (2000). 'Selective serotonin reuptake inhibitors' in B. J. Sadock and V. A. Sadock (eds.) *Kaplan & Sadock's Comprehensive Textbook of Psychiatry* (Philadelphia, PA: Lippincott Williams and Wilkins), 2432–2435.

Kramer, P. (1993). *Listening to Prozac* (New York: Penguin).

Kramer P. (2002). Happiness and sadness: depression and the pharmacological elevation of mood. Available at www.bioethics.gov/transcripts/sep02/session3.html. Accessed 6 May 2005.

Markowitz C. J. (2005). Review of *Prozac as a Way of Life*, by Carl Elliot and Tod Chambers (eds.) *Journal of the American Medical Association* **293**, 237–238.

Orwell G. (1949). *1984* (London: Secker and Warburg).

Pinker S. (2002). *The Blank Slate: The modern denial of human nature* (New York: Penguin).

President's Council on Bioethics. (2002). *Human Cloning and Human Dignity: An ethical inquiry*. Available at www.bioethics.gov/reports/cloningreport/index.html. Accessed 6 May 2005.

President's Council on Bioethics. (2003). *Beyond Therapy: Biotechnology and the pursuit of human improvement* (Washington, DC: Dana Press).

President's Council on Bioethics. (2004*a*). *Monitoring Stem Cell Research*. Available at www.bioethics.gov/reports/stemcell/index.html. Accessed 6 May 2005.

President's Council on Bioethics. (2004*b*). *Reproduction and Responsibility: The regulation of new biotechnologies*. Available at www.bioethics.gov/reports/reproductionandresponsibility/index.html. Accessed 6 May 2005.

Roubenoff R. and Hughes V. (2000). Sarcopenia: current concepts. *Journal of Gerontology A: Biological Sciences and Medical Sciences* **55**, M716–M724.

Rush, J. A. (2000). 'Mood disorders: treatment of depression' in B. J. Sadock and V. A. Sadock (eds.) *Kaplan & Sadock's Comprehensive Textbook of Psychiatry* (Philadelphia, PA: Lippincott Williams and Wilkins), 3432–3455.

Singer P. (ed.) (1994). *A Companion to Ethics* (Malden, MA: Blackwell).

Sweeny, H. L. (2004). Gene doping. *Scientific American* **291** (1), 62–70.

Turner L. (2004). Science, politics and the president's council on bioethics. *Nature Biotechnology* **22**, 509–510.

Wagner K. R., *et al.* (2002). Loss of myostatin attenuates severity of muscular dystrophy in *mdx* mice. *Annals of Neurology* **52**, 832–836.

Chapter 17

The reflectively anxious and depressed: psychotropics and lives worth living

Mark P. Jenkins

17.1 Introduction

This paper explores a philosophical worry involving psychiatry and psychotropic technology. Put most bluntly, the worry is that familiar and widely prescribed antianxiety and antidepressant medications may actually prevent lives worth living. Fully articulating this worry requires unpacking three assumptions. First, that Socrates was right that the unexamined life is not worth living. Second, that there exists both a class of anxious and depressed people and a class of drugs that can effectively treat them. And third, that some not insignificant subset of the first class, call them the reflectively anxious and depressed, finds their anxiety and depression so exacerbated by the very prospect of treatment by some subset of the second class, call them SSRIs,[1] that they refuse any course of therapy that includes psychotropic drugs.

17.2 First assumption: the examined life

In considering Socrates' famous claim at trial that 'the unexamined life is not worth living' (Plato 2002: 41), we might begin by putting it positively as the claim that examination is at least a necessary condition of any life worth living.[2] But what sort of examination are we talking about exactly? At a minimum, self-examination, the ability to adopt a reflective, critical—in a word, philosophical—stance on one's life, that is, on one's dispositions, values, beliefs, plans, actions, motives, relationships, and circumstances; so understood, examination—again, like philosophy—is a fundamentally second-order activity. However, just what does it mean to be reflective or critical here? After all, it is one thing to urge self-examination and quite another to spell out the terms or the criteria by which such self-examination should be conducted.

Here it gets trickier, but one might, for example, reflect on or criticize one's dispositions in terms of consistency, one's values in terms of authenticity, one's beliefs in terms of truth, one's plans in terms of prudence, one's actions in terms of narrative coherence and so forth. On this picture, the examined life consists of unremitting second-order scrutiny of one's first-order existence.[3] A brief contrast with one of literature's most decidedly unexamined lives, that of Tolstoy's Ivan Ilyich, can help us see just what makes Socrates' examined life so worth living.

Great suffering famously attends the death of Ivan Ilyich. Indeed, as Ivan's wife tells it, 'He screamed incessantly not for minutes but for hours on end. He screamed for three straight days without pausing for breath. It was unbearable' (Tolstoy 1981: 43). The physical pain was terrific, but, as the reader knows, Ivan's real suffering is existential. Not until he is literally on his deathbed does it occur to him that 'Perhaps I did not live as I should have' (120). This possibility induces nothing less than 'moral agony,' as Ivan 'suddenly asked himself: 'What if my entire life, my entire conscious life, simply was *not the real thing*?' (126). In this reflective query, of course, we have the bare beginnings of an examined life, albeit arguably too late to do Ivan much good.[4] The fact is that Ivan has never engaged in the sort of second-order scrutiny that characterizes Socrates' and the examined life. From beginning to end Ivan serves but two masters, pleasure and propriety, yet without ever asking himself whether those masters merit subservience. It is only when faced with death that:

> It occurred to him that what had seemed utterly inconceivable before—that he had not lived the kind of life he should have—might in fact be true. It occurred to him that those scarcely perceptible impulses of his to protest what people of high rank considered good, vague impulses which he has always suppressed, might have been precisely what mattered, and all the rest not the real thing. His official duties, his manner of life, his family, the values adhered to by people in society and in his profession—all these might not have been the real thing. He tried to come up with a defense of these things and suddenly became aware of the insubstantiality of them all.
>
> (126–127)

Ivan suddenly realizes that in failing to examine his life as he lived it, he may now have come to the end of a life which, as hard as this may be for him to bear, was simply not worth living.

But what can this really mean, a life that was simply not worth living?[5] A more helpful way of exploring the contrast between examined and unexamined lives or between lives that are and are not worth living may be in terms of happiness. Perhaps what Ivan realizes on his deathbed is that, despite appearances, despite his previous assumptions, despite the testimony of his family, friends, and colleagues, he has never been happy; and perhaps when Socrates recommends a vigorous course of self-examination to his compatriots he does so as one who has found such a course a reliable route to happiness. However, this may seem a stretch; after all, one might be forgiven for thinking Ivan's life, notwithstanding his brink of death doubts, the happier of the two. True, his marriage was a joke, but between the recognition he received from his societal and professional peers, to say nothing of the 'genuine' pleasures of whist, he seems to have carved out a *modus vivendi* that might easily be characterized as happy. Socrates, by contrast, might seem rather unhappy, given the inevitable, incessant frustrations associated with his philosophical mission, a (God-given) mission he at least partly describes as follows:

> I never cease to rouse each and every one of you, to persuade and reproach you all day long and everywhere I find myself in your company…That I am the kind of person to be a gift of the god to the city you might recognize from the fact that it does not seem like human nature for me to have neglected my own affairs and to have tolerated this neglect now for so many years while I was always concerned with you, approaching each one of you like a father or an elder brother to persuade you to care for your virtue.
>
> (Plato 2002: 35)

'All day,' 'each and every one of you,' 'everywhere,' 'always concerned,' Socrates' life certainly seems exhausting, but happy? Happier than Ivan's? No doubt it ultimately comes down to what one means by happiness, and here is may be helpful to take just a moment to consider Mill's famous claim that when it comes to being happy it is 'better to be Socrates dissatisfied than a fool satisfied' (Mill 1979: 10).

Mill's claim arises from his efforts to distinguish his own version of hedonistic utilitarianism, with its qualitative appreciation of higher pleasures, from Bentham's quantitatively oriented 'pig philosophy.' In a valuable assessment of Mill's aims, the philosopher J. J. C. Smart differentiates happiness as contentment, which he associates with Bentham, and happiness as contentment plus some positive evaluation, which he associates with Mill. For Mill, it is not sufficient for happiness that we should be content, we must also be able to judge the quality of the pleasures affording that contentment. As Smart puts it: 'For a man to be happy he must, as a minimal condition, be fairly contented and moderately enjoying himself for much of the time. Once this minimal condition is satisfied we can go on to evaluate various types of contentment and enjoyment and to grade them in terms of happiness' (Smart 1973: 22–23). In other words, for Mill, the very idea of happiness includes an element of examination. And although both Ivan and Socrates meet the minimal condition, only Socrates' life includes something like a reflective endorsement of the pleasures contained therein.

Smart accompanies his analysis with an interesting, if somewhat familiar, thought experiment involving an 'electrode operator.' Suppose we could receive pleasure and contentment reliably and indefinitely through electrical stimulation of the brain; indeed, Smart rather more grandly imagines that 'human arts, such as medicine, engineering, agriculture and architecture will have been brought to a pitch of perfection sufficient to enable most of the human race to spend most of its time electrode operating, without compensating pains of starvation, disease and squalor' (Smart 1973: 20). We attach the electrodes and we are content, we are satisfied, we are enjoying ourselves; the question is: are we happy? The Benthamite, Smart thinks, must say that we are, whereas adherents of Mill will demur. But on what grounds? It must be that on some level we want something more, or something different, than mere contentment. Moreover, it is 'perfectly possible,' as Smart crucially observes, 'that I should be annoyed today if told that from tomorrow onwards I shall be an electrode addict, *even though I knew that from tomorrow onwards I should be perfectly contented*' (Smart 1973: 21, emphasis added). And here we begin to see something of the philosophical precedent for, and the conceptual room occupied by, the reflectively anxious and depressed.[6]

We have no objection to being made happy if we are not, but at the same time we do not want to be made happy any old way; we do not want to settle for a suspect version of happiness, even as we admit that, were we to be made 'suspiciously' happy, we would be content. And just as some would rather be Socrates dissatisfied than a fool satisfied, and some would rather be unhappy than electrode-happy, some, I am suggesting in this paper, would rather be anxious than have that anxiety relieved psychopharmaceutically, even as they willingly admit that, were they so treated, they might well become perfectly content. Ultimately, the unexamined life is not worth living because it is an unhappy life. It may, like Ivan's, be largely contented and full of pleasure, but, as Smart's thought experiment suggests, happiness involves more. It involves the examination, and at some level the endorsement, of the sources and nature of that contentment, even if insisting on the right to make that endorsement places the possibility of contentment, or, in Socrates' case, life itself, in jeopardy.

17.3 Second assumption: the anxious and depressed

A psychiatrist recently complained in the *Journal of the American Medical Association* about the 'temerity' of '[p]undits wielding abstract philosophical opinion,' while 'confus[ing] depression with moral "authenticity" and alienation' (Markowitz 2005: 237). I hope I am not confused in this way. Of course, to the extent that the possibility of lives worth living turns on the practice of reflecting upon and assessing one's values, it will turn on notions of authenticity and avoiding alienation, but as I hope will become clear in the next section, this is in no way to confuse or to identify anxiety or depression with authenticity. The reflectively anxious and depressed do not assert that they are morally authentic in virtue of their anxiety and depression; rather, they assert that antidepressants may undermine the conditions necessary for the possibility of authenticity. In any case, I in no way want to minimize the seriousness of anxiety and depression. I am quite sure that anxiety and depression afflict large numbers of people, interfering with their ability to function and to live normal, balanced, engaged, and otherwise productive lives. Furthermore, I am aware, as apparently the pundits are not, 'that depression can be chronic, subsyndromal, or relapsing...' (237).[7] Drugs, I am sure, can help.

Psychotropic medications, principally in the form of SSRIs, often provide effective therapy and symptom relief for a wide range of conditions related to anxiety and depression. Although it would seem naïve to deny, in an age of non-stop trolling by direct-to-consumer pharmaceutical ads, the plasticity of diagnostic categories, diagnostic criteria, and potential patient population sizes, a certain vagueness at the margins need not obscure our plain view of those who cannot stop crying or worrying or sleeping or lying awake or losing concentration or feeling fatigued or thinking of suicide, nor of the effectiveness of psychotropic medications in treating them.[8] Still, as the work of David Healy so powerfully documents (see, for example, Healy 2004), caution is always appropriate with these drugs, whether because of the disparate effects of identical drugs on similar conditions, or because of the unwholesome relation between drug company research and marketing departments, or because the drugs may have serious side-effects, or simply because they frequently fail to work. As Healy observes on this last point, 'RCT [randomized controlled trial] evidence is used to fuel therapeutic bandwagons. It is sold as evidence that the treatment works (actually does good) rather than evidence that treatments have an effect (which may be put to good use in judicious hands). There is no philosophical or methodological basis for this development' (Healy 2001: 322; see also Healy 2006: 323–324). In other words, effect should not be confused with efficacy, especially statistical effect across a range of subjects with therapeutic efficacy in any particular case. In sum, I take it SSRIs do work, although neither always nor unreservedly.

17.4 Third assumption: the reflectively anxious and depressed

My third assumption basically involves running together the first two. By that I assume that there is some not insignificant number of people who at once suffer from anxiety or depression and are convinced that Socrates is right that the unexamined life is not worth living. Although they are truly anxious and depressed, and although they truly crave relief from their anxiety and depression, they are not so gravely afflicted as to be prevented from entertaining the sincere worry that relief through psychotropic medication might prove more, as it were, life-threatening than, say, cognitive therapy alone or, indeed, no treatment at all, in that such relief might undermine either the conditions or the capacity for the sort of reflection we have located at the core of the examined life. Actually, I can see this worry taking one of two forms. On the one hand, the reflectively anxious and depressed might worry that the object of their reflection or examination might be altered beyond recognition by medication; that is, they might worry that SSRIs will cause the loss of the very self they wish to save. On the other hand, the reflectively anxious and depressed might worry that drug action will block the impulse to or the capacity for reflection or self-examination. In the first case there is no self to examine; in the second there is no examination of the self. Consider, however, two recent efforts to defuse or forestall these worries.

First, take the worry that, say, Prozac or Zoloft will so alter personality as to constitute a loss of self, so that, in effect, there is no longer any there. Framing this worry as ultimately a worry about authenticity, philosopher David DeGrazia counters that, 'However intuitively appealing this reasoning may be, it is undermined by its misleading image of the self as 'given,' static, or something to be discovered' (DeGrazia 2004: 36). Far from losing oneself, 'one can be true to oneself even as one deliberately transforms—to some extent creating—oneself,' and even when such deliberate transformation and self-creation depends upon psychotropic drugs (36). I wonder, however, whether DeGrazia's own analysis might not commit much the same sin he excoriates, in that he 'pictures the self as wood that can be sculpted, "respecting the constraints of natural shape and grain"' (38).[9] Never mind the ease with which seeing the self as wood, natural shape and grain included, lends itself to images of 'the self as "given," static, or something to be discovered,' DeGrazia's metaphor is only as strong as his sculpting tools are weak; that is to say, anyone who has ever tried to sculpt a piece of pine with a rasp will attest to how quickly the wood turns to sawdust. The worry of the reflectively anxious and depressed, then, amounts to the worry that, when it comes to sculpting the self, psychotropic drugs operate more like rasps than emery boards, and that, given the power of these tools, the self's original shape and grain may count for little.

The second form the worry of the reflectively anxious and depressed might take effectively concedes DeGrazia's argument that one may use medication to alter, without completely eradicating, the self. That worry, again, is that the reflective urge itself will wind up a casualty of the pharmacological battle against anxiety and depression. Here one possesses the same self, but without the skills necessary to subject it to the sort of scrutiny required for a life worth living. Rather than allay such fears, one might choose instead to impugn them. This seems to be the course adopted recently by Peter Kramer, whose *Listening to Prozac* more than a decade ago first ignited many of the more philosophical discussions about the increasingly widespread use of antidepressants. In more recent work, Kramer argues that many of the reservations aired about such drugs are best seen as nothing more (or less) than concerns about the deep cultural significance of melancholy and its perceived vulnerability to what are mistakenly taken to be antimelancholic medications: 'I have come to believe that much of the discussion of cosmetic pharmacology is not about pharmacology at all—that is to say, not about the technology. Rather, cosmetic pharmacology is a stand-in for worries over threats to melancholy' (Kramer 2004: 54). Indeed, in his most recent book, Kramer remarks that 'often I had a sense, when I spoke about treating depression, that I was debating two thousand years' worth of elaboration of heroic melancholy' (Kramer 2005: 213). Kramer raises enormous and fascinating issues about melancholy and its relation to clinical depression, the importance of which I can do no more here than acknowledge. However, as I tried to make clear in the last section, the reflectively anxious and depressed are neither candidates for cosmetic pharmacology nor suffering from melancholy.

Remember that Kramer coined his wonderful term 'cosmetic psychopharmacology' in response to his own 'musings about whether it would be kosher to medicate a patient...in the absence of depression' (Kramer 1993: 15). He wondered about people seeking to become 'better than well,' about a brave new world in which 'Some people might prefer pharmacologic to psychologic self-actualization' (15). However, as I have portrayed them, the reflectively anxious and depressed are just that, anxious and depressed. Certainly they want to become self-actualized, who does not? However, they are worried, whether legitimately or illegitimately, not about losing credentials as sensitive, tortured, romantic, melancholic types, but rather about losing the capacity for self-examination, as well as the implications of that loss for the worth of their lives.

Still, at the end of the day, perhaps the two worries I have been attributing to the reflectively anxious and depressed amount to much the same thing.[10] After all, is the first worry, the one that sees a self sculpted into sawdust, really about the obliteration of the self? Or is that worry more accurately described in terms of a psychopharmacologically derived *different* self? But different in what way? For starters: less sensitive to subtleties surrounding the monitoring and regulation of the self; in a word, less reflective. On this view, then, the two worries collapse into one: to worry about losing oneself as the result of medication is equivalent to worrying that one will wind up a different self, one less able to engage in reflection, and *a fortiori* less able to live an examined life.

17.5 **Outcomes**

Assuming that I have said enough at this point to motivate the idea of the reflectively anxious and depressed, that is, to motivate the idea of a group of anxious and depressed patients whose anxiety and depression are exacerbated by the prospect of psychopharmacological intervention, because of fears about a resultant loss of reflective capacity and a belief that such a loss would endanger their chances for a valuable life, it may be helpful to outline what I take to be the four different treatment outcomes open to them. In the first case, the reflectively anxious and depressed succumb to their worries about SSRIs and refuse psychotropic treatment. In the second case, the reflectively anxious and depressed put aside their worries and take SSRIs, but the drugs have no effect whatsoever, either on their anxiety and depression or on their ability to reflect. In the third case, the reflectively anxious and depressed take SSRIs, which work to alleviate their anxiety and depression, while in no way interfering with their ability to reflect. In the fourth case, the reflectively anxious and depressed take SSRIs, which work to alleviate their anxiety and depression, yet their worst fears are realized as the drugs wind up short-circuiting the sort of reflection required for an examined life. I want to say just a little about each of these possibilities.

The last two outcomes assume that psychotropic drugs work. Of course, just what working means in the case of SSRIs turns out to be a fairly complex question, as several different criteria have been used in clinical trials to gauge the effectiveness of psychiatric medications. As Healy writes, 'There are four potential domains of measurement [in clinical trials in psychiatry]: observer-based disease-specific rating scales, such as the Hamilton Rating Scale for Depression (HRSD); patient-based disease-specific rating scales, such as the Beck Depression Inventory (BDI); observer-based non-disease-specific scales of global functioning; and patient-based non-disease-specific scales of global functioning (Quality of Life scale, QoL)' (Healy 2001: 323). The problem, Healy continues, is that 'there is not a single antipsychotic or antidepressant that has been demonstrated to have treatment effects across all these domains' (323). This is indeed a problem, but one that, for present purposes, must be put aside.[11]

Beginning with the last two outcomes, then, both feature psychotropics working to alleviate anxiety and depression. The third case, of course, represents the best of all possible worlds: formerly reflectively anxious and depressed patients are no longer, or no longer as severely, anxious and depressed, and their capacity to engage in reflective self-examination is in no way pharmacologically stymied. Indeed, one might reasonably expect that capacity to become significantly enhanced. Certainly it seems possible, even probable, that whatever self-examination the reflectively anxious and depressed engage in before treatment may prove sub-optimal because of the deleterious consequences of anxiety and depression. By contrast, it would be foolish to dismiss the possibility that more perspicacious reflection and more penetrating self-examination are just exactly what SSRIs allow; indeed, some claim that precisely what they allow is (at long last) access to one's 'real self' (see, for example, Kramer 1993: 18–21). Under this preferred outcome, patients are able to successfully re-engage with both the world and themselves.

Just how negatively one should characterize the fourth outcome, whereby the reflectively anxious and depressed lose both their anxiety and depression and the power to examine their lives, depends in no small measure on one's reaction to Smart's electrode operator. Certainly this is the worst case from the point of view of the reflectively anxious and depressed; after all, fear about its likelihood effectively constitutes their condition. They worry that, although psychotropic medications may well make them better able to *live* their lives, they will simultaneously be made less able to *lead* them, a distinction of enormous importance. However, if, as the parallel case of the electrode operator seems to suggest, psychotropics induce not simply the desired effect of psychic well-being and (*ex hypothesi*) the undesired effect of loss of reflective capacity, but also a third, more ambiguous, effect, the incapacity to appreciate that loss, then whether and just how the patient has been made worse off becomes a subject for heated philosophical debate. It is a debate that this chapter certainly does not settle, although it does try to make clear which side the reflectively anxious and depressed are on and why.

The first two outcomes both assume, in their own way, that SSRIs do not work: the first, analytically, so to speak, because the patient refuses to take them; the second because they are simply, for whatever reason, clinically inefficacious. In this latter case, one might be tempted to conclude that the reflectively anxious and depressed are no worse off. I think this would be a mistake. After all, for this outcome to occur the reflectively anxious and depressed must have made some effort, at some psychic cost, to overcome their reflective anxiety and depression, at least to the point of acquiescing to psychopharmacological treatment. However, this psychic cost, I suggest, may be far from trivial. Frustrated in the face of drug inaction at the persistence of their anxiety and depression, their affliction may actually intensify owing to regret, resentment, and the perception that they have now compromised themselves—psychically, physically, philosophically—for nothing.

If this is a real possibility, then it counts, from the point of view of the reflectively anxious and depressed, as a reason against something like Pascal's wager applied to antidepressants. The idea would be that the reflectively anxious and depressed might as well *try* antidepressants, for the amount of harm (however construed) they can possibly suffer is, if not quite infinitesimal, then certainly trivial compared with the potential benefits.[12] Although I hope I have said enough by now to show that I in no way underestimate those benefits, I also believe that, again from the reflectively anxious and depressed's point of view, the potential consequences of drug inaction, not to mention the consequences of, so to speak, drug over-action, simply rule out assigning either a tiny coefficient or a tiny probability to calculations about whether to accede to treatment by psychotropic drugs. In fact, one might say that the reflectively anxious and depressed have gone ahead and formulated a wager using the terms above, but in something like reverse order. As a result, they cannot see the (even quite likely) good SSRIs might do them amounting to much in the face of the almost incalculable harm they would suffer in the (no doubt quite unlikely) loss of the ability to philosophically scrutinize their lives.

Finally, as far as outcomes are concerned, the reflectively anxious and depressed, in refusing treatment, will be arguably made no worse off, which is just to say they will still be anxious and depressed. In which case it is possible they may come to take a rather ironic view of themselves. This is because in living both an examined life and an anxious and depressed life they may well be living a life that both is and is not worth living. However, is their prognosis necessarily bleak? After all, in rejecting antidepressants they do not reject psychiatry per se. Certainly I would expect the reflectively anxious and depressed to avail themselves of all manner of psychological counseling in an effort to alleviate their anxiety and depression. But perhaps someone might wonder as follows: if both psychotropic medication and psychological counseling are capable of alleviating anxiety and depression such that their treatment outcomes, however measured, are virtually indistinguishable, then cannot one assume, despite obvious differences in form, that both treatments succeed by (putting it very roughly) manipulating the same content? However, if this is so, then should the reflectively anxious and depressed be just as concerned about talk therapy undermining their capacity for reflection as they are about drug therapy? Why not worry that *any* form of therapy that succeeds in relieving anxiety and depression will pose a serious threat to the examined life?

In considering this question, we need to remember that the worry of the reflectively anxious and depressed is about what drugs may do *besides* alleviate anxiety and depression, about the possibility that one might become, so to speak, unreflectively well. Part of their worry is no doubt associated with the sheer power and scope of the drugs, but another part of it, perhaps even a larger part, is connected to the speed with which these drugs are said to work, especially when compared to psychotherapy. Perhaps they recall Kramer's testimony that 'I was used to seeing patient's personalities change slowly, through painfully acquired insight and hard practice in the world. But recently I had seen personalities altered almost instantly, by medication' (Kramer 1993: xiv–xv). Anything but instantaneous, here the very nature of psychotherapy may seem particularly well suited to allay the worry of the reflectively anxious and depressed, and not just in the obvious and negative sense that, however it works, its effects will be gradual (although this is where I do think DeGrazia's metaphor of therapeutically sculpting the self fits quite nicely). There is also a positive sense in which psychotherapy, being inherently dialogic, mirrors Socrates' own pursuit of a life worth living. Moreover, self-examination and self-transformation through psychotherapy may seem to feature a degree of control and, probably more importantly, a degree of transparency that drugs can never match. In sum, to the reflectively anxious and depressed, psychotherapy may well appear as much more than merely the anti-antidepressant consolation prize.

17.6 **Conclusion**

What about someone who complains that at the end of the day my analysis amounts to so much spun gold, for in actuality the set of the reflectively anxious and depressed is empty? Although, as Kramer points out, 'Patients often have extreme fears about drugs, stemming from their apprehension that medication will take over in a way that cannot be reversed, that drugs will obliterate the self' (Kramer 1993: 13), such fears are easily dissolved through psychiatric or other expert counseling. There simply are, the complainant concludes, no anxious and depressed individuals who would sooner endure anxiety and depression than take SSRIs. Although I must admit I know of no studies documenting a reflectively anxious and depressed patient population, absence of evidence is not necessarily evidence of absence. My own conversations, anecdotal and limited to be sure, with physicians, academics, mental health professionals, people who are taking or have taken psychotropic medication and, of course, people who have refused to do so on, so to speak, philosophical grounds, lead me to insist on the reality of the reflectively anxious and depressed.

What about what might seem to be a related complaint, one that concedes the existence of the reflectively anxious and depressed, but simply refuses to take them seriously, on the ground that their worry is so obviously misplaced? Although antidepressants may ruin your sex life, they will in no way keep you from philosophizing on that unfortunate turn of events—and everyone knows this.[13] Although I readily agree that psychotropic drugs may not prevent philosophizing and may, as I suggested in the last section, even facilitate the task, it should be clear by now that the question of whether they actually do interfere with self-examination is off point; the point being that certain people with anxiety and depression refuse psychiatric treatment for what are ultimately philosophical reasons. Perhaps I need not add that if it did turn out that (whatever this might mean) the concerns of the reflectively anxious and depressed were empirically validated, say, because someone somehow conclusively demonstrated that SSRIs deactivate certain neural networks known to be necessary for self-examination, it is the entire population of anxious and depressed people who would then be threatened with a real and significant loss by psychotropic medications, and not just the subset of that population I have termed reflective. In any case, and for the last time, it is the fear of loss, and not necessarily the loss itself, that has been my concern.

Having said that, consider, by way of conclusion, this invaluable caution by Iris Murdoch: 'It is frequently difficult in philosophy to tell whether one is saying something reasonably public and objective, or whether one is erecting a barrier, special to one's temperament, against one's own personal fears' (Murdoch 1970: 72). Parenthetically she adds, 'It is always a significant question to ask about any philosopher: what is he afraid of?' (72). In my own case I might answer, not presuming to speak for the reflectively anxious and depressed, a world in which philosophy has become a casualty of contentment.[14]

Endnotes

1 SSRIs is short for selective serotonin reuptake inhibitors, of which the three best-known brand names in the USA are Paxil (paroxetine), Zoloft (sertaline), and, of course, Prozac (fluoxetine). Because it is these types of drug that are currently so widely prescribed for anxiety and depression, it is these types that I am generally associating with reflective anxiety and depression. However, I do not mean to rule out the possibility, indeed, the likelihood, of similar worries attaching to other drugs prescribed for the same or similar conditions: tricyclic antidepressants, for example Elavil (amitriptyline), or antidepressants like Wellbutrin (bupropion), held to target neurotransmitters other than serotonin. For details on these and other psychotropic drugs see Healy (2005).

2 With this famous claim, Socrates gives us one of the earliest pictures of philosophical practice, and still one of the most powerful. Like Kraus's psychoanalysis, however, philosophy may itself be the disease for which it purports to be the cure. At the very least philosophy's own self-image appears expansive enough to accommodate metaphors of

both illness and treatment; or as I should better suggest in this context, both anxiety and therapy. Philosophy as a form of therapy is perhaps most naturally associated with Wittgenstein, whose method of analysis aims to dissolve pseudo-problems, whereas philosophy as a form of anxiety may be most clearly seen in the case of Socrates. Not that Socrates himself necessarily appears particularly anxious. Yet the gadfly of Athens' preferred philosophical method of elenchus seems almost invariably to increase, where it does not itself create, the mental and emotional agitation of his interlocutors. As philosopher Jonathan Lear wryly notes, 'It seems to me no accident that Socrates went to jail and Wittgenstein went to the movies' (Lear 1984: 148).

3 Of course, nothing prevents iterating perspectives—meta-scrutiny, if you will; for example, a third-order examination of the standards used during second-order reflection on our first-order lives. For classic discussion of such issues see Frankfurt (1988) and Watson (2003).

4 Just how much good Ivan's eleventh-hour philosophical turn does him is a matter of interpretation; there is some chance that in causing him to literally 'see the light' it does him all the good there is (see Tolstoy 1981: 132). Such interpretive issues have little bearing on my invocation here of Ivan as the anti-Socrates.

5 See Kraut (2006) for extended discussion of this question as it relates to Socrates.

6 For a somewhat similar (and decidedly more famous) thought experiment, see Robert Nozick's 'experience machine' (Nozick 1974: 42–45). Note how Nozick effectively discounts Smart's annoyance: 'Would you plug in? *What else can matter to us, other than how our lives feel from the inside?* Nor should you refrain because of the few moments of distress between the moment you've decided and the moment you're plugged. What's a few moments of distress compared to a lifetime of bliss (if that's what you choose), and why feel any distress at all if your decision *is* the best one?' (43).

7 Certainly this point deserves emphasis. As Judd *et al.* conclude: 'The long-term weekly course of unipolar MDD [Major Depressive Disorder] is dominated by prolonged symptomatic chronicity...The symptomatic course is dynamic and changeable, and MDD, MinD [Minor Depressive Disorder], and SSD [Subsyndromal and Subthreshold Depression] symptom levels commonly alternate over time in the same patients as a symptomatic continuum of illness activity of a single clinical disease' (1998: 694).
At the same time, it seems to me interesting ontological and epistemological, not to mention clinical, issues arise about so-called subthreshold depression and its symptoms.

8 I have selected these symptoms for general illustrative purposes from among the diagnostic criteria for major depressive episode and generalized anxiety disorder in the *Diagnostic and Statistical Manual of Mental Disorders*, 4th edn (American Psychiatric Association 2000: 356, 476).

9 DeGrazia attributes the embedded quote, indeed, the entire metaphor, to Glover (1988: 136).

10 A point suggested to me by Marya Schechtman.

11 I thank David Healy for providing me with copies of some of his papers, and for clarifying his views on the effectiveness of SSRIs. His many publications speak for themselves, of course. However, one point may be worth emphasizing here: Healy emphatically believes that, under conditions of caring, attentive clinical supervision, drugs work.

12 I am grateful to Maura Tumulty for pressing me on this point, although she did not raise it in quite this form.

13 Alternatively, they might just save it. As Healy somewhat disturbingly points out, 'sexual functioning may be more reliably affected by an SSRI than mood.' Citing Waldinger *et al.* (1994), he continues, 'Where up to 200 patients may be needed to demonstrate a treatment effect for an SSRI in depression, as few as 12 may be needed to demonstrate efficacy for premature ejaculation' (Healy 2001: 325).

14 I thank Alexa Tullis for arguing me through (read: never agreeing with me about) these issues on several occasions, as well as Marya Schechtman and, especially, Maura Tumulty for commenting on earlier drafts.

References

DeGrazia D. (2004). 'Prozac, enhancement, and self-creation' in C. Elliott and T. Chambers (eds.) *Prozac as a Way of Life* (Chapel Hill: University of North Carolina Press), 33–47.

American Psychiatric Association. (2000). *Diagnostic and Statistical Manual of Mental Disorders*, 4th edn., text revision (Arlington: American Psychiatric Association).

Frankfurt H. (1988). 'Freedom of the will and the concept of a person' in *The Importance of What We Care About* (Cambridge: Cambridge University Press), 80–94.

Glover J. (1988). *I: The philosophy and psychology of personal identity* (London: Penguin).

Healy D. (2001). The dilemmas posed by new and fashionable treatments. *Advances in Psychiatric Treatment*, **7**, 322–327.

Healy D. (2004). *Let them Eat Prozac* (New York: New York University Press).

Healy D. (2005). *Psychiatric Drugs Explained*, 4th edn. (Edinburgh: Elsevier).

Healy D. (2006). The antidepressant tale: figures signifying nothing? *Advances in Psychiatric Treatment*, **12**, 320–328.

Judd L., Akiskal H., Maser J., *et al.* (1998). A prospective 12-year study of subsyndromal and syndromal depressive symptoms in unipolar major depressive disorders. *Archives of General Psychiatry*, **55**, 694–700.

Kramer P. (1993). *Listening to Prozac* (New York: Viking).

Kramer P. (2004). 'The valorization of sadness: alienation and the melancholic temperament' in C. Elliott and T. Chambers (eds.) *Prozac as a Way of Life* (Chapel Hill: University of North Carolina Press), 48–58.

Kramer P. (2005). *Against Depression* (New York: Viking).

Kraut R. (2006). 'The examined life' in S. Ahbel-Rappe and R. Kamtekar (eds.) *A Companion to Socrates* (New York: Blackwell), 228–242.

Lear J. (1984). 'Moral objectivity' in S. C. Brown (ed.) *Objectivity and Cultural Divergence* (Cambridge: Cambridge University Press), 135–170.

Markowitz J. (2005). Review of *Prozac as a Way of Life*. *Journal of the American Medical Association*, **293**, 237–238.

Mill J. S. (1979). *Utilitarianism* (Indianapolis: Hackett).

Murdoch I. (1970). *The Sovereignty of Good* (London: Routledge).

Nozick R. (1974). *Anarchy, State, and Utopia* (New York: Basic Books).

Plato. (2002). *Apology* (G. M. A. Grube, tr.) in *Five Dialogues*, 2nd edn. (Indianapolis: Hackett), 21–44.

Smart J. J. C. (1973). 'An outline of a system of utilitarian ethics' in J. J. C. Smart and B. Williams (eds.) *Utiltarianism: For and against* (Cambridge: Cambridge University Press), 3–74.

Tolstoy L. (1981). *The Death of Ivan Ilyich* (L. Solotaroff, tr.) (New York: Bantam).

Waldinger M., Hengeveld M., and Zwinderman A. (1994). Paroxetine treatment of premature ejaculation: a double-blind randomized placebo-controlled study. *American Journal of Psychiatry*, **151**, 1377–1379.

Watson G. (2003). 'Free agency', in G. Watson (ed.) *Free Will*, 2nd edn. (Oxford: Oxford University Press), 337–351.

Index

Please note that references to endnotes will be followed by the letter 'n'. US spellings are used.

ACT (standardized aptitude test) 45
ADD (attention-deficit disorder) 156–159, 161
  compensatory strategies in 158
  'design', and 'intentional' stances 157
admissions committees, colleges 36
Adorno, Theodor W. 39, 40, 41, 44
aesthetic explanations
  and causal explanations 77
  psychoanalysis 80
  questions, origins 77–79
  relation to object of study 79–81
  therapeutics, aesthetics in 82–83
  types 75–77
  validation 81
affective disorders 161–164
affectivity 60, 61, 65
African-American/womanist and racial/ethnic feminism 93–96, 109
AIDS research 130–131
air bag fiasco, US auto industry 90–91
America by Design: Science, technology, and the rise of corporate capitalism (Noble) 127
amitriptyline (antidepressant) 128
ancient Greeks 62, 193
Angell, Marcia 128
animals, psyches of 63
antidepressant trials, children and adolescents 215–228
  additional criticisms 222
  Boyle–Hobbes controversy 226–228
  double-blind 217, 218–219
  economic context 219–221
  failed, public disclosure 221–222
  overview of hearings/presented data 216–218
  placebos 218, 219
  suicidal thoughts and behavior 217, 222–225
antidepressants
  see also antidepressant trials, children and adolescents; psychotropics
  gender differences 97
  homogeneity of, questioning 117
  market interests 128
  as one of many possible depression treatments 103
  SSRIs *see* SSRIs (selective serotonin reuptake inhibitors)
  trials *see* antidepressant trials, children and adolescents
  use of in less developed countries 105
  women, differences in response to 101
anti-psychotic medication 206
anxiety
  assumptions 296–300
  panic attacks, personal experience of 189–191, 195
  primordial 192
  reflectively anxious and depressed 297–300
Aristotle 3, 11, 273
art, mass-produced 41
artifacts 12, 25, 26, 30
artificial intelligence, rationality 9
Asperger syndrome (AS) 14, 159–161, 165
astronomy 10, 11
attention-deficit disorder (ADD) *see* ADD (attention-deficit disorder)
Augustine 60, 67–68
aura 41–42
authenticity
  and flexibility 62, 63
  moral 296
  and truth 67–68
  as uniquely human concern 62–63
automobiles, role in contemporary society 40
avarice 60
awareness 32
Awareness of Social Inference Test (TASIT) 256, 257
Axys Pharmaceuticals 93

Bacon, Francis 3–4
Baron-Cohen, Simon 251, 252, 253
Beck Depression Inventory (BDI) 300
Being-in-the-World (Dreyfus) 190
Benjamin, Walter 41, 42
Bentham, J. 295
benzodiazepines, withdrawal from 126
Beutler, L. E. 50
Beyond Therapy: Biotechnology and the pursuit of happiness (report) 279, 280, 281, 282, 285
  Argument from Repugnance 283
biological determinism 98
biology and feminist theories
  African-American/womanist and racial/ethnic feminism 93–94
  cyberfeminism 107–108
  essentialist feminism 95–96
  existentialist feminism 97
  liberal feminism 89–90

biology and feminist theories (*cont.*)
post-colonial feminism 105
postmodern feminism 103
psychoanalytic feminism 99
radical feminism 100–101
socialist feminism 91–92
biomedicine 107
biopsychiatry
bad politics 187–189
bad rhetoric 186–187
bad science 185–186
dominance of 187
and hegemony 185
postpsychiatry 189
state-of-the-art (2006) 182–184
bipolar disorder 163
boredom, profound 15, 189, 193–198
Borgmann, Albert 7–8, 31–32, 172
Boyle–Hobbes controversy, and clinical trials 226–228
The Boy Who Couldn't Stop Washing 128
Bracken, P. 51, 187, 189
brain 62, 137
Brave New World (Huxley) 281
BRCA1 and *BRCA2* cancer genes 95, 99
Brentano, F. 253
Broome, Carole 94
Buber, Martin 237, 238
Bush, George W. 280

Cacioppo, J.T. 37
capitalism 91
Captains of Consciousness: Advertising and the social roots of the consumer culture (Ewen) 128
Caputo, J. D. 196
cardiovascular disease, and existentialist feminism 97
caring values 100
Caro, R. 93
CASP (Child and Adolescent Social Perception Measure) 255, 256, 257
castration complex 98
categorical imperative 123
CATIE (Clinical Antipsychotic Trials of Intervention Effectiveness) 188, 198
CBT (cognitive behavioral therapy) 206, 207
CCC (Community Cancer Care), quality of life program 231, 233–234, 243
Chaitin, Gregory 140
Charland, Louis 29, 30, 31
Chiarugi, Vincenzo 65
Child and Adolescent Social Perception Measure (CASP) 255, 256, 257
Chodorow, N. 98
Cioffi, F. 73, 76, 77, 79
Citalopram (antidepressant) 187
citizen participation, psychopharmacology 129–131
client-centered approach, psychiatric rehabilitation as 208
Clinical Antipsychotic Trials of Intervention Effectiveness (CATIE) 188, 198
clinical psychology and technical methodology 35–36
Code, Lorraine 242
cognitive behavioral therapy (CBT) 206, 207
collaborative empiricism 207
commodities 2, 8, 51
Community Cancer Care (CCC), quality of life program 231, 233–234, 243
conceptual confusions, Wittgenstein on 74
congruence 271
consciousness-raising 101
contractual trustworthiness 266, 270
Copernicus 4, 11
cosmetic psychopharmacology 279, 284–290
Cosmopolis (Toulmin) 10
critical theory
Habermas on 123, 128
and identity thinking 40–41, 44
psychopharmacology 115–132
CSM (computer-automated system) 236, 243
cultural artifacts 12, 25, 26
cyberfeminism 106–108, 109
CyberPsychology and Behavior (journal) 29
cyborgs 107
cyclicity, concept 100–101

Darkness Visible (Styron) 195
Darwin, Charles/Darwinian theory 39, 52, 155
and mental disorders 165
publications 60
Davidson, A. 51
Dawkins, R. 95
de Montaigne, Michel 10
Declaration of Independence, as example of immanent critique 41
DeGrazia, David 298–299
Dennett, Daniel 157, 252, 253
depression
antidepressants *see* antidepressant trials, children and adolescents; antidepressants; psychotropics; SSRIs (selective serotonin reuptake inhibitors)
assumptions 296–300
Beck Depression Inventory 300
chronic 101
gender differences 97
Hamilton scale for 117, 125, 300
major, general concept 40, 189
melancholic subtype 194
SSRIs as one of many possible treatments for 103
STAR*D study 182–184, 185, 186–187, 196, 198
derealization 190, 191

Descartes, René 4, 10, 65
on passions 56, 57, 58, 59, 63
on truth and authenticity 67
Description of the Retreat (Tuke) 66
Design Stance 157, 252–253
despair 196
determinism, scientific 38
device paradigm 7, 8, 203
Dewey, John 12, 35, 43
Diagnostic and Statistical Manuals of Mental Disorders (DSMs) 29
diagnosis criteria 28
hyponarrativity, guiding assumption of 30, 31
major depression, general concept 40
maps analogy 47, 49
panic attacks 190
psychiatry, examples from 46–47
revision, subject to 47
technical methodology, and clinical psychology 36
Digby, Ann 67
Dinnerstein, D. 98
discipline 32
Dixon, Thomas 60
double-blind studies
antidepressant trials, children and adolescents 217, 218–219
liberal feminism 89
Drane, James 272
dreams 78, 82
Dresser, Rebecca 131
Dreyfus, Hubert 9, 25, 190
DSMs (Diagnostic and Statistical Manuals of Mental Disorders) *see* Diagnostic and Statistical Manuals of Mental Disorders (DSMs)
dualism 57, 58, 102, 120
Dunston, Georgia 94
Durkheim, Emile 39

Easlea, B. 96
EBM *see* evidence-based medicine
ECT (electroconvulsive therapy) 184
Edwards, J. 83
either/or dichotomy 43, 120
Ekman, P. 256
electroconvulsive therapy (ECT) 184
Eliot, George 241
Ellul, Jacques 4, 6–7
Emanuel, Ezekiel 123
emotional awareness, assessment 249–258
empathy, developing 253–254
intentionality, understanding 252–253
knowing emotions of another 250
mind reading 250–252, 254–257
emotional intelligence 63, 64
emotions
lack of identification 26
new technologies 55–57
passions 56, 57–59
regulation of 61–65
new technologies 55–57
secular 60–61
empathy, developing 253–254
enframing concept (Heidegger) 161, 182, 192, 195
engagement 32
Enlightenment, and immanent critique 42
epidemiology 44, 224–225
epistemological approach to knowledge, symptom management systems, technology-driven 240–243
epistemology
psychopharmacology 120–121
revised considerations 124
social 116, 121
essentialist feminism 94–96
ethical issues in technology and psychiatry 16–17
principles approach to ethical analysis 287
technical/technological expert model 265–267
evidence-based medicine 9, 48–50
evidence-biased medicine 119
Ewen, Stuart 128
examined life 293–296
existential paradox, Heideggerian 144, 146, 147
existentialism 177–178
existentialist feminism 96–98, 109
expertise, qualified 45–46
explanation, understanding distinguished 84
Exploring the Biological Contributions to Human Health: Does sex matter? (Institute of Medicine) 90
The Expression of Emotion in Man and Animals (Darwin) 60
extraversion–introversion 288
Extravertia 288, 289

FDA (Food and Drug Administration)
on depression 184
antidepressants for children and adolescents 216, 223
on randomized controlled trial 117
regulations, amendment of 1962 116
Fee, Elizabeth 97
Feenberg, Andrew 8–9, 129
Feighner criteria, schizophrenia 48
feminist theories 87–88
African-American/womanist and racial/ethnic feminism 93–96, 109
andocentric bias 88
and computers 100, 102
cyberfeminism 106–108, 109
essentialist feminism 94–96
existentialist feminism 96–98, 109
liberal feminism 89–91, 102, 109
postcolonial feminism 104–106, 109

feminist theories (*cont.*)
postmodern feminism 102–104, 109
psychoanalytic feminism 98–100
radical feminism 100–102, 109
and reproductive technologies 109
socialist feminism 91–93, 109
Feynman, Richard 147
film, and technological rationality 42
Fink, M. 194
Firestone, Shulamith 108
First, Michael 47
first-generation philosophic analyses 5–7
flexibility 62, 63
fMRI (functional magnetic resonance imaging) 13
access to 93
cyberfeminism 108
essentialist feminism 96
'norm' for 94
postcolonial feminism 106
radical feminism 101
sex differences 98
folk psychology 253
formulas, technical 36
Foucault, Michel 135, 187
Frankfurt school of critical social theory 9, 12, 35
French Moralists 59, 63
Freud, Sigmund 78, 80, 98
Wittgenstein on 74, 81
frontal fatigue
prefrontal cortex 167, 175–176
human 169–172
technology 172–175
Fulford, K.W.M. 120
functional magnetic resonance imaging (fMRI) *see* fMRI (functional magnetic resonance imaging)
functionalism 136–137
'fuzzy logic' 141

Galileo 4, 10, 11
gauge fields 142, 143, 145
'extreme' 148
generic clinician 9–10, 31
genetic counselors 99
genetics, socialist feminism 91–92
genome research 108
geometry, analytical 4, 10
Gestell (enframing) 182, 192, 195
Ghaemi, Nassir 28, 84
Giere, R. 47, 49
GlaxoSmithKline 216–217
grade point averages, students 44
Greenspan, Miriam 196
grieving 80
Grundstimmungen (fundamental moods) 191

Habermas, J.
and critical theory 123, 128
and symptom management systems 237, 239, 240
Hacking, Ian 38, 39, 43, 51
Hamilton scale, depression 117, 125, 300
happiness 295, 296
Haraway, Donna 107, 108
Harding, S. 100
Haynes, B. R. 49
Healing through the Dark Emotions (Greenspan) 196
Healy, David 13
on authenticity 62, 63
criticism of 119
critique of psychopharmacology 115, 124–125, 131
on evidence-biased medicine 119
on ideology 119
on rating scales 300
on RCTs 118, 297
on science 119, 122
technological reform advocated by 116
Hearing Voices Network 189
hedonism 295
hegemony 135–137, 185
Heidegger, Martin
on boredom 15, 189, 193–198
compound words, use of 191
conservatism of 50
on embeddedness of human in the world 9
enframing concept of 161, 182, 192, 195
existential paradox 144, 146, 147
and Jonas 6
ontological semantics of 148
and primordial moods 191–193, 198
publications 6, 24
on pure science and technology 2
on role of technology in modern life 191–192
spirituality of 196
Heisenberg uncertainty 148
Held, Klaus 191, 192, 194
HGI (Human Genome Initiative) 90, 95
hit rate analysis 44
Homo erectus 36
Homo sapiens 36
Horkheimer, Max 39, 40
Human Genome Center, Harvard 94
Human Genome Diversity Project 93
Human Genome Initiative (HGI) 90, 95
Hume, David 60
Husserl, Edmund 143–144
Huxley, A. 281
hypermodern, defined 107
hyponarrativity 30–31
hysteria 80

'identity thinking', and critical theory 40–41, 44
Ihde, Don 9, 84
I-it relationship and I-Thou relationship (Buber) 237
Ilyich, Ivan (Tolstoy's character) 294–295
imipramine (antidepressant) 101, 117
immanent critique 12, 41–44, 47
INCPAD trial 244
inevitability, notion of 115
information
  defined 138
  intentionally intrisic, and subjective existence 143–147
  ontologically meaningful 147–149
  theory *see* information theory, post-technological
  treatment decisions 49
information technology, and feminist theory 100, 102
information theory, post-technological
  computational algorithm 140
  instrumental, and bad faith in psychiatry 138–141
  intentionally intrinsic information, and subjective existence 143–147
  'intrinsic', meaning 140
  symmetry 141–143
  techno-psychiatry, current hegemony 135–137
instrument metaphor 12, 30
instrumental reasoning *see* technical reason
instrumentalism, Dewey on 43
instrumentality/instrumental thinking 24–25, 37
'The Instrument Metaphor, Hyponarrativity and the Generic Clinician' (Sadler) 12
Intentional Stance 157, 252, 253
intentionality, understanding 252–253
interactive voice response (IVR) 236
interpretation, in psychoanalysis 81–82
IVR (interactive voice response) 236

Japanese teacup, artifact of 25
Jaspers, K. 84
Johnson, Mead 126
Joint Primary Aircraft Training System 98
Jonas, Hans 3, 4, 5–6
Journal of the American Medical Association 296

Kaiser, David 193, 196
Kant, Immanuel 30, 123
Kaplan, David 124
Kass, Leon 282
Keller, E. F. 99, 100
Kendler, Kenneth 47, 48
Kirk, S. A. 51
Kitcher, Phillip 120, 124
knowledge
  and Aristotle 3, 11
  contextual 242
  epistemological approach 240–243
  obtaining in rational manner 88
  pluralistic approaches to acquiring 242
  as socially constructed 91
  technical reason 9
  theoretical and practical 11
Kramer, Peter 279, 286, 303
  Listening to Prozac 284, 285, 299
Kroenke, Kurt 244
Kutchins, H. 51

Lebenswelt (life-world) 239
Lectures and Conversations (Wittgenstein) 76
Leong, F. T. L. 50
Les Passions d l'Âme (Descartes) 57, 67
Leslie, Alan 253–254
Levinas, E. 238
Lewis, B. 187
liberal feminism 89–91, 109
  and postmodern feminism 102
Listening to Prozac (Kramer) 284, 285, 299
Lomas, Peter 56
Longino, H. 88, 122
low need for cognition, concept 37

Mackey, R. 6
MacKinnon, C. 101
Mad Pride 189
madness, benevolent affections untouched by 66
Magill-Evans, J. 256
magnetic resonance imaging (MRI) 94, 96
Malcom, Shirley 90
map metaphor 47, 49
Marcuse, Herbert 39–40
market ideology, psychopharmacology 127–129
Marx, Karl/Marxism 39, 104
Maslow, Abraham 38
McDonald, Skye 256
MDASI (MD Anderson Symptom Inventory) 236
means and ends 37–38, 64
Meehl, Paul 35–36, 48
Megamachine 5
mental disorders/illness 168–169
  see also specific disorders such as ADD (attention-deficit disorder)
  actuarial approach 48
  affective 161–164
  Asperger syndrome (AS) 159–161
  attention-deficit disorder 156–159
  causes, contemporary theories 137
  classification 47
  concept of mental illness, critique 51
  essentialism 95–96

mental disorders/illness (*cont.*)
  research 48
  and stress 167
  and technology 153–165
  validators 47, 48
mental health
  example of technological rationality in mental health profession 38
  internet phenomena 29
  and self, engagement of 31
  standardization procedures 28–29
metarepresentations 254
Middlemarch (Eliot) 241
Military Standard 1472, use of 97–98
Mill, J. S. 295
Millar, M. 107
mind 62, 136–137
mind and body, as organic unity 57
Mind Freedom 189
mind reading
  development 250–251
  empathy, developing 253
  failures 251–252
  measuring competence at 254–257
Mitcham, C. 6
modernism/modernity 167, 168, 172
monotechnics 5
A Mood Apart (Whybrow) 194
moods
  boredom, profound 15, 189, 193–198
  fundamental 191–192, 193
  ontological status 191
  primordial 191–193, 198
moral skepticism 116
Moral Theory and Medical Practice (Fulford) 120
moral treatment, technological reason 56, 57, 65–67
Moses, Robert 93
motion, analysis of 11
MRI (magnetic resonance imaging) 94, 96
Mumford, Lewis 5
Murphy, D. 51

narratives, reasonableness of 10
National Comprehensive Cancer Network (NCCN) 232, 236
National Institutes for Health (NIH) 90, 130–131
National Institutes for Mental Health (NIMH) 182, 217
nature 4, 5–6
Nausea (Sartre) 190
NCCN (National Comprehensive Cancer Network) 232, 236
Nelson, C. A. 250
neo-colonialism 104
neurons 137
neuropsychiatry 137
neuroscience 279
NIH (National Institutions for Health) 90, 130–131
NIMH (National Institutes for Mental Health) 182, 217
Noble, David 127, 129
noble lie 46
Nozick, Robert 305n

object relations theory 98
objective truth, concern for 120, 121
obscurantism 81
Oedipus complex 98
Ordering Diversity by Taxonomy 38
The Origin of Species (Darwin) 60
Other, woman as 96
Oudemans, Wooten 193, 194

panic attacks, personal experience of 189–191, 195
paroxetine (Paxil) 188, 217
passions, regulation of 56, 57–59
  Descartes on 57, 58, 59, 63
path integration concept 147, 148
pathological phenomena 120
patient-reported outcomes (PROs) 231, 233, 240, 244
patriarchal bias, in science 88–89
Paxil (paroxetine) 188, 217
Penrose, R. 148, 149
perception, real and illusory objects of 143–144
Petty, R.E. 37
PFC (prefrontal cortex) 167, 168
  basic functions 170, 175
  capacities 171
  human 169–172
  integration with neocortex and subcortical areas 176
  and stress 171
  and world 175–176, 178
pharmaceutical industry 119, 126
  market interests 127–129
philosophic analysis 5–11
  contemporary analyses 7–9
  first-generation analyses 5–7
  technical reason 9–11
  technologically assessed psychiatric and oncology symptoms 237–240
philosophical technology 51
phronesis (practical knowledge) 11
physical enhancement, and biotechnology 283–284
Pinel, Philippe 65
placebos 218, 219
positivism 88
postcolonial feminism 104–106, 109
postmodern feminism 102–104, 109
postpsychiatry 189

Postpsychiatry (Bracken and Thomas) 191
pragmatism
  Darwinian emphasis of 52
  Dewey on 12, 35
  evidence-based medicine 49
prefrontal cortex (PFC) *see* PFC (prefrontal cortex)
President's Council on Bioethics 279, 280–283, 285, 286–287
  flawed method of 290
pride 60
primary representations 254
primordial moods 191–193, 198
'probability', concept of 38–39
problem solving, scientific approaches to 51
professional ethics 265
professionalism, as remedy 267
PROs (patient-reported outcomes) 231, 233, 240, 244
Prozac 1
  benefits of 287
  case study 286
  commodity of 2
  and suicidality 125–126
psyche 62, 63
psychiatric disorders, and technology 14–15
  see also mental disorders/illness
psychiatric nosology 158
psychiatric patients, abnormal findings in brains of 137
psychiatric rehabilitation 203–211
  notion of technology in 208–210
  technologies and notions of technology in psychiatry 205–207
psychiatry
  academic 136, 184
  bad faith in, and instrumental information theory 148
  dimensions of philosophy and technology 11–17
  ethical issues in 16–17
  examples from 46–48
  instrumentalist thinking/instrumentality 12, 24–25
  multiple perspectives, need for 84
  neuropsychiatry 137
  plurality in 84
  psychiatrist–patient relationship 270
  and psychotropic technology 293–304
  residency training accreditation requirements 27–28
  science replacing art or craft of 10
  technical reason in 12–13
  technological instruments in 15–16
  technology in
    achievements 1, 2
    critical approaches to 13–14
    de-humanization of medicine 204, 205
    notions of, in psychiatry 205–207
    reciprocal nature 2
    threats to identity 1
  techno-psychiatry, current hegemony 135–137
  treatment as mechanical procedure 9
psychoanalysis
  see also psychoanalytic feminism
  Freud's ideas, development 80
  interpretation types 81–82
  object relations theory 98
  pseudoscientific nature of, alleged 211n
  technical reasoning, use of 74
  therapy 206
  and Wittgenstein 80
psychoanalytic feminism 98–100
psychologists, scientist and practitioner differences between 50
psychopathology 31, 147–149
psychopharmacology
  agents, as technological things 8
  citizen participation for better technology 129–131
  cosmetic 279, 284–290
  critical theory 115–132
  defined 205
  epistemology 120–121
  Healy's critique of 115, 124–125, 131
  market ideology 127–129
  normative considerations 118–119
  rational argumentation 121–124
  social benefit of 115
  social contingencies, in technological development 116–118
psychotherapy 62, 206
psychotherapy pill 28
psychotropics 8, 293–304
  see also antidepressant trials, children and adolescents; antidepressants; SSRIs (selective serotonin reuptake inhibitors)
  assumptions
    anxious and depressed 296–297
    examined life 293–296
    reflectively anxious and depressed 297–300
  outcomes 300–303

Quaker values 66, 67
quantum field theory 147
'The Question Concerning Technology' (Heidegger) 6, 24

radical feminism 100–102, 109
randomized controlled trial (RCT) 117, 118, 297
rational argumentation, psychopharmacology 121–124
rationality, technological
  clinical psychology and technical methodology 35–36

rationality, technological (*cont.*)
  critical theory and 'identity thinking' 40–41, 44
  criticism 44–45
  definitions 35, 74
  evidence-based medicine 48–50
  example, in mental health profession 38
  expertise, qualified 45–46
  and film 42
  immanent critique 12, 41–44, 47
  means and ends 37–38
  norms of rationality 39
  in psychiatry 35–52
  psychiatry, examples from 46–48
  technological domination 39–40
  technological understanding, advantages 36–37
  trenchant external criticism, role 50–52
RCT (randomized controlled trial) 117, 118, 297
RDC (Research Diagnostic Criteria) 48
realism, versus antirealism 38
Recognising the Depressed Patient 128
reductio ad absurdum 140
reductionism 191
reform, and re-engagement 31–33
reformatting 175
regimes of truth 187
repetitive transcranial magnetic stimulation (rTMS) 184
res extensa, physical world as 4
Research Diagnostic Criteria (RDC) 48
restraint 273
Retreat for the Insane, York 65, 66, 67
Return to Reason (Toulmin) 10
Ricoeur, Paul 148
Rocha Barros, Elias Mallet da 82, 85
Rogers, Carl 271
romanticism 50
rTMS (repetitive transcranial magnetic stimulation) 184
Rush, A. John 183

Sartre, Jean-Paul 190
Schaffer, H. R. 251
Schaffer, S. 215
schizophrenia
  anti-psychotic medication prescribed for 206
  cross-cultural studies, WHO 154–155
  diagnostic categories 47, 48
  and dopamine 117
  felt needs of patients with 211n
  non-compliance rates, drug treatment 188
  user groups 189
Schrag, Calvin 122
Science, Truth and Democracy (Kitcher) 124
science, value-neutral 116
scientific reasoning
  myth engendered by 40
  styles 38, 39, 43, 51
'scientific revolution' 3, 4
secondary representations 254
secular emotions 60–61
selective serotonin reuptake inhibitors *see* SSRIs (selective serotonin reuptake inhibitors)
self-control 273
self-examination 296
self-understanding 77
sertraline (antidepressant) 101, 126, 127
Shannon, Claude 135, 138
Shapin, S. 215
Sharfstein, Steven S. 1–2
Smart, J. J. C. 295, 296
Smith, Adam 60
social constructionism 153, 158
social contingencies, in technological development 116–118
socialist feminism 91–93, 109
Society for Women's Health Research, proposals of 90
Society of Friends 65
Socrates 293, 294, 295, 296, 304n
Sorenson, K. 99–100
specialization 50
SSRIs (selective serotonin reuptake inhibitors) 13
  Beyond Therapy: Biotechnology and the pursuit of happiness (report) 285
  birth defects associated with 188
  brand names 304n
  and essentialist feminism 96
  and existentialist feminism 97
  and racial/ethnic feminism 93
  and radical feminism 101
  self, loss of 298–299
  and socialist feminism 92
  STAR*D results 182–184, 185, 186–187, 196, 198
  therapy and symptom relief 297
  withdrawal from 126
  worries about 300
standardization procedures, mental health care 28–29
STAR*D (Sequenced Treatment Alternatives to Relieve Depression) 182–184, 185, 186–187, 196, 198
statistical prediction, advantages 36
Statistically Analyzing Regularities Using Probability 38
Strauss, Leo 46
strengths of character 273
stress 167, 171
Styrofoam cup, artifact of 25, 30
Styron, William 195–196

subjective existence, and intentionally
intrinsic information 143–147
Suchman, L. 102
suicidality
in children and adolescents 217, 222–225
epidemiology and suicide 224–225
and paroxetine 217
and Prozac 125–126
Summers, Larry 87
symmetry
broken 145, 146
defined 141–142
global and local 142
of Heidegger 144
and information theory 141–143
symptom management systems 231–246
Community Cancer Care quality of life
program 231, 233–234
epistemological approach to knowledge
240–243
mixed methodology, objective and
qualitative research inquiry
243–245
technologically assessed psychiatric and
oncology symptoms 237–240
technology applied to 234–237
Symptom Monitor (CSM) 236, 243
symptoms, and dreams 78
Szasz, T. 51

TADS (Treatment of Adolescent Depression
Study) 217
TASIT (Awareness of Social Inference Test)
256, 257
technical methodology, and clinical
psychology 35–36
technical processes, defined 55
technical reason
see also rationality, technological
and modern rationalism 11
origins 10
philosophic analysis 9–11
practical experience of practitioner,
omission 10
in psychiatry 12–13, 74
psychoanalysis 74
rationality and reasonableness
distinguished 10
technical/technological expert model 263–274
and ethics 265–267
as misleading and inapplicable 267–271
omissions 271–274
professional, as technical/technological
expert 264–265
technological approach to life 2
technological development, social
contingencies in 116–118
technological instruments, in psychiatry
2, 15–16
technological procedures, as rules for action
36–37
technological rationality, in psychiatry *see*
rationality, technological
technological reason
moral treatment 56, 57, 65–67
new technologies, emotion regulation
55–57
passions, regulation of 56, 57–59
secular emotions 60–61
truth and authenticity 67–68
'technological society' 4
technology
citizen participation 129–131
defined 55
ethical issues in 16–17
faces of 2
feminist theories
African-American/womanist and
racial/ethnic feminism 94–96
cyberfeminism 108
essentialist feminism 96
existentialist feminism 97–98
liberal feminism 90–91
post-colonial feminism 105–106
postmodern feminism 103–104
psychoanalytic feminism 99–100
radical feminism 101–102
socialist feminism 92–93
and frontal fatigue 172–175
historical background 3–4
and mental disorders 153–165
notion of, in psychiatric rehabilitation
208–210
philosophical 51
philosophical characterization 211n
in psychiatry *see* psychiatry: technology in
and pure science 2
revealing of Being 6
as set of devices 203
symptom management, applied to 234–237
as a value 225–226
values
revealed/made subject to consideration 45
technological and poietic 25–29, 32
Technology and the Character of Everyday Life
(Borgmann) 31
techno-psychiatry, current hegemony
135–137
The Technological Society (Ellul) 6
theory of mind 254
therapeutic science, notion of 119
therapeutics, aesthetics in 82–83
Thomas, P. 51, 187, 189
thought experiments 296
Tolstoy, Leo 294
Toulmin, Stephen 10, 11
traits 273
treatment algorithms, and technical reason 9

treatment manuals 9
Treatment of Adolescent Depression Study (TADS) 217
Trevarthen, C. 251
Trivers, R. L. 95
trustworthiness 273, 274
truth and authenticity 67–68
Tuke, Samuel 65
Tuke, William 65, 66

utilitarianism 295

vagal nerve stimulation (VNS) 184
values
  caring 100
  either/or dichotomy 43, 120
  Quaker 66, 67
  technological and poietic 25–29, 32
Values and Psychiatric Diagnosis (Sadler) 24, 30
virtual speculum, image of 108
virtues, prudential 273
VNS (vagal nerve stimulation) 184

Waits, Tom 37
Watts, James 4
Webster, J. 103–104
When Science Offers Salvation (Dresser) 131
Whybrow, Peter 194
Wilson, E. O. 95
Winner, Langdon 9
Wittgenstein, Ludwig 74–81
  on aesthetics and psychoanalysis 73, 76, 84
  on causes and reasons, mixing 85
  on conceptual confusions 74
  on dreams 78
  on empirical propositions and philosophical pseudo-propositions 75
  on Freud 74, 81
  on intermediate cases 83
  lamp metaphor 79
  method of doing philosophy 83
  and therapeutic method 83
Wolin, R. 42
wonder and awe, fundamental moods of 197
'The Work of Art in the Age of Its Technological Reproducibility' (Benjamin) 41

Zachar, P. 50
Zen Buddhism 197
Zimmerman, Michael 191, 192, 197